HEALING BY HAND

HEALING BY HAND

Manual Medicine and Bonesetting in Global Perspective

KATHRYN S. OTHS
SERVANDO Z. HINOJOSA, EDITORS

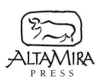

A Division of Rowman & Littlefield Publishers, Inc.
Walnut Creek • Lanham • New York • Toronto • Oxford

ALTAMIRA PRESS
A division of Rowman & Littlefield Publishers, Inc.
1630 North Main Street, #367
Walnut Creek, California 94596
www.altamirapress.com

Rowman & Littlefield Publishers, Inc.
A Member of The Rowman & Littlefield Publishing Group
4501 Forbes Boulevard, Suite 200
Lanham, Maryland 20706

PO Box 317
Oxford
OX2 9RU, UK

British Library Cataloguing in Publication Information Available

Library of Congress Cataloging-in-Publication Data

Healing by hand : manual medicine and bonesetting in global perspective / edited by Kathryn S. Oths and Servando Z. Hinojosa.
   p. cm.
 Includes bibliographical references and index.
  ISBN 0-7591-0392-5 (hardcover : alk. paper) — ISBN 0-7591-0393-3 (pbk. : alk. paper)
  1. Chiropractic. 2. Manipulation (Therapeutics) 3. Medical anthropology. I. Oths, Kathryn S., 1959– II. Hinojosa, Servando Z., 1904-

  RZ242.H436 2004
  615.5'34—dc22

                                                        2004006864

Printed in the United States of America

♾™ The paper used in this publication meets the minimum requirements of American National Standard for Information Sciences—Permanence of Paper for Printed Library Materials, ANSI/NISO Z39.48-1992.

CONTENTS

Foreword

I APPROACHED THIS BOOK with heightened anticipation because anthropologists' disinterest in manual medicine always struck me as wrongheaded—and I was not disappointed. Much more than a loose collection of essays on a common theme, *Healing by Hand* offers a coherent overview and in-depth examination of some time-tested healing arts. It also takes on the nettlesome issue of how to assess the efficacy of traditional medical treatments.

While most anthropological work on "embodiment" has focused only on metaphoric or representational dimensions, *Healing by Hand* presents a richly documented systematic analysis of practitioners at work—several of whom are both clinicians and scholars—revealing fascinating common principles that transcend the conventional categories of "traditional" and "modern."

Healing by Hand persuasively demonstrates that manual medicine is much more than the simple manipulation of bone and tissue. This book will certainly stimulate new and much-needed dialogue among clinicians, researchers, and social and medical scientists.

C. H. Browner
UCLA School of Medicine

Preface

MY PROFESSIONAL ASSOCIATION with other enthusiasts of musculoskeletal medicine began at the American Anthropological Association (AAA) Meetings in Washington, D.C., in 1985. I had just delivered my first academic paper based on original research of practitioner–patient communication in a chiropractic clinic when I was approached by Bob Anderson. We exchanged introductions. He was both a senior anthropologist at Mills College and a chiropractor. I was a lowly Ph.D. candidate in medical anthropology at Case Western Reserve University. We quickly decided we must be the only two anthropologists alive who were interested in manual medicine. Shortly after that, I was fortunate to meet Hans Baer, who had similar interests in osteopathy. My colleagueship with both men took root and has grown until today.

Many years later, in much the same vein, I approached Servando Hinojosa after hearing a conference paper of his on Maya bonesetters. This time we decided that, with the attention in the social sciences to issues of embodiment, not to mention the public's growing interest in and professional practice of bodywork, indeed there just might be a modest groundswell around the topic of musculoskeletal healers within anthropology. With the assistance of Bob and his far-flung contacts in the manual medicine field, we pooled enough names to start an informal bonesetters interest group. We were amazed and delighted to discover so many with dual training both as social scientists and body workers.

As an outgrowth of the interest group, Servando and I organized the first conference panel in known history devoted to the topic, *Making Some Bones about It: Toward an Ethnography of Manual Medicine*, at the Society for Applied Anthropology meetings in Merida, Mexico, in 2001. What is more, as a corollary to the session we staged a workshop, *Of Bonesetters and Body Workers: An Open Demonstration of Various Musculoskeletal Healers,* which was *certainly* unparalleled in the history of anthropology. Sue Walkley and Marc Weill, both contributors to this volume, stationed at opposite ends of a conference room, lectured to avid audiences while demonstrating their therapeutic skills on volunteers. A hotel staffer caught sight of outstretched bodies on the conference table and fetched the manager, who ordered us to desist for fear we would damage the furniture! (However, the crowd was not to be denied. We posted guards outside the door and continued with the demonstration for a full two and a half hours.)

The snowball kept rolling and soon we had all the presenters from the session (minus Caroline Peterson, Oregon-based chiropractor and Ph.D. candidate in anthropology, who had moved to South America) plus several more researchers who were willing to contribute to an edited volume that would bring together the disparate studies of manual medicine into a useful, readable, and seminal primer. Rosalie Robertson, a perspicacious acquisitions editor at AltaMira, expressed early and consistent enthusiasm for the project. Two years later, the volume was complete.

I wish to express my deepest appreciation to Bob Anderson. Without his moral support and sage advice at every step of the process, this work would never have come to fruition. He has served as a mentor of the highest caliber across my entire academic career. Rosalie Robertson has been an indefatigable supporter of the project from its inception. She and her staff have been a delight to work with. Servando Hinojosa is an ideal coeditor in every sense of the term, from his keen editing eye, to the formulation of ideas, to the structuring of the book. He has the patience of Job. The contributors, to a fault, have been punctual and pleasant to work with. Their humor, grace, and wit in the face of our endless exchanges to get everything just right have been truly remarkable. Many along the way, having edited their own books, asked if I had yet come to regret the frustrations involved in a decision to publish an edited volume. On the contrary, the process was enriching and invigorating throughout, with no exceptions. Both the department of anthropology at the University of Alabama and the department of psychology and anthropology at the University of Texas–Pan American are to be thanked for their support of our efforts over the past several years. Finally, I wish to personally thank Bill Dressler, my husband and closest colleague, who has enabled this project in ways too numerous to count.

Kathryn S. Oths

Like with so many other conference papers, I thought my paper at the 1999 American Ethnological Society Meetings would be presented, briefly discussed, and, once I got home, shuffled to the end of a long line of papers to be later developed. I was surprised, then, months after the meetings, to receive a call from someone named Kathy Oths, who requested a copy of my paper. I was intrigued by Kathy's interest in bonesetters. As any anthropologist interested in manual medicine knows, it is difficult enough finding research on bonesetters, let alone other people who are also looking for it. Needless to say, I looked forward to learning about Kathy's work. Following our first phone conversation, I found we were of a mind when it came to bonesetting.

We were both puzzled by the lack of research on bonesetters, especially given the substantive coverage given to other healing specialists. Having reviewed the literature, we knew the existing work on bonesetting was spotty, but the writings of Ben Paul and Robert Anderson encouraged us. They underlined the cultural importance of bonesetting, which was the aspect of the craft that most interested me. I had thought especially about Paul's work with Mayas when I did my 1992 master's fieldwork in Guatemala, and included interviews and observations of three Kaqchikel Maya bonesetters. He and Anderson reminded me that it was legitimate and necessary to meet those people with manual vocations who might lack a high public profile. Their example was well taken, and it continues to the present.

To have worked with the bonesetters when I first did proved auspicious. They became most valued teachers. I was reminded of this every time I visited them in their homes or went with them when they visited clients, and would hear them explain that their hands would find the problem in people's bodies. They couldn't necessarily say *how* their hands did this, but expressed great confidence that they *did*. It was enough to watch their interaction with ailing clients to know that the bonesetters did more than provide only manual therapy: By letting people describe the circumstances of the injury and guide them through their bodily limitations, they also helped people participate in their own healing. Bonesetters taught me that the healer must listen through his own body to the sufferer's body, and in this way find what needs to be done.

This collection grew from the input of people who, in their own ways, have also found bonesetters and manual medicine workers to be great teachers. Kathy and I were fortunate to come into contact with so many contributors who appreciated body workers as teachers *and* as people who could augment their own healing work. Their perspectives reminded us of the possibilities of dialogue between

Western health workers and informal manual practitioners. We hope these chapters will further this dialogue.

Numerous people helped make this volume possible. Among those who helped my personal research along, few made as big a difference as Judith M. Maxwell, Victoria R. Bricker, and the late Munro Edmonson. In the field, Guatemalans such as Chuti' Hunahpu' and his mother in San Juan Comalapa, and Aj Pub' and his father in San Pedro la Laguna helped me meet the bonesetters who would become the cornerstone of my work. For his welcome input and creative perspective, I also thank Vincent Stanzione. Before this collection was ever assembled, Kathy Oths led the charge in drawing together a community of manual medicine researchers. She then initiated the linkages with our helpful and insightful editor at AltaMira Press, Rosalie Robertson. Rosalie appreciated the uniqueness of our project and, fortunately for us, had the chapters reviewed by very capable individuals. My work on the manuscript was facilitated by release time afforded by my institution, the University of Texas–Pan American. Support from my family has been constant, and I especially appreciate the artwork my father, Servando G. Hinojosa, patiently created for my chapter. Last, I would acknowledge the central role my wife, Nihan Kayaardı, has played in my life as I have put this volume together. She has kept me mindful of how learning and living can both be quality experiences.

Servando Z. Hinojosa

Introduction

KATHRYN S. OTHS AND SERVANDO Z. HINOJOSA

ANTHROPOLOGISTS, WITH FEW EXCEPTIONS, have summarily overlooked the practice of "bonesetters," or manipulative therapists, one of the primary providers of both "traditional" and professional medicine. One of the main motivations for this volume has been to fill a gap in anthropological scholarship by providing a body of systematic, accessible research on manual medicine. By discussing specific bonesetter practices and how they are expressed institutionally, this volume presents manual medicine as a field of study of local and global importance. Through situated analyses of musculoskeletal therapy, much can be learned about human experience in terms of lifeways and injuries resulting from them, in terms of ethnoanatomy, and even in terms of phenomenological dimensions of healing. Close attention to localized experience and macro-level considerations yields insight into, among other things, how knowledge is created and authorized, the strengths and weaknesses of technology and the constraints on its use, and how structures beyond the community condition local practice.

Given recent anthropological discourse on the body and how bodies remember, the study of manual therapies assumes a much larger theoretical significance than simply its ethnographic description. Despite current anthropological interest in the phenomenon of embodiment (Csordas 1994; Dejarlais 1992; Halliburton 2002; and others), little attention has been directed to the actual practice of bodywork by healers. This volume can provide a needed corrective to the focus on the metaphorical and representational aspects of embodiment to the exclusion of biocultural and biomechanical aspects of it.

In manual traditions, the body is recognized as having important capacities for self-healing as well as an instrumental importance in healing others. A volume on manual medicine that treats these issues in depth is long overdue. Its timeliness in part stems from the growth of different types of manipulative therapies as options in the modern world. Thus, modern therapies (such as chiropractic, Rolfing, and osteopathy) also have a place in this volume alongside more traditional forms of bonesetting.

Those who have seen the workings of manual traditions in urban and rural, Western and non-Western contexts know the vital role bonesetters play in the lives of individuals and communities. Though frequently overshadowed and challenged by allopathic practitioners, they continue to engage with the sick and injured, helping them reach their health goals and lead productive, satisfying lives. Manual medicine takes numerous forms, both lay and professional, across the world's communities, and through each of these forms it validates its presence and methods by helping clients. Importantly, manual medicine has reached the level of popularity and importance it has because practitioners have not disavowed the role of the human body in healing.

Bonesetters are unquestionably the least studied of healers. While all other categories of health care specialists have received adequate, if not ample, anthropological attention—herbalists, midwives, shamans, and curers (along with their respective biomedical cognates, pharmacists, obstetricians, psychiatrists, and general practitioners)—manual practitioners rarely figure in the social science literature. Explanations for this deficit might include a culturally constructed revulsion toward touching others' bodies, stemming from emotional defenses, inhibitions against feeling good (Walkley, chapter 2), or a fear of ritual or actual pollution (Jervis 2001:95). A Cartesian dualism favoring the mind over the body may also be implicated. Or, possibly, social science's ambivalence toward bodywork is a cultural product that mirrors biomedicine's own bias, evidenced by its near total lack of training of physicians in the area of musculoskeletal health and its institutional competition with other specialties who do treat the corporeal body. The long history of turf battles between the American Medical Association (AMA) and osteopathy and chiropractic bears this out (see Baer, chapter 4).

From another perspective, one might argue that because manual medicine is by and large devoid of exoticism or ritual content, it has not captured the imagination of researchers in the same way that the spectacle of shamanism has. However, this would not account for the interest afforded the mundane herbalist and midwife, practical healers not generally viewed as expressive or colorful. Besides, a few types of bonesetter, such as the *balian uat* (Klein, chapter 8) and the Mayan bonesetter (Hinojosa, chapter 6), in fact do incorporate supernatural elements. As Anderson and Klein (chapter 8) state, "The time has come for anthropologists to balance their extensive documentation of exotic, supernatural healing practices with studies of healing based on the pragmatism of ordinary human anatomy, physiology, and pathology."

The dearth of systematic observation of manual practitioners cannot be attributed to the recentness of the practice. Despite the origin myth of modern chiropractic, which claims the profession of moving bones was invented in 1895 when D. D. Palmer adjusted a cervical vertebra of a Midwestern janitor and cured his deafness, its roots are much deeper. Wardwell (1987) may locate bonesetting's beginnings in ancient times and Fabrega (1997) at a somewhat later time with the advent of chiefdoms and early state societies, but without dispute the practice is at least several millennia old (Minor, Warburton, and Black, chapter 5). The application of manual medicine by Hippocrates' adherents, for instance, is well known (Lloyd 1983), and scholars have inferred its importance among ancient Egyptian physicians (Nunn 1996) as well.

In the scant literature on current bonesetters, one finds that epidemiologists, health service researchers, and until recently, social scientists have focused on the efficacy of one indigenous U.S. modality, chiropractic—whether or not it works and who it serves; its deviance; its medical professionalization; and the status and role of the chiropractic doctor, especially vis-à-vis physicians. Later anthropologists and sociologists have explored the political underpinnings of chiropractic's "deviant" label and put more emphasis on the patient's experience and understandings of chiropractic treatment (Coulter, chapter 3). Going beyond, this book explores uncharted territories of Western and non-Western bonesetting alike, such as the evolution of various manual medical traditions, embodiment and experience, the degree of technological innovation, and wider public health ramifications.

Oths (2002) finds a great deal of variability in the labeling of indigenous musculoskeletal practices, especially throughout North, South, and Middle America, with "bonesetter" the preferred English translation for them all. For instance, Huber and Anderson (1996:31) have deemed a bonesetter a manual therapist who does joint manipulation in addition to massage. As another example, in the Andes a distinction is made between the *componedor*, the rough equivalent of a lay chiropractor, and the *huesero*, or bonesetter, the more skilled of the two practitioners, who sets broken bones and performs the skeletal manipulation of the *componedor*. A systematic study of bonesetting requires that a precise classification of manual therapists and a working definition of "bonesetter" be established.

To help sort out the ambiguity in the literature on the topic, we attempt here a provisional taxonomy of those who work physically upon bodies to ease distress. Manual therapists, popularly called *body workers*, can be divided into two types: those who primarily emphasize bioenergetics, sometimes called *energy healers*, and those who are musculoskeletally oriented, sometimes called *structural body workers*. Both are noninvasive, hand-centered modalities. The first type, energy healing—a burgeoning sector represented by well-known practices such as reiki, polarity therapy, craniosacral therapy, and acupuncture—operates on the general theory that illness is caused by imbalance or restriction in the body's meridians, energy fields, or patterns of motion. Their methods of treatment entail a gentle touch or no-touch technique (that is, simply passing the hands over all or part of the client's body). There is little to no penetration of tissue involved. The second type, musculoskeletal therapists, the subject of this book, operate on the theory that illness, pain, and dysfunction—often emotional as well as somatic—are fundamentally the result of the impacted or displaced matter of bones, muscles, connective tissue, and organs, and their sequelae of pinched nerves and inhibited blood flow. In this sector, it is useful to identify three levels of practice that correspond to the depth of tissue worked on—in essence, the level of complexity of the treatment procedures. The levels are: 1) soft tissue, 2) soft tissue and joints, and, 3) soft tissues, joints, and broken bones. At the first level, one finds massagers who work primarily with the outer layers of muscle. At the second level are situated those such as chiropractors and Danish *kloge folk* who manipulate muscle, joints, and organs to reposition them and alter bodily structure. At the final level are those such as Peruvian *hueseros* and Kenyan *chiressa* who, in addition to possessing the aforementioned skills, set broken bones. Each level of practice, then, subsumes all levels above it. All three levels are represented in this volume.

To follow conventional social science use and retain a manageable moniker, all musculoskeletal healers described in this volume are loosely considered to be bonesetters, whether they do massage, adjust bones, set fractures, or any combination of the three.[1] The normative glossing of the various levels of musculoskeletal therapist simply as "bonesetters" probably has as much as anything to do with the poverty of the English language for describing the domain of bodily illness and its treatment. An expanded definition of "bonesetter" that captures all three levels would be: a healer who may set fractures, mobilize joints, and reposition the minor movements or major dislocations of the vertebrae, joints, muscles, and even organs (see Oths 2002:64).

In the chapters that follow, manual practitioners draw on their respective traditions to move the body's parts in ways valued by those they serve.

Outline of the Chapters

The researcher of manual medicine can fully expect to encounter practitioners whose work is neither fully old nor entirely new. Over time, manipulative therapy has been adapted to a multitude of modern settings, and in each of these it assumes distinct forms. While the different bonesetting traditions in this volume all evidence the melding of the ancient and the modern to some degree, the first five chapters covered in part I, "Past Meets Present in Manual Medicine Practice," foreground the phenomenon. The contributors write about time-proven manual medicine forms that, if not already professionalized, seem well on their way to acquiring this status. Robert Anderson, for example, bringing his anthropological, medical, and chiropractic knowledge to bear, outlines an ostensibly "traditional" bonesetting practice in Denmark, reporting how inherited healing traditions have over time become more structured and regularized. Current bonesetters perform roles previously the domain of those remembered as "wise people," enjoying the respect that comes from an association with them, all the while supplementing their practices with cliniclike waiting rooms and adjustments learned from watching chiropractors.

The status of massage, as documented by Susan Walkley, has oscillated repeatedly over time between disreputable and respectable. Its current high level of acceptance in the United States has hinged on its developed professional status and demonstrated place amid mainstream health care providers. The practice now finds itself in the unusual position of regularizing its training and licensing procedures while trying to promote respect for its own noninvasive approach to healing. As a practitioner and anthropologist, Walkley appreciates the centrality of hands in bodywork, but is also aware of how the intimacy and pleasure of bodily contact in massage has at times impeded its acceptance as a serious therapy by health industry gatekeepers.

Sociologist Ian Coulter explores the coverage of chiropractic in both the epidemiological and social scientific literature from the 1950s to the present. Public health scholars have tended to focus on service provision and efficacy, while sociologists and anthropologists generally focus on the status and holistic nature of the healing paradigm. Early on, the medical establishment's challenge to bonesetting strongly influenced its treatment by researchers. That discussions of chiropractic became more balanced in later decades was in no small way a function of chiropractic's tenacity in the marketplace and clinic. Coulter explains why epidemiologists and social scientists pursued the divergent lines of inquiry they did, providing a thought-provoking chapter on how a manual modality can be officially misperceived, even persecuted, and yet remain viable.

The contribution by Hans Baer then illustrates not only how some aspects of manual medicine have taken institutional form in osteopathy, but also how this institutionalization itself takes different paths. Osteopathy has become a very distinct practice in the four English-speaking countries he reviews, an outcome attributable to the various social, political, and economic conditions under which it operates. In the United States, for example, competing institutional pressures have distanced osteopathy from its original musculoskeletal focus. The American practice now bears little resemblance to osteopathy in Canada, Britain, and Australia, where manual manipulation remains the field's distinguishing trait.

The following chapter by Jennifer Minor, Miranda Warburton, and H. Vincent Black provides a look at a very different institutional situation, deriving from a unique set of historical circumstances. In China, manual therapeutics have a long and respected history. Evolving out of age-old understandings of balance, harmony, energy, and movement, manual medicine in the *Tuina* form has undergone successive moments of development over the millennia. In part thanks to Mao's revitalization of Traditional Chinese Medicine, *Tuina* is currently regarded as an effective diagnostic and treatment modality, one encouraged by a state also supportive of Western medicine.

As mentioned earlier, a surprisingly undervalued feature of musculoskeletal therapy, at least in the scholarly literature, is bodily experience. While relatively few efforts have been made to study bonesetting, even fewer have been directed at the deeper levels of engagement experienced by bodies during the healing encounter. In part II, "Experience and Embodiment in Practitioner–Patient Encounters," attention is placed on how the healer learns and applies his or her skill through the hands, and how the patient responds in kind. The four contributors to this section reiterate that physical contact between bodies enables the knowledge underwriting diagnosis and healing, and ultimately serves as the vehicle for change. The Guatemalan Maya bonesetters in Servando Z. Hinojosa's chapter thus understand manual medicine as an outcome of hand-based knowledge derived from working with suffering bodies. They regard their abilities, for the most part, as secular, although some practitioners do attribute a divine quality to them. However they view their abilities, bonesetters operate in a world in which changing therapeutic resources and professional tensions force them to rethink their approach to care. Hinojosa finds that Maya bonesetters remain committed to their healing mandate while also responding creatively to change.

The account of *hilot* bonesetting in the chapter that follows puts a similar emphasis on learning through the body. Working from his own perspective as a chiropractor and scholar, John O'Malley explicates how he and his Filipino counterpart have each acquired skills in the healing arts, and demonstrates that while each healing model provides a basis for learning, skilled manipulation is ultimately a function of experience. This case suggests that different manual practitioners bring something similar to their work because their knowledge begins with and rests on an embodied basis. Because the indigenous healer demonstrates considerable manipulative know-how, it is possible to argue that he should be seen as a useful part of skilled health care delivery.

Utilizing what might be called "comparative revisitation," anthropologist–chiropractors Robert Anderson and Norman Klein next make a rapid ethnographic assessment of a Balian manual therapist. At different points in time, each researcher created a video documentary of bonesetters in Bali, and each consulted with and experienced the therapeutic hands of one particular bonesetter using their own bodies as evaluative media. They did not reach similar conclusions about the bonesetter, however. With great collegiality and a desire for intellectual discovery, Anderson and Klein attempt to understand why their conclusions are, in fact, starkly opposite. At work may be how each researcher unknowingly "telegraphed" to the bonesetter what he was most interested in seeing and hearing, resulting in their receiving distinctive, incomplete, but not unfaithful renderings of the bonesetter's practice and worldview.

The author of the next chapter also draws on his backgrounds in manipulative therapy and anthropology to formulate a clearer understanding of the healing experience. Eric Jacobson's long clinical experience in Rolfing and craniosacral therapy, forms of structural bodywork indigenous to the United States, prepares him especially well to confront the deficits in anthropology's theoretical discussions of embodiment. He cogently argues for the inclusion of myofascial elasticity alongside psychological and neurological constructs as a source of disordered bodily states. He posits that the manual therapist is actually privileged to a rich phenomenology of the patient's bodily experience, which at times is quite revealing of the patient's somatic and psychic health. What is more, he recognizes that this kind of bodily engagement takes place in different manual medicine traditions, raising stimulating questions about the bonesetter as a technician of both the body and self.

With or without the active endorsement of Western practitioners, it is clear that manual medicine practitioners attend to people of all walks of life, and do so even when formal institutions oppose them. Perhaps because bonesetters have been adaptable and willing to modify their tool kit, their efforts have remained timely and sought-after nearly everywhere. In part III, "A Wider Lens: The Bonesetter's Contribution to Community Health," four contributors writing about vastly different places show how bonesetters, though they may be reluctantly acknowledged or even resisted by authorities, nonetheless have an impact on how people seek treatment and regain health.

Kathryn S. Oths provides a needed look at how bonesetters serve a highland Andean population. Using nine case studies, she describes the variety of healing methods that Peruvian musculoskeletal therapists use in addition to hand-based manipulation, and how bonesetters are utilized alongside other healers as part of a comprehensive health care strategy. Because of the constant assault on the body by highland agrarian life, inhabitants of the region experience a high frequency of bodily ailments. This fact, complicated by factors of access, modesty, and a chronically underfunded public health sector, make the continued service of bonesetters in local communities quite necessary.

Turning to the little studied experience of bonesetting among pastoralists, Isaac K. Nyamongo details how northern Kenya's Borana people seek care for bone injuries. Because they are frequently on the move and constantly on guard against neighboring groups, the Borana must avoid bodily debility at all costs and treat it quickly when it does occur. While they prefer traditional bonesetters, Borana sometimes resort to hospitals when their pastoral schedule permits. Nyamongo demonstrates how bonesetters avail themselves of whatever resources they deem useful, including x-rays that patients can surreptitiously acquire from clinical facilities. His chapter highlights how enduring and complex kinship ties bind Borana both to each other and to those among them with trusted healing abilities.

The section's next contributor considers how a local-level bonesetting experience in Wales intersects with many aspects of life in a working-class industrial town. Scholar–chiropractor Simon Leyson's portrait of a veteran bonesetter at once deepens our appreciation for how a single person can commit to a life of healing, and challenges assumptions about bonesetting in the British Isles. Unlike other bonesetters of the region, the Welch practitioner did not come from a long line of bonesetters, nor did he keep a purely secular outlook on his work. During his sixty years of practice, though, he more than proved his importance to his community. Leyson's chapter reminds us of how, even in places where Western medicine has long been established, local people often entrust their injuries to individuals whose humility, accessibility, and competence physicians can only hope to emulate.

In his reflective account, Marc Weill, nutritionist and Rolfer, reveals that the healer's work must begin with astute observation of the body and its movement, acknowledge the client's complaint, and correct the structural underpinnings of the problem. Well aware that North American clients harbor misunderstandings about Rolfing and expect quick solutions to chronic problems, Weill knows he must clarify his method and achieve results on the initial encounter if he has any hope of seeing the client again. Perhaps most importantly, though, his practice relies on the family and friends of his clients providing referral and social support for Rolfing, the professional exchange between himself and the local community of alternative and biomedical practitioners, and the creation and maintenance of his good reputation in the community at large, enabled nowadays by the Internet.

Beyond the three larger topical considerations into which the chapters are subdivided, a dynamic convergence occurs across chapters around certain themes. The first is a documentation of the breadth of the *materia medica* used by bonesetters, offering a correction to the stereotype of the bonesetters' treatment as limited in scope (Coulter). Whether trained in a professional school or receiving their knowledge as a "gift from God," manual medicine specialists, beyond simply using their hands to manipulate bone and tissue, may employ other noninvasive means as an adjunct to diagnosis and healing such as: sacred objects (Hinojosa); visual assessment (Jacobson, Weill); lubricating and warming agents (Anderson and Klein, Hinojosa, Oths); herbs and poultices (Anderson, Oths, Nyamongo, Leyson); bandages and splints (Hinojosa, Nyamongo, Oths); nutritional supplementation and exercise (Weill, Coulter); over-the-counter pharmaceuticals (Oths, Hinojosa); drugs and vaccines (Baer); psychosocial intervention (Coulter, Nyamongo); and even x-ray technology (Hinojosa, Nyamongo, Baer), bioenergetic testing machines (Weill), and electrical muscle stimulation (Coulter). Also, bonesetting may be practiced by a healer who integrates other modalities such as herbalism or mediumship (Oths, Klein), or as a necessary component of a more general medical tradition such as Traditional Chinese Medicine (Minor et al.). Simultaneous resort to different practitioners (bonesetter, physician, and so on) may occur when one has a musculoskeletal disorder (Jacobson, Nyamongo, Oths). Additionally, the clientele of bonesetters, contrary to myth, represents the full socioeconomic spectrum, though several authors (Leyson, Nyamongo, Oths, Minor, Hinojosa) make the point that bonesetters provide a critical resource for those with limited access to physicians and clinics.

Across distinct manual medicines of similar theories and techniques, the apparent independent invention to address the myriad forms of disordered body structure might be attributed to an unvarying morphology in humans, both between healer and client and across culture groups (Laughlin 1961; O'Malley, Jacobson). In their explanatory models, for example, both the Danish *kloge folk* (Anderson) and U.S. Rolfers (Weill, Jacobson) are concerned with correct balance—or the orientation of all segments of the body, especially the hips and legs, to the ground—as the true solution to problems in other parts of the body such as the back. O'Malley, likewise, finds theoretical divergence but substantially equivalent techniques between himself, a chiropractor, and the Phillipine *hilot* he observed (also see Jacobson).

Other salient themes discussed by more than one contributor also merit our attention. Several found that while healers have a routine approach to their maneuvers, each healing session is a creative act, with the precise adjustments calibrated to the specific condition of the client's body (Jacobson, O'Malley, Oths, Leyson). In anthropological accounts of healing, the efficacy of treatments is an issue usually sidestepped by researchers, given the logistical difficulty of carrying out objective measurements (Coulter). Anderson and Nyamongo, while recognizing the benefit of their respective healer's therapies, nonetheless question the soundness of some practices, while Oths, using a random sample and epidemiologic methods, finds a high success rate and no negative outcomes. Relations between the bonesetter and the biomedical physician are the subject of several accounts (Baer, Hinojosa, Anderson, Oths). Commentaries regarding the effects of local sociopolitical power on bonesetting come from two quite distinctive essays: Jacobson notes the social and moral implications of body carriage and how these can complicate successful treatment, while Baer shows the different shapes that osteopathy took as it evolved under various governmental and cultural regimes. Finally, three authors touch on the role of faith in healing (Coulter, Leyson, Anderson and Klein).

This volume forms part of a growing body of work that speaks to the relation between culture and health. By understanding how manual medicine develops and unfolds in particular places, readers will be better able to understand how these traditions change over time in response to different conditions, and in many cases emerge as institutions and professions. Another important outcome of this volume, we hope, will be a heightened quality of discussion between the social sciences and the health-centered disciplines. Many anthropologists and field researchers have learned to negotiate the maze of health knowledges and practices, equipping themselves to communicate, to a certain degree, with persons in the health field and with a public interested in health. In turn, an increasing number of health professionals are finding ways to learn from the healing practices of different peoples, including past peoples, to improve their own practices.

Conclusion

The vast range of manual medicine modalities indicates, in the end, the pragmatic importance of bonesetting to human lives. There is little question that it has been important since antiquity—human bodies have demanded it—nor is it likely to disappear as invasive biomedical technologies expand their global reach. A likelier scenario is that the official health sector will take more notice of manipulative therapies and, in those places where it has legal strength, attempt to regulate those forms whose practice appears to threaten the existing medical market. Some forms of bonesetting may gravitate toward the official sector, while others may recede, situating themselves where they have always been influential—in rural settings and among clients able to discern effectiveness from conventionality.

One of the unique and innovative features of this edited medical anthropological volume is that, for the first time, a majority of the contributing scholars are or have been themselves practitioners of the bodily arts. This ability to wear both hats, to cross the emic–etic divide and integrate theoretical with clinical insight, greatly enlivens the materials in the collection. For this alone it will appeal to researchers and health care specialists across many fields. Because most manual medicine is largely considered pragmatic and natural rather than religious or supernatural by its practitioners, Western health professionals can relate to it quite directly. It is hoped that after reviewing the contributions in this volume, students of culture and health will recognize how manual medicine represents an area of study with yet many possibilities, and one to which they might contribute.

Note

1. The term "bonesetter," while not commonly understood by the general public, does have a history of use in the English language. Andrew Still, a medical doctor and father of osteopathy, referred to himself as a "Bone Setter" in the late nineteenth century (Baer, chapter 4). And we see that Jack Leyshon of Wales considered himself a bonesetter throughout the twentieth century, even though the better understood occupational title would have been physiotherapist (Leyson, chapter 12).

References

Csordas, Thomas, ed.
  1994 *Embodiment and Experience: The Existential Ground of Culture and Self.* Cambridge, England: Cambridge University Press.
Dejarlais, Robert R.
  1992 *Body and Emotion: The Aesthetics of Illness and Healing in the Nepal Himalayas.* Philadelphia: University of Pennsylvania Press.
Fabrega, Horacio
  1997 *Evolution of Sickness and Healing.* Berkeley: University of California Press.
Halliburton, Murphy
  2002 Rethinking Anthropological Studies of the Body: *Manas* and *Bodham* in Kerala. *American Anthropologist* 104(4):1123–35.
Huber, Brad R., and Robert Anderson
  1996 Bonesetters and Curers in a Mexican Community: Conceptual Models, Status, and Gender. *Medical Anthropology* 17:23–38.
Jervis, Lori L.
  2001 The Pollution of Incontinence and the Dirty Work of Caregiving in a U.S. Nursing Home. *Medical Anthropology Quarterly* 15(1):84–99.
Laughlin, William S.
  1961 Acquisition of Anatomical Knowledge by Ancient Man. Pp. 254–72 in David Landy, ed. *Culture, Disease, and Healing.* New York: Macmillan.
Lloyd, G. E. R., ed.
  1983 *Hippocratic Writings.* London: Penguin Books.
Nunn, John F.
  1996 *Ancient Egyptian Medicine.* Norman: University of Oklahoma Press.
Oths, Kathryn S.
  2002 Setting It Straight in the Andes: Musculoskeletal Distress and the Role of the *Componedor.* Pp. 63–91 in Joan D. Koss-Chioino, Thomas Leatherman, and Christine Greenway, eds. *Medical Pluralism in the Andes.* New York: Routledge.
Wardwell, Walter I.
  1987 Before the Palmers: An Overview of Chiropractic's Antecedents. *Chiropractic History* 7(2):27–33.

PAST MEETS PRESENT IN MANUAL MEDICINE PRACTICE I

TO PRESENT A BALANCED OVERVIEW of hand-based healing, it is imperative to examine the origins of the various traditions and how these origins condition the modern-day practices of each. In part I, we assess the change over time in five unique manual medicine modalities: Danish bonesetting, massage, chiropractic, osteopathy, and the Chinese musculoskeletal therapy, Tuina.

The five chapters are organized along a continuum from those having the shortest history of professionalization to those with the longest—that is, the manual practices are plotted by the degree to which their knowledge is currently internalized (nonsystematic, passed down through apprenticeships) compared to externalized (accumulated, reproduced in texts, characterized by accredited schools, degrees, certifications, and governing associations) (Young 1976). Coincident with this, each chapter explores the individual trajectory of a specific healing tradition diachronically along the same continuum. All five therapies can be seen to have evolved across time from modest origins to a greater degree of complexity, acceptance, and respectability.

With the Danish bonesetters we have a case of a centuries-old tradition of musculoskeletal therapy that may (or may not) be at an incipient stage of institutionalization. In part, the familial inheritance of the vocation keeps it from becoming standardized and broad-based, though the reputation of the Danish bonesetter's skill at manipulation is as high as that of any certified practitioner. Former "masseuses" are now "massage therapists," almost entirely free of an earlier association with brothels and back alleys, and now promoted by the mainstream health care system as an effective physical therapy and antidote to stress. In the late-twentieth century, chiropractors have finally escaped from the dual disparagement of the biomedical and scholarly communities to emerge with an earned reputation as a valid, efficacious provider of needed health care services. Practitioners who were once called "osteopaths" are now "osteopathic physicians" who provide a system of medical care parallel to that of primary care biomedicine. The tradition has found a different professional niche in each of four Western countries, at times by jettisoning its very foundation as a form of manipulative medicine. Tuina arose in rural China two millennia ago as a mode of musculoskeletal treatment for farmers, gradually becoming incorporated as the third leg of Traditional Chinese Medicine (TCM), the dominant indigenous professional medicine in the country today.

Interestingly, with each of the four fully professionalized traditions—osteopathy, chiropractic, massage, and TCM, we see a practice that has grown so wide in its appeal that it has transcended the boundaries of its country of origin and established roots in new soil, with each case, of course, adapting and transforming to meet local sociocultural needs. The case of the Danish *kloge folk* is the exception. While popular with patients, the number of practitioners is declining precipitously. "The symbol of family tradition supports their claims to high virtue and respected status, but it may prove not to be enough to ensure a long-term future for their way of providing health care," laments Anderson, adding that "demise of the tradition is apparently well underway."

According to Robert Anderson, the present Danish bonesetting tradition can be clearly traced along distinct family lineages through a few generations at most, despite its undoubtedly greater antiquity (see chapter 1). Though parents with whom they apprenticed were called *kloge folk*, or wise people, Danish bonesetters now shun this identity in favor of "masseur." Anderson concludes, "The appearance of being traditional is misleading and they are best thought of as a variant of contemporary alternative styles of bodywork differentiated from all others by virtue of their descent from historically recent autodidacts." Their styles have changed over the past generation, with many taking on the trappings of biomedicine by adopting clinical settings, regular appointments in place of a more informal, first-come first-served schedule, and a more hurried pace. They tread a fine line, however, between emulation of and differentiation from other practitioners such as doctors, chiropractors, and physical therapists, with their claim to uniqueness stemming from their attention to deep tissue as well as bones and joints.

In chapter 2, Susan Walkley highlights the recent history of the four-thousand-year-old practice of massage, showing the shift in cultural perceptions of it across the twentieth century in the United States, which is now rejoining the rest of the world in its appreciation of the healing potentialities of massage. U.S. biomedicine eschews physical contact with patients, preferring to rely on high technology diagnostics rather than physical exam. Walkley finds it "sometimes disconcerting to patients [to] have their muscle pain diagnosed from a distance," and the result has been to create a therapeutic opening in which massage has flourished. While massage therapy continues to face a challenge from skeptics who demand to see verifiable health benefits from controlled clinical trials, it has meanwhile embraced the route of professionalization as a survival strategy. It is interesting to note that the rise in legitimacy of massage in the United States has tracked with the scientific development and entrenchment of the "stress and disease" hypothesis.

In chapter 3, Ian Coulter shows that though chiropractic is more extensively used in the United States than osteopathy—with use doubling in the past two decades—it took longer to professionalize. "From the late 1940s, when some chiropractors were being prosecuted and jailed for practicing medicine without a license, to the 1990s, a radical transformation occurred in the way chiropractic was perceived," finds Coulter. Since the 1950s, health services researchers have considered chiropractic a limited neuromusculoskeletal specialty and focused on its efficacy and utilization, while social scientists have viewed chiropractic as a more broad-based paradigm and focused on the clinical encounter. Basing their ideas on conventional wisdom rather than empirical data, the tendency of sociologists and anthropologists to label chiropractic as "deviant" or "marginal" insured that it would continue to be viewed as such for some time. The result was that it came to be judged, rather oxymoronically, as a stigmatized profession. Only later did researchers shift their emphasis from social structural issues such as status and role to one of systematically studying the clinical encounter and the beliefs of patients. Subsequently, over the course of a century, chiropractic changed status "from a marginal to a *limited* medical profession" (not *parallel*, as is seen below for osteopathy); their treatment in the literature helped define this trajectory. The debate still remains: Will the chiropractic of the future be a specialist's role or a broad-based form of health care? We are left to ponder to what degree scholars and public observers of a practice influence its present and future trajectory.

In chapter 4, Hans Baer traces the meioticlike fissioning of one manual therapy into four entities, each shaped by the cultural matrix in which it became embedded. The rapid diffusion of osteopathy across the United States, Europe, and Australia shortly after its Midwestern inception in the late 1800s was aided by the close collaboration of physician William Smith with its founder, Andrew Still, also trained as a doctor. Ironically, while Still envisioned a scientific manual medicine and strongly rejected the use of drugs, surgery, and technology, the modern-day version is virtually indistinguishable from biomedical primary care, suffering from "an 'osteopathic invisibility syndrome' in that the . . . public is generally unaware of the profession." It has not only professionalized, but now specializes as well, with only one percent of its practitioners choosing manipulative therapy as a specialty. The sociopolitical contexts of each of the four countries featured—the United States,

Canada, Britain, and Australia—have influenced the evolution of osteopathic medicine within their borders. In contrast to the United States, where osteopathy has accommodated to biomedicine and filled the primary care physician shortage created by a free market system, in the other three countries, which have national health care systems, manipulative therapy has continued to be its signature feature. Baer shows why in the first of these three countries osteopathy has lost ground to chiropractic, in the next it has won out, and in the final it has formed an easy alliance.

The aim of Jennifer Minor, Miranda Warburton, and Vincent Black's chapter 5 is to derive an understanding of Tuina's present structure and function from the ancient social and cultural values that engendered it. One can trace its transformation over the millennia from its humble start as a peasant practice to a cumulative, systematized dominant practice influenced by the written word, philosophy, and other aspects of increasing cultural complexity. Founded on Daoist principles of universal flow such as yin-yang, the five elements, and qi, Tuina is an integral part of a Traditional Chinese Medicine that diagnoses, treats, and prevents sickness. The world's oldest surviving medical texts, dating back thousands of years, set out some of the foundational principles of present day Tuina. The folk musculoskeletal treatment of Anmo gradually developed into a learned Tuina, which itself was later synthesized into the state-authorized TCM. Today's TCM education consists of formalized rigorous training that includes the study of classical texts as well as elements of Western biological sciences. "The effects of Tuina manipulations on the body clearly reflect the underpinnings of the cultural beliefs of holism, balance, and the connection to the natural environment that guided the development of the medical system, its diagnostic and treatment procedures, and even how students learn the system," states Minor.

What Walkley notes for massage can be said of each of the modalities under examination: "'East' and 'West' are problematic categories. . . . [T]oday's global variety of practices has been created through multiple cross-cultural interactions, reflecting the same early historical contacts between peoples and pragmatic blending of cultures that have characterized human history." Each chapter here demonstrates the vitality of the musculoskeletal methods employed. But perhaps the unavoidable conclusion to be drawn is that in large-scale contemporary society, a tradition must professionalize if it hopes to survive and compete in the modern world, despite the inherent risk of losing what is unique and powerful about itself.

Reference

Young, Allan
    1976 Internalizing and Externalizing Medical Belief Systems: An Ethiopian Example. *Social Science and Medicine* 10:147–56.

Indigenous Bonesetters in Contemporary Denmark

I

ROBERT ANDERSON

Old Tradition or Modern Innovation?

IN DENMARK TODAY, practitioners of alternative medicine successfully compete with physicians and other conventional medical clinicians just as they do in the rest of Europe and in the United States. The variety of alternative practitioners in Denmark, although similar to that found elsewhere, is unusual in that it includes a small number who are said to perpetuate a centuries-old Danish folk healing tradition. My curiosity was aroused because I thought they were extinct.

In 1999 and 2000 I flew to Denmark to engage in blitzkrieg ethnographic research lasting a couple of weeks on each trip. Carried out against years of living and working in Denmark and based on my being clinically qualified in both medicine and chiropractic, those brief incursions provided time enough to interview and observe the work of five bonesetters said to perpetuate the tradition of Danish folk healers known as *kloge folk*. It was time enough to learn that only the designation as *kloge folk* is old. Their methods and theories are recent.

The designation *kloge folk* defies translation; no English word seems to quite convey the meaning it once had for Danes. The most widely used translation is "wise people" (singular, *klog mand*, "wise man," or *klog kone*, "wise woman"), although many would argue that *kloge folk* were not so much wise as they were clever. Whether wise or clever in the past, in our time it would be more meaningful to designate the ones I observed and interviewed as bonesetters, manual therapists, or massage therapists because they make no claim to being wise or cunning; they think of themselves as *masseurs* (Danish singular, *massør*) rather than as all-purpose healers, which in their view might imply a touch of magic or prayer that has no place in their completely pragmatic, hands-on treatments (Tangherlini 2001:4). For cross-cultural comparisons they meet my definition of bonesetting because they practice both massage and joint manipulation (see Huber and Anderson 1996:31). I traveled to Denmark to study them because they reputedly still employ some of the curative strategies of *kloge folk*.

I first heard about these indigenous practitioners from Kaj Brandt Thomsen, a retired middle school teacher who happens to be my cousin. He told me that years earlier he had himself been successfully treated on two different occasions for acute, incapacitating low back pain by two different *kloge folk* in or near the small city where he lives in rural Jutland. We agreed to meet the following year when he would take me to meet the successors of each of the two wise men who once treated him.

I found that the *kloge folk* are modern practitioners of noncertificated, nonstandardized kinds of naturalistic, nonmagical bonesetting. Although it is legal for them to diagnose and treat musculoskeletal disorders using hands-on methods, they are treated with benign neglect by the biomedical community and their care is not reimbursed under the national health care system. They are distinctive within Denmark, however, in that they learned their craft by means of apprenticeship. Each was trained by a close relative and they all trace their origins to a founding parent, grandparent, or great-grandparent who was self-taught, having acquired skills by combining personal experimentation with information adopted or adapted from books, hearsay, and casual observation. They thus differ from chiropractors, physical therapists, acupuncturists, massage therapists, and others who also treat musculoskeletal problems but who acquire their skills and concepts by successfully completing courses of study and passing qualifying examinations.

Wise People in the Danish Folk Tradition

It appears that the *kloge folk* who provided health care in earlier centuries often relied heavily on occult knowledge. Although we have very few details about them, we know that their practices were by no means uniform (Kæseler 1998). Among those who were burned at the stake as witches in the seventeenth century, for instance, Old Anne Kruse reportedly claimed to cure animals and people made ill by the machinations of witches or the sorcery of elves by uttering an incantation over the victims. But we know neither the origin of her theory of disease nor how she acquired her magic spell. We do know that the spell concluded with the words, "In the name of God the Father, the Son, and the Holy Spirit." These power words from the formulae of Christian prayers were tacked onto what otherwise appears to be an older pagan conjuration (Henningsen 1978:70–71).

Old Anne Kruse may represent a hoary peasant tradition passed on from one generation of *kloge folk* to the next. Indeed, traditions of modest antiquity and continuity (a century or two) are evident in some lineages that lasted well into the twentieth century. Petra Mosegaard, for example, produced magical cures as a *klog kone* until her death in 1976. The founder of her tradition, Christen Rasmussen Skov, established himself five generations earlier in the latter part of the eighteenth century (Henningsen 1978).

A *klog mand*, referred to as *Majeribestyrer Svenstrup*, also represented a family tradition. He was active until at least 1927 as the last in a succession of eight *kloge folk* who traced their descent from Maren Haaning, a *klog kone* who lived from 1781 to 1853 (Rasmussen 1927:80–82). This lineage, which historians refer to as the "wise women of Vindblæs"—since only the last was a man—made medicines from herbs, liquors, and other substances based on formulae and instructions passed on from one generation to the next.

For the most part, however, twentieth-century *kloge folk* have been autodidacts, inventors without predecessors who often left no successors. Marie Kjærgaard Nielsen, better known as The Fladbro Woman (*Fladbro konen*), was active from the mid-1930s until the mid-1950s. She said that her teachers were angels who early in her career visited her three nights in a row as apparitions in a jail cell where she was imprisoned on charges of being a quack. After a quarter of a century as a *klog kone*, she died without either training or authorizing a successor. Her modus operandi was to fall into a trance, place her hand on the patient, and reputedly draw the sickness into her own body. Witnesses say that the transfer made her body and limbs thicken and grow hard until she either shook off or vomited the extracted disease (anonymous 1976:129–34; *Demokraten* 1955; *Berlingske Tidende* 1949).

Klog Mand Arno Wolle's long career stretched from about 1920 to 1979, when he likewise retired without training a successor. He taught himself to make herbal remedies beginning in 1920 when he was only seventeen years old. In that first instance he acquired a recipe for long life allegedly from a Chinese temple priest whom he encountered in Germany. At the height of his career he imported hundreds of different herbs from around the world which he used to prepare elixirs and compounds in his home laboratory (Randers town library archive, unidentified clipping).

The five bonesetters I got to know descended from twentieth-century, self-taught health care providers of this type who differed from practitioners such as Nielsen and Wolle only in that they passed their skills on to younger members of their families. They therefore constitute indigenous, family traditions. Only the designation as *kloge folk* is old. Their methods and theories are relatively recent innovations.

The Dilemma of Anthropology versus European Ethnology

When I was a student at the University of Copenhagen half a century ago, I moved easily between two related but separate ethnographic traditions. In the anthropology department, under the aegis of Professor Kaj Birkit Smith, students were taught how to do research in other parts of the world, while in the Danish ethnology program of Professor Axel Steensberg, the goal was to document Danish cultural history. In both anthropology and European ethnology at that time, an enormous amount of research was dedicated to the study of peasant culture—hence the overlapping of disciplines. However, one prominent difference relevant to the bonesetters I report on here has to do with identifying individuals, families, and communities by name when one writes about them. As a matter of ethics, anthropologists are usually constrained to preserve anonymity by using pseudonyms and disguised locations that will protect the privacy of people they write about. A contrary obligation dominates European ethnology. Because it is a way of writing history, the practice whenever possible is to clearly name people and places, the way Marie Kjærgaard Nielsen and Arno Wolle are named, in order to acknowledge their contributions to a contemporary national identity.

I have always tended to favor the approach that names. I did so several decades ago when I published a book about the community of Dragør in the vicinity of Copenhagen, and I shall do so now (Anderson and Anderson 1964). But note the potential dilemma. I would never want to publish anything that might embarrass or harm people who generously admit me into their lives. Yet, especially when dealing with medical issues, I have an obligation to discuss practices that I fear might do harm to others. Fortunately, from my observations as a medical doctor and a chiropractor, no practitioner observed and interviewed in this study performed harmful or dangerous manipulations, so that aspect of the dilemma is only potential rather than actual. But there are further considerations. It can be intrusive to discuss the popularity, efficacy, or income of individual practitioners. It must be acknowledged that, in order to avoid possible embarrassment, I am inclined toward writing appreciatively rather than critically, and selectively rather than thoroughly. Readers will want to take this possible bias into account as I discuss the practitioners I came to know.

Four Family Traditions

Laust Nielsen in Randers

This *massør* is a third generation bonesetter. His great-grandfather (his father's father's father), the original Laust Nielsen, lived from 1867 to 1955 and was widely known in eastern Jutland as the *Klog Mand* in Auning. The elder Nielsen started out as a farmer who discovered that he had a knack for treating musculoskeletal problems in animals and people. With practice he developed this skill. Success with his own animals and family led neighbors to seek him out. By roughly 1920 he was so busy taking care of people in pain that he handed the farm over to his son, and from then on earned his living solely by practicing as a *klog mand* in the village where he lived. It is said that his technique was to offer deep massage combined with the manipulation of joints. For example, if he diagnosed a shoulder as being "out of place" (*sætter forkert*), he would treat it with heavy rubbing combined with a maneuver to set it back in place (*sætter den på plads*). He was a "bonesetter" in this sense.

The old Laust Nielsen in Auning passed over his son on the farm to teach his skills to three grandsons, Kristian Laust Nielsen in Randers (the second bonesetter to be known professionally as "Laust Nielsen"), Knud Nielsen, who still practices in Odense, and Martin Nielsen, who is located in Aarhus. As I write, Knud and Martin are quite old and frail, although still able to care for one or two patients a day, and Kristian Laust Nielsen has retired. Neither Knud nor Martin trained a successor, so the tradition will not continue in those parts of Jutland. Kristian Laust Nielsen in Randers, on the contrary, was succeeded several years ago by his son, Søren Laust Nielsen, the current practitioner known professionally as "Laust Nielsen." Søren's twenty-three-year-old son, Mikel Laust Nielsen, is studying to be a master machinist and denies any interest in taking over his father's practice as a fourth "Laust Nielsen"—but, of course, one never knows what may happen in the future, especially since he occasionally will give a treatment to his father. All three of the Laust Nielsen's to date began in other professions, the first as a farmer, the second as a dance instructor, and the third as a schoolteacher. The third is only in his early fifties, so there is time enough for his son to change career goals and take up the family's traditional occupation.

As to terminology, only the great-grandfather was consistently referred to as a *klog mand*. Laust number two identified himself as a *massør*. However, when the local newspaper acknowledged his sixtieth birthday in 1983, the caption to the article identified him as a "*klog mand*," the use of quotation marks implying that it was already old-fashioned to refer to a modern massage therapist in that way. Yet, within the article it says, "When he moved to Randers it was both as a *klog mand* and as a dance instructor," with no quotation marks at all.

Henning Vad and Annette Vad in Fårup

This family line also comprises three generations, but the family history is more recent. It began with Henning Vad's mother, who started in a small way by assuaging her husband's sore muscles and those of others in the family. Little by little neighbors realized that she had a talent for healing and began coming by for aid. Her reputation grew by word of mouth and by 1948 she was working full-time in this career.

Her practice flourished until the mid-1960s when she suffered a shoulder injury and had to cut back; Henning then began to take over. It is ironic that shortly after I first observed Henning's work in 1999, he fell down a flight of stairs and tore ligaments in his shoulder, which required surgery and a long recuperation. Since the accident he can only handle a small part of his former workload. History repeated itself as his daughter Annette largely took over for him in the last year or two. Fortunately, Annette had already begun to work part-time with her father from 1992 and was therefore well-qualified to carry on.

Their style of practice is very similar to that of Laust Nielsen. Although Henning never apprenticed to Laust's father, they were good friends in the old days and accustomed to talk shop when they occasionally met. It appears that what Henning was taught by his mother has been modified in the direction of old Laust's techniques.

Was Henning's mother a *klog kone*? The answer is yes and no. By the 1950s it was already more appropriate for her to be spoken of as a *massør*. However, it was customary for many in the rustic environment of that part of Jutland to refer to her by the old term, and even Henning is sometimes thought of that way, although the usage is now clearly archaic, as is apparent in the following conversation among Henning, a sixty-eight-year-old pensioner named Jonas, and me. Henning was instructing Jonas, who comes periodically to be treated for low back pain, on how to bend over to put on his pants. As Henning finished, Jonas caught my eye to say, "He really is wise (*Han er da klog*)."

Henning interjected: "No, I'm not *klog*, but . . . (pausing)"

Jonas: "He is good at giving advice, but it's hard to remember afterwards."

Bob: "But he is a *klog mand*, isn't he?"

Jonas: "No, one wouldn't say that. He is only skilled (*dygtig*)."

Bob: "Why wouldn't you say he's a *klog mand*?"

Jonas: "That was the usage in the old days. In the old days, my oh my, then they were *klog mand* and *klog kone*. But they don't do that now. Well, a few do. There are a few."

Henning: "In those days it was about 'medicines,' charms, herbs, and all of that. This here, it's, shall we say, more a kind of craft (*et stykke handværk*)."

Bob: "Yeah, *massør*."

Jonas: "Yeah, that's what's on his business card, *massør*, and it's these here [opening and closing his hands and fingers]."

Bob: "But your mother? Wasn't she called a *klog kone*?"

Henning: "More then than now. That's right."

Martin Haakonsen in Ringkøbing

The business card that Mr. Haakonsen handed me also reads *massør*, but his waiting room unambiguously identifies him with the *kloge folk* tradition. A plaque prominently displayed on the wall reads, "*Kloge folk* in Jutland," under which is written, "In thankful memory of the wise men (*kloge mænd*) who sustained so many (*vor af mange bleve bevaret*)." It is flanked on both sides and underneath by the framed pen and ink drawings of eleven *kloge mænd* from all over Denmark, each identified by the man's name and home community. Lowest down on this display, symbolizing his descent from all of the old "wise men" displayed above, hangs a solitary portrait, that of Richardt Haakonson, the father of Martin. But the drawing is of a man quite different in appearance from the other *kloge mænd*, because, unlike all of them in their old peasant costumes, Richardt had his hair cut in an urbane fashion and he was wearing a suit and tie.

Richardt did not apprentice to any of the old bonesetters displayed in his waiting room. Martin says that the family tradition began with Richardt's mother and his mother's brother, but I was unable to elicit any information at all about what kind of patient care they offered or how they practiced. Their father before them, Martin's great-grandfather, was also said to be a *klog mand*, but Martin couldn't tell me anything about him. He couldn't even remember his name, and his picture is not displayed on the wall. I finally concluded that just about all that was passed on to Richardt from these forebears, as from the eleven unrelated healers pictured on Martin's waiting room wall, was the sense that an innate gift for healing was transmitted from generation to generation in a family line. In a 1958 newspaper clipping that Martin let me read in his kitchen, it was said of Richardt: "There is a tradition in Haakonsen's lineage of having a touch of supernatural power (*at have en smule overnaturlige evner*)." Richardt apparently drew on that somewhat occult family history as an inspiration or authentication, but he seems to have learned on his own how to do bodywork.

As a youth Richardt worked as a bricklayer and a backyard butcher (*murarbejdsmand og hjemmeslagter*). He did not inherit a place to work or any clientele from his mother or uncle. However, at the beginning of World War II, while doing manual labor, he began to treat people for rheumatism. Within a year or two he set himself up to practice full-time in his home as a *massør*. His son Martin, born in 1944, apprenticed to him, and Martin hopes that his daughter Johanne will carry on the tradition. At the time we spoke, she was only thirteen and too young to do more than affirm that she liked the idea.

In the 1958 clipping Richardt was asked, "Do you call yourself a *klog mand*, Haakonsen?" His answer was, "No, one doesn't do that." But according to the reporter, he smiled in a self-conscious way when he responded to the question, adding, "I say *massør*. You have to have some way of describing your work." His

son Martin also does not refer to himself as a *klog mand*, but others are not so inhibited. An article about Martin in a 1996 edition of Denmark's most prestigious
national paper, *Berlingste Tidende*, identified him as "Martin Haakonsen . . . who for
miles around is known as the *klog mand* in Ringkøbing."

Tove Carstensen in Ørsted

In 1929, an eighteen-year-old farmer (*landmand*) named Kristian Nygaard was
painfully injured when a large workhorse crushed him against a stall door. The local chiropractor failed to make him better, even after repeated visits, but young
Nygaard paid close attention to how the chiropractor performed spinal and peripheral joint adjustments. More than a decade later, in 1940, when he was working on his grandfather's farm, his wife injured her finger while milking the cows.
Kristian treated her successfully. He subsequently treated his father for an injury.
News of his success spread to neighbors and friends. Years later he told his daughter Tove that he was not a bit interested in doing bodywork. He wanted to be a
landmand, but he could not refuse the many farming people who came to him for
help, and soon it was a major part of his work.

His method of treatment combined massage with joint manipulation. Judging
from how two former patients and his daughter described his methods, it is clear
that he taught himself to do lumbar, thoracic, and cervical adjustments in somewhat the way he saw the local chiropractor do them in his youth, but with a startling difference. Except for having a patient sit on a chair while he manipulated
the neck, he positioned his patients on the floor, where he kneeled next to them
to massage and manipulate spinal and peripheral joints. Now ninety years old and
retired, until a few years ago he still got down on the floor with his patients. I was
told that in those last years he was so old and stiff that when he finished he would
have to ask the patient to pull him back up onto his feet.

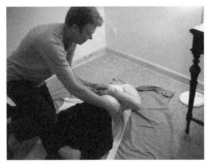

Figure 1.1.   Tove Carstensen administering
a chiropracticlike manipulation in an unchi-
ropracticlike way on the floor. (Photo by
Robert Anderson.)

His daughter Tove Carstensen, her husband, and their two grown sons continue the agricultural tradition, living in an old, half-timbered, straw-roofed farmhouse at the edge of the small east Jutland village of Ørsted. She recalls that as a teenager she was not interested in apprenticing to her father, but he liked to have her with him and they eventually agreed that he would teach her, which resulted in her working with him daily for a whole year to learn the trade. Shortly after that, Kristian became sick for six months and she temporarily took over his entire practice. However, she gave up bonesetting when she married and found herself fully occupied with raising two boys and managing a farm with her husband. But now her sons are adults and her father has retired, so a couple of years ago she began to offer care to her father's former patients. More and more, such people sought her out, so in the year between my visits she had two rooms at one end of the old farmhouse remodeled to serve as a proper clinic. Her treatment room is distinctive. It looks quite empty. Instead of a treatment table it features wall-to-wall carpeting and a straight-backed chair, the only equipment she needs.

People who remember Kristian Nygaard typically refer to him as a well-respected *klog mand*, but, of course, his daughter is not usually described as a *klog kone* because she is too much a modern woman, even though she lives in a very old house. She is a *massør*. "Will either of your sons take up massage therapy?" I asked one afternoon. "They are not interested," she said, "and I would never push them into it. If one of them should want to learn, however, I would certainly be willing. But I don't think it will happen."

On Identity and Differentiation

Alternative practitioners, including Danish *kloge folk*, compete for patients in a pluralistic health care marketplace. In order to build a successful practice, a practitioner must create a professional identity that is competitive. To understand how that is accomplished, I found it helpful to use an approach that can be applied more broadly both within and beyond health care. In fact, I first found it useful years ago when the challenge was how to identify certain cultural patterns that underlay the complexities of European history.

In the late 1960s I was attempting to write an ethnographic overview of preindustrial Europe, but I wanted to break with the practice then common in anthropology of writing only about peasant cultures. I had done a small amount of work on the persisting land-based aristocratic culture in Denmark and knew that in Europe, as a whole, one could identify uniformities of aristocratic culture that cut across national boundaries. The same was true of town cultures. As I struggled with how to write about premodern Europe as a culture area when it was shot through with the diversities of peasant, aristocratic, and town cultures, I found that a simple analytic concept was of enormous value: imitation versus differentiation. Whereas uniformities seemed to reflect in part a strong tendency for people of like social status to mimic one another using culture traits (clothing, housing, dialect, values, and so on) as symbolic markers of identity, they also seemed to select or modify culture traits to be as different as possible from those they did not want to identify with. In an ongoing process of culture change, they tended to differentiate as well as emulate (Anderson 1971:9–18; see also Anderson 1973:12–15; Anderson 1975).

The concept of cultural differentiation versus imitation can be applied within medicine (Anderson 1990). For example, alternative practitioners emulate selected aspects of the practice of biomedicine as a way to communicate similarities they share or aspire to with the power brokers of institutionalized health care (Anderson 1996:288–90). The bonesetters in this study, for example, acknowledge the importance of being knowledgeable about anatomy and physiology and they designate their places of work as "clinics" within which they have waiting rooms and treatment rooms. They post regular hours and all but Mr. Haakonsen schedule patients for routine time slots. Of course, to do so is practical, but it also has symbolic importance. The present Laust Nielsen, for example, works very differently from his great-grandfather, whose clients simply turned up at his farm unannounced and waited, or returned if the *klog mand* was too busy with other patients or with farmwork.

But imitation is not the dominant process for bonesetters. On the contrary, what seems very important to them is to portray how different they are from all other kinds of health care providers who specialize in musculoskeletal disorders. I have indicated that these bonesetters are distinctive and think of themselves as such by virtue of completing apprenticeships to predecessors who were self-taught. However, when asked more specifically how they distinguish themselves from others who also specialize in musculoskeletal pain and dysfunction, I found that they hinge their identity very importantly on being able to offer a service that no competitor can match. It is clearly important in practical and symbolic terms to justify an identity that sharply differentiates them and what they do from others who diagnose and treat musculoskeletal disorders. To be an alternative practitioner is to be recognized as sharply differentiated.

When Laust and I first discussed similarities and differences relating to chiropractic he made a statement that did not fit with what I observed when he was with patients. He freely confessed, "I also use some chiropractic here and there" (*Jeg bruger også noget kiropraktik in imellem*). But that statement was misleading. In his usage, the term "chiropractic" is simply generic for joint manipulation, and to the extent that he does manipulate, it hardly resembles chiropractic in the least. Above all, it is ancillary to heavy massage. When he said that he uses some chiropractic, he added a basis for differentiation by stating, "That is to say, I manipulate. If it is a shoulder, for example, I pull it out and sort of set it in again, but I massage it first, with very heavy (*meget kraftigt*) massage." His separate identity is especially obvious when a patient presents with low back pain, for which the signature procedure of chiropractors is to perform spinal adjustments based on the theory that a vertebral joint is misaligned (subluxated). As he explained, "I prefer to take off from where the problem really is, because the problem is not in the back (*rygen*). It is in the hips (*hofterne*). People have bad backs because their hip and thigh muscles are not as they should be. Back muscles are only used to hold the back straight. When the hip and thigh muscles are not correctly oriented to the ground we are forced to hold the back wrong, and so we get a back problem." His procedure, then, is to do deep massage of the buttocks and legs as well as of the powerful paraspinal muscles of the back. For Laust, the two professions are complementary. In his view, chiropractors work with bones and joints while he works with muscles and tendons.

Although Tove Carstensen's technique of doing spinal manipulation originally grew from her father's imitation of the chiropractor who adjusted him for a crush injury, her approach to back pain and other joint disorders ended up being thoroughly different from that of formally trained chiropractors. The difference is most obvious in the habit of working with the patient and practitioner positioned directly on the floor. In addition, however, insofar as I was able to observe the work of Tove, two other differences are equally striking. First, she spends most of the twenty minutes or so performing a gentle massage of the back, buttocks, and legs. Second, only at the very end of the treatment session does she perform spinal manipulations, and they are quite nonspecific. Chiropractors characteristically attach great importance to adjusting in a highly "specific" way. That is, whereas a chiropractor identifies each single vertebra as being misaligned or hypomobile in a precisely defined position or characteristic of motion, and administers a thrust to the spinous or transverse process by applying the piseform bone of the wrist in a calculated way, Tove administers her "adjustments" to vaguely defined areas on the lumbar, thoracic, and cervical spines with what appear to be generic manipulative moves. In her defense, it should be noted that no experimental research has ever demonstrated that the difference between specific and nonspecific adjustments results in any differences in outcomes. In fact, one famous teacher and practitioner of spinal manipulation, James Cyriax, insists that the joint that needs to release will do so spontaneously if one performs a nonspecific maneuver under traction (Cyriax and Cyriax 1983:156–57).

Tove's clear sense of the importance of being different emerged when we were talking about chiropractic adjustments one morning. "My father and I offer a mixture of physical therapy and chiropractic. First we warm up the muscles the way [she imagines] a physical therapist would do. The warmer the muscles are, the more they relax, and the easier it is to move things. Only after that do we perform manipulations." I pointed out that many chiropractors begin with heat and massage whereas others simply go directly to the adjustment. "Too many chiropractors do not warm the muscles," she countered, "at least not in Denmark. There are so many different kinds of practitioners now," she added. "The worst is, they all want to make money. It's up to the patient to figure out who can or cannot offer a cure." In another conversation she added that because she is first of all a farmer and only does bodywork as a sideline, she doesn't need to make money from her practice.

Annette Vad explained to me that certificated massage therapists perform what she characterizes as a completely different kind of massage. Of that, more below, but for the moment I would only point out that while the difference is justified in strictly anatomic and physiological terms—hard, deep massage is said to achieve what the gentle massage of physical therapists fails to do in treating severe pain— the difference can also be said to serve an important symbolic function. The same is true of Laust Nielsen's explanation for how physical therapy is totally different from what he does. That is, to describe these differences is to advertise that the bonesetter offers efficacious care for conditions that chiropractors, massage therapists, and physical therapists cannot successfully treat.

Efficacy and Time

But are these bonesetters successful in treating back pain and other musculoskeletal problems? Is it more than merely a claim? It is important in doing an ethnography of alternative medicine to document as precisely as one can the health benefits such practitioners confer or the harm they may do (Anderson 1991). Efficacy can be measured in several ways, but the only measure I am able to offer from this rapid ethnographic study is that of patient satisfaction, and that only in an impressionistic way (on efficacy, see Anderson 1997:563). On the whole, patients appear to value the care they receive from each of the five bonesetters I observed, as demonstrated by their well-attended waiting rooms. Yet, from that admittedly subjective observation it is possible to challenge one nearly universal explanation for why alternative practitioners are popular.

It is widely assumed on the basis of no systematic research at all that alternative practitioners attract patients because the interaction of medical doctors with patients tends to be hurried and impersonal, whereas alternative practitioners devote much time and attention to their patients and thus make them feel well cared for (see Anderson 2000:12, 2002:197).

To challenge that assumption about "cultural and psychological strengths," I would offer the observation that time and attention do not appear to be determinative of patient satisfaction in this study of Danish bonesetters. That had already been my conclusion some years ago based on my professional involvement with chiropractors, but it seems verified by what I learned from Martin Haakonsen, who has earned an enviable reputation as a *massør*. In interviews with a convenience sample of twelve patients encountered in his waiting room, I asked about their experiences with Martin. Their consistent responses were that they liked him and felt that they had received excellent care. His waiting room is always filled. Yet Martin only spends five to ten minutes with each patient, a practice in which he deviates markedly from what his father taught him.

All of the other bonesetters in this study spend twenty to thirty minutes with each patient, mostly doing massage, but chatting all the while. A treatment is always accompanied by an unhurried conversation. Old Richardt did the same. Massage was so central to his practice that during World War II he required his patients to bring lard or ration coupons when they came for treatment, because it was a time of food shortages and he could not massage without an emollient. His son Martin does no massage at all. "I had to give it up," he told me. "It took too much time. It takes half an hour if I do massage." So he moves rapidly, although in a friendly manner, from one patient to the next, limiting his treatments to quick thumb jabs, rapid finger probes, light slaps with his fists, pinches, grasping moves with his hands and fingers, and, only in certain cases, gentle pressure adjustments of one or another of the peripheral joints (e.g., shoulders, wrists, fingers). Unlike all of the others, he does not maintain a schedule of appointments because he moves too fast and unpredictably for that. His reception room always has several people waiting, but the wait is never very long because each patient requires only a few minutes. Evidently an alternative practitioner can be highly effective by the measure of patient satisfaction, even if he or she moves very rapidly from one patient to the next.

Efficacy and Pain

Some bonesetters cause a lot of pain when they do massage and manipulation. The techniques of others are very gentle and nearly pain-free. The deep, friction massages performed by Laust Nielsen, Henning Vad, and Annette Vad leave trails of hot, red marks on the skin of their patients, who often groan and wince. In contrast, the treatments of Martin Haakonsen and Tove Carstensen cause scarcely any pain at all. Because all five practitioners are equally successful, this difference on the pain dimension raises an interesting question. How do Nielsen and the Vads justify pain to themselves and to their patients?

Annette is in a particularly good position to offer an explanation. She is not only an experienced registered nurse but has also completed a six-month massage school course where she "learned about the muscles and their functions, what they do and don't do," as she put it. I asked how that training changed her approach to

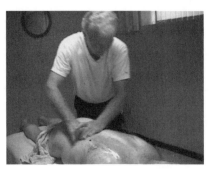

Figure 1.2.   Vad performs a deep knuckle
massage, leaving visible red marks on skin.
(Photo by Robert Anderson.)

bodywork. She said it led to no change at all. "It is a very different kind of massage from what we do here." How so, I asked. "You are taught there to use the flat of your hands and fingers, which I found was more exhausting, because you have to use your body in a way that stresses your wrists, elbows, and shoulders." She, Henning, and Laust all have enormous calluses on the proximal interphalangeal joints of their fingers from the hours they spend each day leaning their bodies onto those finger knuckles to apply heavy pressure when they do massage.

I asked if she was taught to do deep massage at the massage school. "No," she emphasized. "They say if the massage hurts the muscles will cramp and it doesn't help, but I say something different, because how are you going to get through the muscle if you can't use some strength?" And that approach is painful, as attested to by Else, a sixty-seven-year-old patient with chronic, diffuse musculoskeletal pains who seeks care every month or two from Annette. "The first time I came here, Bob, I was completely yellow and blue over my whole body," she told me as she was dressing. "Some days I think, I don't want to come. But I know how good it is."

Laust, too, has a good basis for explaining and justifying the pain. In addition to graduating from teacher training school, he was trained as a physical therapist. "How did physical therapy change your way of working with patients when you took over your father's practice," I queried. "I benefited from the anatomy and physiology. It's important to know that. But I make no use of their treatment methods." Do you use heat? "No." Muscle stretching or passive exercises? "No. I find no use at all for the purely practical physical therapy."

A year later the subject of pain came up in a three-way conversation that included his friend and patient, Mr. Sørensen. "You told me that people will not tolerate the pain of treatment the way they used to," I interjected. "Yes. It's harder for people to accept it. It's harder for people to understand that it will hurt more in order to get better. Sometimes after the first treatment there is a reaction. The problem changes. Sometimes it changes in such a way that people feel they are worse than they were. They don't come to me to have it get worse. They come to have it get better. But that is a transition. It will get better." Sørensen agreed that subsequent treatments are increasingly less painful. Laust continued, "Sometimes a patient will telephone to cancel because the first treatment hurt too much. But that's dumb, because the second treatment won't hurt nearly as much, and third will hurt even less. By quitting after the first she doesn't get anything out of it. It's kind of sad, because she cheated herself by not listening carefully to my explanation that the first treatment is the worst. If she continued she would see that what I say is right." Sørensen offered this concluding observation: "Sometimes you get such bad advertising because they only went half way."

What then do Haakonsen and Carstensen have to say about treatments that cause pain? They provide painless treatments in quite different ways, so pain-free cannot be attributed to any single technique. I have already referred to Martin's abandonment of massage to rely only on quick and gentle probes and pinches in combination with gentle joint manipulations. Tove, in contrast, spends twenty to thirty minutes with a patient. Most of that time is devoted to a very soft and gentle massage. "I do massage that warms the muscles," she told me. "Deep massage can do harm. I just use the flat of my hand. My rule is, never too hard and you will never have a problem." Similarly, although she routinely performs lumbar, thoracic, and cervical adjustments, they, too, are done cautiously.

Although Tove has not reestablished her father's high-volume practice in the short time since she quietly reentered the field, Martin demonstrably maintains a high-volume clinic. Patient satisfaction is high, and that puzzles me. If one can be effective in a painless way, how can one justify causing pain? The answer in part is that patients simply accept what is offered, not being aware that other practitioners offer relatively painless treatment. In addition, patients are taught that pain is good for them, and apparently it is if the patient sticks it out. But it requires stoic patients. When one of Laust's patients, a young marine machinist, stepped down from the treatment table, I said, "You feel better, huh?" "Yes." "Did it hurt?" He paused before saying, "You can definitely notice it (*man kan godt mærke det*)," and as he spoke his lips formed a Mona Lisa smile and he glanced at Laust in a self-conscious way. Responding to this obvious reticence to appear unmanly, Laust clarified for my benefit. "Now he's a good Jutlander, so he isn't about to complain." "Yeah, I know," said I, and we all chuckled.

Conclusion: Is the End in Sight?

The epoch of the original *kloge folk* is gone. The bonesetters I encountered are an epiphenomenon of that old tradition. The appearance of being traditional is misleading and they are best thought of as a variant of contemporary alternative styles of bodywork differentiated from all others by virtue of their descent from historically recent autodidacts. They also tend to differ dramatically from one another, particularly along the dimensions of treatment time and pain. Yet they have one thing in common. Although they imitate biomedical practitioners in maintaining clinics and, in the case of Laust Nielsen, wearing clinic coats, they differentiate themselves in their hands-on methods and biomechanical explanations.

The symbol of family tradition supports the bonesetters' claims to high virtue and respected status, but it may prove not to be enough to ensure a long-term future for their way of providing health care. They appear to be dying out as alternative practitioners in the health care marketplace. As Laust Nielsen lamented and as Martin Haakonsen illustrates in his waiting room pictures, recent decades have witnessed a precipitous decline in the numbers of these practitioners. Why are they dying out?

Is it how they use their time? It is taken as a truism that alternative practitioners have created a niche in the health care marketplace because they give a lot of personal attention to their patients, including a lot of time during visits. This assumption is unconvincing. Martin Haakonsen maintains a busy practice in which he spends very little time with each patient.

Is it because they are painful? Some Danish bonesetters cause a lot of pain. Laust Nielsen believes that his practice is falling off because contemporary people are not willing to endure pain of treatment the way they once were. Yet, Henning and Annette Vad also cause intense pain during treatment, and their practice is thriving. It would appear that pain is not decisive in survival or failure.

Why then is the bonesetting tradition of Denmark apparently on the verge of extinction? I do not know, but perhaps it is because the tradition of entering a family trade or business is no longer attractive to young people (Anderson 2002:201). A successful bonesetter earns a good living and considerable social respect, but family cultures have changed and economic opportunities are more abundant now. Laust Nielsen's son is studying to be a master machinist. Tove Christensen's sons are well into careers as agriculturalists. Demise of the tradition is apparently well under way. Now, in the whole of Denmark, as far as I could determine, only five *kloge folk* are still active, and perhaps soon there will be none. And perhaps not!

Note

I am deeply indebted to Kaj Brandt Thomsen for introducing me to four bonesetters and for warm friendship. I am equally indebted to George Nellemann, a specialist in Danish ethnography and a colleague since we were fellow students at the University of Copenhagen (1949–1951). Nellemann arranged for me to meet a fifth bonesetter. I am grateful to Niels Clausen, chiropractor, who carefully briefed me on how he and Martin Haakonsen, bonesetter, complement each other in what they offer patients in the town of Ringkøbing. I especially want to acknowledge Kathryn S. Oths and Servando Z. Hinojosa for organizing the symposium in which my findings were first presented and for their dedicated and skillful attention to editing, and to Holly Robinson of Mills College for administrative support. To all of you, my most heartfelt thanks.

References

Anderson, Robert
  1971   *Traditional Europe: A Study in Anthropology and History.* Belmont, Calif.: Wadsworth Publishing Co.
  1973   *Modern Europe: An Anthropological Perspective.* Pacific Palisades, Calif.: Goodyear Publishing Co.
  1975   *Denmark: Success of a Developing Nation.* Cambridge, Mass.: Schenkman Publishing Co.
  1990   Chiropractors for and against Vaccines. *Medical Anthropology* 12:169–86.
  1991   The Efficacy of Ethnomedicine: Research Methods in Trouble. *Medical Anthropology* 13:1–17.
  1996   *Magic, Science, and Health: The Aims and Achievements of Medical Anthropology.* Fort Worth, Tex.: Harcourt Brace College Publishers.
  1997   Is Chiropractic Mainstream or Alternative? A View from Medical Anthropology. Pp. 555–78 in Dana J. Lawrence, J. David Cassidy, Marion McGregor, William C. Meeker, and Howard T. Vernon, eds. *Advances in Chiropractic*, vol. 4. St. Louis, Mo.: Mosby.
  2000   Alternative and Conventional Medicine in Iceland. *Public Health in Iceland. Supplement 2000* nr. 1. Reykjavik, Iceland: Directorate of Health.
  2002   The Fugelli Tactic. *The Journal of Alternative and Complementary Medicine* (8) 2:197–205.
Anderson, Robert, and Barbara Gallatin Anderson
  1964   *The Vanishing Village: A Danish Maritime Community.* Seattle: University of Washington Press.
Anonymous
  1976   *Kloge Folk og Skidtfolk - Kvaksalveriets Epoke I Danmark.* Copenhagen: Politikens Forlag.
Berlingske Tidende
  1949   Randers town library.
Cyriax, James, and Patricia Cyriax
  1983   *Illustrated Manual of Orthopaedic Medicine.* London: Butterworths.
Demokraten
  1955   Randers town library.
Henningsen, Gustav
  1978   Kloge Folk og "Kloge Søren." Pp. 70–86 in Gustav Henningsen and George Nellemann, eds. *Det Farlige Liv.* Copenhagen: Nationalmuseet.

Huber, Brad R., and Robert Anderson
  1996 Bonesetters and Curers in a Mexican Community: Conceptual Models, Status, and Gender. *Medical Anthropology* 17(1):23–38.
Kæseler, Arnold
  1998 *Hekse-Tro og Hekse På Mors.* Bjergby: Forlaget Fortiden.
Rasmussen, Louise
  1927 *De Kloge Koner I Vindblæs—Maren Haaning.* Copenhagen: Woels Forlag.
Tangherlini, Timothy R.
  2001 Ghost in the Machine: Supernatural Threat and the State in Lars von Trier's Riget. *Scandinavian Studies* 73(1):1–24.

When the Body Leads the Mind: Perspectives on Massage Therapy in the United States

2

SUSAN WALKLEY

TOUCHING OR KNEADING OF TISSUE IS a primal activity for humans and the rest of the mammalian world. Given the unique design of human hands, with their long, opposable thumbs that can mold to muscular surfaces, the importance of early physical contact in social adaptation, and the propensity of animals to touch painful areas, it seems clear that massage in some form has always been a human activity. This chapter examines the current practice of therapeutic massage in the United States and how it can be related to ideas of stress and mind-body connections. As a medical anthropologist and massage therapist, I will explore the history of massage as a therapeutic modality, including the recent shift in cultural perceptions of it, the cross-cultural context of touch therapy, the professionalization of American massage, the experience of the practitioner, and how massage therapy illuminates anthropological discussions of embodiment.[1]

Massage therapy can be defined as systematic, skilled manual manipulation of the soft tissue of one person by another that is intended to promote positive physical changes and relaxation. As a manual therapy, by definition it involves the precise, manipulative capacities of the fingers to effect change in the body (Hinojosa 2002:22). Massage is clearly a body-oriented healing system under Anderson's categories (1996: 391) and distinct from spinal manipulation techniques such as chiropractic, which moves bones. Currently in the United States, massage therapy includes contemporary Western massage (including Swedish, deep tissue, sports, and medical), reflexology, neuromuscular therapies and various myofascial techniques.

This list does not include certain Eastern, energy and/or light touch techniques such as shiatsu, Tui Na, craniosacral therapies, zero balancing, and Reiki. While these techniques are practiced in the United States, they are based on Traditional

Chinese Medicine and focus on balancing *chi* (shiatsu and Tui Na), attempting to affect cerebrospinal fluid flow (craniosacral), addressing structural and energetic imbalances (zero balancing), or utilizing light or no touch techniques and minimal training (Reiki). While "East" and "West" are always problematic categories, they retain some usefulness in discussing broad categories of bodywork techniques. However, today's global variety of practices has been created through multiple cross-cultural interactions, reflecting the same early historical contacts between peoples and pragmatic blending of cultures that have characterized human history (Wolf 1997:xv). It would be an impossible task for an anthropologist to identify the original sources of a particular American massage therapist's craft. It would involve analysis of formal massage school curricula, their teacher's experiences and travels, and the individual practitioner's idiosyncratic training, treatment experiences, travels, and innate sensitivities.

History of Massage

Skilled manipulation of soft tissue as a form of therapy is discussed specifically in ancient Egypt, Greece, Rome, China, and India, and has appeared in Thai statuary for at least four thousand years. Notable early Western physicians such as Asclepiades, Hippocrates, and Galen advocated its use as well (Greenman 1996:3). Since early-sixteenth-century Europe, Western medical proponents of massage have appeared periodically. The Enlightenment brought the first great modern Western revival of manual therapies and was of interest to people such as Rousseau and Tissot (Ackerknecht 1982:196). The practice of massage continued in Europe in different settings and has been a part of hydrotherapy, the German "*kur*" and French therapeutic spa traditions for over two hundred years (Maretzki 1989). Then as now, skeptical attitudes toward drugs and invasive therapies (such as bleeding practices in the eighteenth century) increased popular use of folk physical therapies and remedial exercises. Today, massage therapy continues to benefit from the general allure of alternative medicines that are low technology and understood as "natural" and "pure" (Kaptchuk 1998:1061), attributes Rousseau would have also appreciated.

One of the most famous early proponents of Western or Swedish massage was the Swede P. H. Ling (1776–1839) who developed his own system of "Swedish Remedial Massage and Exercise" (Calvert 2002:84–94). He organized the basic strokes of European based massage that would later be given French names such as *effleurage* (a gliding or light touch stroke) and *petrissage* (kneading), which are still in use. The oldest massage school in the United States, established in 1916, is located in New York City and still called The Swedish Institute. What the American public pictures as a massage (with crisp white sheets and oil) would probably still fall under the category of Swedish massage.

Mainstream medical acceptance of massage has been periodic and cyclical. As part of the late-nineteenth-century revival of ancient Greek philosophies of physical and mental development, dozens of books were written promoting massage as a medical treatment (Calvert 2002:100). The proponents included prominent mainstream physicians such as S. Weir Mitchell (1877) and George Taylor (1860), as well as alternative health care theorists Douglas Graham (1890, 1902) and John Kellogg (1895). So massage has appeared in specific American medical contexts from Civil War battlefields (Calvert 2002:108) to Midwestern health sanitariums at the turn of the century to New York City hospitals, where "massage operators" from the Swedish Institute obtained most of their training in the 1920s and 1950s. Field suggests that massage "disappeared from the American medical scene at approximately the time of the pharmaceutical revolution of the 1940s" (2000:xi). By the 1960s and 1970s, massage had developed a more marginal, unprofessional, counterculture reputation among the general public. Legitimate therapeutic massage devolved into short, adjunctive physical therapy sessions directed by specific physician prescription.

Contemporary biomedicine is a historical anomaly, where physicians have less of a diagnostic need to touch their patients than perhaps any other time in human history. While Western physicians have rarely ever had the time or inclination to perform long, intensive manual therapies like massage, now for the first time data from high technology diagnostics provide the central evidence of disease and suffering, not physical exams or subjective patient reports. This lack of a physician perceived need for physical examination is still sometimes disconcerting to patients who have their muscle pain diagnosed from a physical distance. As with the Mayan bonesetters that Hinojosa describes, the centrality of practitioner embodied knowledge gained through direct touch so important to manual therapies is absent from biomedicine (2002:23). The direct intimacy of massage therapy helps fill a certain void in the United States, where even surgery is being performed by machine.

Massage in Cross-Cultural Perspective

While massage therapy is still negotiating a new role in mainstream American biomedicine, a cross-cultural perspective demonstrates that touch therapies have been unproblematically viewed as legitimate medical practices for millennia. This legitimacy is recognized in most European health care systems, particularly the Swedish and German, traditional Chinese, and Indian medicine, and appears in a variety of highly evolved and unique forms in areas as diverse as Russia, the South Pacific, Thailand, Hawaii, Japan, Poland and the Yucatan Peninsula

Though the introduction of "Western" medicine to other cultures has often been accompanied by subtle or explicit attempts to marginalize and suppress traditional therapists of all kinds, localized manual therapy traditions continue to survive at a grassroots level. Occasionally, large political events even touch on the practices of indigenous manual therapists. After World War II, American forces under General MacArthur tried to ban traditional medical practices like shiatsu in Japan, but professional and public resistance (including blind practitioners for whom Helen Keller advocated) ensured their survival (Birch and Junko 1998:6–7). The Chinese Communist government has also attempted to promote and develop Traditional Chinese Medicine and in 1950 Chairman Mao adopted a specific official policy to promote both Western treatments and a traditional medical system that included massage (Xinnong 1987).

Beyond Jordan's documentation of maternal massage in the Yucatan Peninsula (1993:24–28), there has been little discussion of massage in an anthropological context, aside from scattered offhand mentions in ritual and symbolic healing ceremonies (e.g., Fabrega 1997:81; Finkler 1994). It is interesting to consider the overlap between massage and the "anointing" of many religious and shamanic ceremonies around the world. A few more anthropologists have commented on the amount of touching in general between parents and children, often finding Western societies in some sense "touch deprived" (Konner 1976; Doi 1973; Mead 1935).

Cross-cultural comparisons of touch practices and manual therapies reveal the complexity of human interaction and the range of types of health professionals around the world. It is important to note that the current American version of a massage therapist is not the only model for a manual practitioner. For example, in Russia, massage therapists are closer to physical therapists and orthopedists and receive over two thousand hours of training, including certain aggressive, deep manipulation, and adjustment techniques that are simply not done by American massage therapists or physicians. In nearby British Columbia, massage therapists must take three thousand hours of training and a licensing exam that has an extremely high failure rate. Perhaps surprisingly, chiropractors, physiatrists and physical therapists in the United States already receive some training in massage, which has opened the way for some scope-of-practice legal skirmishes over who does what (Calvert 2002:213-14)

It may be that a new category of manual practitioner with a different range of techniques and education will yet emerge in the United States, or is here and has yet to be labeled. Massage practitioners can take a wide range of continuing education classes and be inspired by body theorists like Alexander, Rolf, Feldenkrais, Pilates, Travell, Chaitow, and Trager.[2] Individual therapists inevitably develop eclectic and unique hybrids of styles and movements that make it very difficult to generalize what a massage *is* in the United States. Using myself as an example, my own massage work combines elements of massage school training that included

Western and Eastern techniques, selective elements of continuing education classes, the overarching body philosophies of Alexander and Rolf, and my experiences as a receiver of massage. I personally could not even identify the source of many of my movements.

Furthermore, like any manual trade there are widely varying levels of competence of practitioners. Years of training cannot make some people gifted massage therapists and there are others whose anatomical knowledge, years of observation, and kinesthetic sensitivities create a profound, unmistakable tactile virtuosity. A visit to a mediocre massage therapist can be an extremely unsatisfying waste of money while a visit to a superb practitioner can demonstrate how massage can be both a craft and an art. Superior therapists command a specific tactile knowledge and skill that clients will return to for decades, particularly for treatment of chronic painful conditions like sciatica or low back pain, for which physicians offer little help.

Interestingly, the medicalization of massage also inevitably frames the therapists' experience of giving a massage and understanding what they feel in their hands. Massage therapists find tight muscles, not energy imbalances or wayward spirits. Unlike other manual practitioners in the world who may speak of meridians or energy centers, American massage therapists would be overwhelmingly likely to speak of massage in terms of muscles, blood vessels, and maybe myofascia (fibrous coverings of muscles). This follows the basic linguistic insight that how we label the world tends to construct how we experience it (Sapir 1968[1929]). One location on the body can be understood very differently in separate bodywork philosophies, just as one ailment would be treated differently (see O'Malley, chapter 7).

Massage as a Therapeutic Modality

Today massage has emerged once again as a semilegitimate health care treatment in the United States and its medical efficacy is again proposed, questioned, and examined by the reigning medical establishment. The current effort to disentangle the specific physiological effects that accompany the global, positive feeling of receiving a massage is in its initial stage. It faces daunting methodological and theoretical challenges, even in establishing basic research about treatment outcomes (Kahn 2001; Field 2000). Yet the very existence of these new studies attests to a rapid change in the perception of massage in the United States, from harmless indulgence to its being seen as an alternative medical modality. In fact, times have come full circle, as massage therapists in New York City again work in hospitals. Mt. Sinai Hospital offers classes for massage therapists working with cancer patients and practitioners work in settings like Beth Israel Hospital's alternative health center. Noting the recent addition of "therapy" to the label "massage therapy," massage has embraced (or renewed) a connection to mainstream medicine and has consciously worked to become medicalized, so to speak. The practice continues to attain greater professional legitimacy and relevance through its recent association with medicine and wellness (Eisenberg 1993, 1998).

Now that massage is tentatively accepted as a therapeutic modality, research is exploring how it actually affects the human body. Current findings demonstrate massage can lower heart rate, lower blood pressure, increase blood circulation and lymph flow, break down fibrous adhesions, reduce scar tissue formation, reduce edema, relax muscles, improve range of motion, and reduce pain (Fritz 2000:143–70; Rattray and Ludwig 2000:8–16). It does not enhance muscle strength or cardiovascular capacity, but it can increase circulation in inactive muscles. Massage also appears to improve immune system function, as demonstrated by increased numbers of natural killer cells, and reduce stress, as shown by reduction of the hormone cortisol (Fritz 2000:146). The broader implications of these results and the apparent efficacy of massage treatment for chronic back pain are discussed below.

An important element of the shifting popular perceptions of massage is the fact that without physician referral or advice, Americans seek out massage for a broad variety of health maintenance and wellness reasons, including stress reduction, illness prevention, and treatment of various tangible, medically diagnosable painful conditions (Eisenberg 1993, 1998). In a survey commissioned by the American Massage Therapy Association, 35 percent of people receiving treatment from a massage therapist did so for an explicitly medical reason. The reasons included muscle soreness or spasm, pain reduction, wellness and prevention, improvement of joint flexibility or range of motion, improvement of blood circulation, and injury recovery and rehabilitation (American Massage Therapy Association 2001). Arguably, the very fact that people are going to a massage therapist for treatment of pain and/or dysfunction demonstrates it is a type of American health care or ethnomedical practice.

Massage is a particularly relevant treatment for chronic back pain, as it seems to offer therapeutic benefits and also because alternative medical treatments are often sought for chronic conditions (Eisenberg 1998; Astin 1998). One controlled randomized study found massage to be more effective than acupuncture or self-care education for treating low back pain. The authors concluded that therapeutic massage "was effective for persistent low back pain, apparently providing long lasting benefits. . . . Massage might be an effective alternative to conventional medical care for persistent back pain" (Cherkin 2001:1081).

Lower back pain is certainly ubiquitous, as demonstrated by Kostuik's statement that "all Americans experience some degree of low back pain, and more than

70 percent will seek help for the condition at some point during their lives" (2002:19). From my own experience as a therapist, many first time back pain sufferers become extremely frustrated by a nonchalant physician who only seems to suggest analgesics (and doesn't even touch them where it hurts). The physicians know that back pain will probably resolve itself without treatment and the true cause will probably never be identified. However, many educated, proactive persons want to do something besides take pain relievers. Indeed, Astin found that more education and a holistic orientation to health predicted alternative medicine use (1998:1548). And while dissatisfaction with conventional treatments has not been reliably shown to predict alternative medical use, it seems that chronic pain, poorer health status, and/or a higher number of health problems does (Astin 1998). In any case, back pain sufferers are entering the United States' version of the "contested terrain of musculoskeletal disorders" (Hinojosa 2002:23), where questions of biomedical surgical intervention remain hotly debated in and outside of the profession (Groopman 2002).

Massage as Ethnomedicine

As a health care practice sought out by Americans, massage is appropriately studied as an ethnomedicine—that is, as part of the medical beliefs and practices of a given population. This follows Nichter's exploration of ethnomedicine as involving all health-related experiences within a "multidimensional and meta-medical" approach. He adds that inquiry "is based on the interpretation of bodily experience as well as the embodiment of ideology, discourse as well as disease, and accommodation as well as resistance. . . . It entails a study of the full range and distribution of health-related experience, discourse, knowledge, and practice among different strata of a population" (1991:137).

This ethnomedical perspective includes "the situated meaning . . . at a given historical junction" of medical behavior and "the outcome of health related ideas, behaviors and practices" (1991:137). Massage therapy is thereby intriguing for its sudden appearance on the health care scene and can be viewed in the cultural context of rapidly changing attitudes about health, fitness, and the body (Conrad 1994).

The recent growth of the field is apparent in the statistic that twice as many adult Americans reported having a massage in 2001 as in 1997, at 17 percent compared to 8 percent (American Massage Therapy Association 2001). However, while the idea that massage has therapeutic value may be increasingly accepted, it should be noted that massage is only rarely covered by health insurance and remains largely a service for the upper-middle and higher classes who can afford generally expensive out-of-pocket fees. Massage thus forms part of the medical pluralism that characterizes American society and reflects class, racial, and gender divisions (Baer 1989, 2001). Still, the rise in the number of people receiving a massage reflects the increase in alternative medicine use across all American populations (Eisenberg 1998).

The practice of massage in the United States can be located within popular, folk, and professional domains of health care (Kleinman 1980). However, this chapter focuses on professional practitioners of massage in the United States, not a backrub between family members at the popular level or the variety of unlicensed massage and bodywork practitioners in the folk sector. (In New York City alone, this unlicensed folk sector would include nationals of China, Thailand, Japan, Korea, Russia, and Poland. Their marginal, illegal employment reflects language barriers, class divisions, and idiosyncrasies of New York City immigration.)

The Professionalization of American Massage Therapists

Most legally practicing American massage therapists have completed at least five hundred hours of training, which includes human anatomy and physiology, have passed a state board exam or national certification test, and pay some form of liability insurance. Currently, there is an uneven patchwork of laws in the United States regarding massage, but as part of the effort to have it acknowledged as a legitimate health profession, a national member-funded organization is working to create specific state and federal professional accreditation standards for massage therapists. Massage laws vary from the requirement of a thousand hours of education and passage of a state board exam for licensure (New York State) to the requirement of fifty hours of school and registration with the health department (California). A challenging National Certification test requiring five hundred hours of training has been introduced, but it is not professionally or legally applicable in all states.

In a way, one problem massage faces in the struggle for medical legitimacy is that it feels good. There is something that makes biomedicine and insurance companies uneasy about a "medical treatment" that one would perhaps do for fun or pleasure as well. For centuries there was an idea in Europe and the United States that medical treatments had to be painful or uncomfortable to be effective (Pernick 1985). However a recent survey found that 27 percent of Americans think of massage as something that is both therapeutic and feels good (American Massage Therapy Association 2001). Perhaps as part of a wellness–holistic paradigm shift, there is a growing acceptance of the idea that therapeutic acts can feel good; also, the recent attention to therapeutic benefits may help justify the seeking out of a pleasurable experience.

Just ten to twenty years ago, massage in the United States was much more associated with "massage parlors" and prostitutes. In some idiosyncratic municipalities like Redwood City, California, massage therapists still work under vice laws that require a test for venereal disease. The connection between massage and prostitution goes back at least as far as the Roman baths (Calvert 2002:145) and despite all efforts to sever it, the physical intimacy and privacy of the treatment makes it likely the connection will never fully disappear. Periodically there are incidents, such as the "massage scandals" of the late 1800s, when nurses were lured into working in houses of "ill-repute" and the reputation of massage in England was marred for decades (Rattray and Ludwig 2000:4; also Fritz 2000:18). Still, the general trend toward more education requirements and the increasing medical orientation of the field will help limit future associations with prostitution.

While I have met some elderly individuals who have used massage for specific medical purposes throughout the twentieth century, until recently there has been little mainstream perception of massage as a health practice in the United States. It is in fact quite surprising how quickly mainstream perceptions have changed, or from another perspective, how quickly the United States has rejoined the rest of the globe in viewing manual therapists as a type of health care provider. Massage therapy in the United States could be said to have embraced medicalization, the process whereby events or practices previously considered nonmedical are brought under medical control. This medicalization process is generally viewed positively by massage therapists and therefore is quite different from the usual medicalization examples found in social theory discussions that criticize increased medical control, surveillance, and bureaucratic alienation (Conrad 1992). However, certainly some massage therapists deeply resent ever-increasing regulations and large impersonal organizations speaking for them that simultaneously limit their independence and seem to discount nonmedically oriented treatments and the role of intuition. Indeed, Calvert comments that the exclusion of massage from mainstream medicine in the twentieth century nurtured this independent spirit, which is now perceived to be threatened (Calvert 2002:201). Yet it appears that given the choice between an association with prostitutes or doctors, massage therapists consciously chose medicine to change public perception of the work, as well as to legitimate and articulate the benefits therapists felt they were giving their clients.

The recognition that massage has therapeutic value and can play a special role in a comprehensive physical rehabilitation is a source of tremendous satisfaction to practitioners. Furthermore, many massage schools have taken it upon themselves to thoroughly prepare their students for biomedical contacts. In my training, the anatomy, physiology, pathology, and medical massage classes were consciously designed to allow massage therapists to understand medical language, talk to doctors, make intelligent treatment decisions in a variety of situations, and conduct themselves professionally as health care practitioners. As mentioned before, this shift can also readily be seen in just the change of professional titles over the past two decades; "massage therapist" has replaced "masseuse" and "masseur."

Still, massage is rarely covered by health insurance in this country, although it is in many European countries. While some massage therapists are working for insurance coverage and biomedical recognition of massage, many massage therapists do not want to be involved with insurance compensation. This is not surprising given the popular level of dissatisfaction with health insurance companies. Ironically, many medical practices are now starting to see massage therapy as both an additional source of income and of new patients. The new "integrative medicine" model, in which cutting-edge technological treatments can unproblematically be combined with complementary ones in the most prestigious hospitals of the country, perfectly reflects a historical pattern of "annihilation, restriction, absorption, and even collaboration" that has characterized the relationship of biomedicine and alternative medical practices in the United States (Baer 1989:1103). Pictures of massage sessions have already appeared in the advertisements for major hospitals (such as Mt. Sinai) and the development of the interdisciplinary pain clinic model has also helped to both theoretically and logistically create a new place for massage in the medical environment (Bonica 1990).

An Embodied Practice

Based on experience, a massage therapist has a unique, preverbal, intimate knowledge of what feels normal and what does not. As one of the bonesetters that Hinojosa talked with said, "The hand knows well the injuries and the healthy bones" (2002:26). Maya bonesetters located that knowledge very explicitly in their hands themselves, such that the hands guide the practitioner and not the other way around (2002:26). The basic insight that "the hands know" by "apprehending the problem directly" (2002:23) powerfully intrigues me, although leaves me struggling to connect it with ideas of "muscle memory" which I have never seen well-explained physiologically.

The bonesetters insist that this knowledge cannot be taught, but can only be realized "as the hands make contact with the suffering bodies" (2002:27). It is knowing something in "a bodily, multisensorial way, lacking the language and categories of human experience" (Hinojosa 2002:27; see also Csordas 1990). The idea reminds me of an offhand remark by one of my teachers in massage school, that some things you could not understand until you had done at least one thousand massages. After six thousand, I understand that she was getting at the type of experiential learning you can only get from doing something (see also Jordan 1993:192–93). It is the *praktognosis* or practical, embodied knowledge that Lindsay (1996) develops in taking a hand drumming class or the "feel for the game" that Bourdieu describes (1980:66).

Following Bourdieu's adaptation of Proust's phrase, the hands of massage therapists and bonesetters are filled with numb imperatives (1980:69). The ways that experienced massage therapists intuitively *know* how a given body will respond or resist involves "practical anticipation of the 'upcoming' future contained in the present" (1980:66), "the pre-verbal taking-for-granted of the world that flows from practical sense" (1980:68) and "an immanence in the world through which the world imposes its imminence, things to be done or said, which directly govern speech and action" (1980:66). Finally, relevant to the practice of massage is Bourdieu's idea of "practical sense," which "converted into motor schemes and body automatisms, is what causes practices, in and through what makes them obscure to the eyes of their producers, to be *sensible*, that is, informed by a common sense. It is because agents never know completely what they are doing that what they do has more sense than they know" (1980:69).

Giving a massage is an embodied experience that demonstrates "how the body can constitute a source and starting point of knowledge" (Hinojosa 2002:22). It is a strange type of extended interbody communication. In fact, sometimes when I am massaging someone in a dark, quiet room and they surprise me by suddenly starting to talk after a long period of silence, I almost feel as if they are interrupting a conversation I am having with that person's body. Bodies communicate an extreme amount of information to my hands that is quite difficult to verbalize and categorize. Literally and theoretically, naked and exposed, the body can communicate volumes about pain, anxiety, strength, flexibility, long-term tension, and the ability to relax and cannot lie to the massage therapist's touch.

The Embodiment of Stress

While massage can be a direct treatment for physical pain and dysfunction, from vague, ubiquitous back pain to specific joint injuries, it is also used to treat certain more complicated contemporary American conditions. This side of massage therapy is still too nebulous to be discussed in quantitative studies and yet relates to everyday practices and the native understandings of this activity. When I ask clients about any relevant physical conditions they might have before giving them a massage, the most common answer I receive is "stress" or "just stress."[3] What has become clear to me is that stress is a rich, multivocal, and confused concept.

A basic medical definition of stress refers to a process whereby a stimulus taxes or exceeds the adaptive capability of an individual, creating an imbalance in the internal environment (Tortora and Grabowski 1993:10). As it is popularly understood, stress could also be considered a native illness category in the United States and essentially functions as a folk illness. The classic definition of a folk illness is a "syndrome[s] from which members of a particular group claim to suffer and for which their culture provides an etiology, diagnosis, preventative measures, and regimens of healing. I apply the prefix "folk" to those illnesses of which orthodox Western medicine professes neither understanding nor competence" (Rubel 1977: 20).

Americans routinely suffer from and diagnose themselves and others as "stressed" because of work or relationships, and know how to treat themselves without a doctor's prescription. I do not deny the genuine experience of stress by any means, but want to look at it as a culturally constructed category. Relevant here are the implications of the popular idea that massage can "treat" stress and that persons essentially act on the idea by making it to a massage therapist's office and identifying stress as the main problem.

The history of the stress concept is fascinating in itself, in its rise from a laboratory term in the 1950s to a ubiquitous popular description and metaphor. Anthropologically, stress could be considered an "idiom of distress" describing a mindful body, acknowledging physiological, cultural, environmental, emotional, and intellectual domains and interactions (Nichter 1981). Stress has many parallels with the extensive anthropological work on nerves (*nervios*) and can be similarly viewed as a "large and expansive folk diagnostic category of distress . . . literally seething with meanings (some of them contradictory) that need to be unraveled and decoded for what the terms reveal as well as what they may conceal" (Scheper-Hughes 1992:230). Like nerves, stress functions as an "emically derived, popular, variable, multipurpose complaint which transcends mind, body and culture and is best understood through anthropological investigation and analysis" (Davis and Guarnaccia 1989:2).

Ultimately stress is experienced in both mind and body. The way the word is used in the United States suggests it can simultaneously spring from intellectual or emotional causes and inhabit various locations in the body (such as the neck, heart, stomach, or intestines). The ways people physically "feel" stress reflect personal histories and also Taussig's (1992:86) comment that the "body responds with a language that is as commonplace as it is startling" and Nichter's notion of the "multivocality of somatic communication" (1991:138). The idea of massage (as well as exercise, yoga, and meditation) "treating" stress perfectly exemplifies both the paradoxes created by Cartesian dualism and the commonsense strengths of the holistic mind/body/spirit health paradigm. More importantly, if a wide range of diseases are currently thought to be caused by stress and massage reduces stress, massage's possible significance and application as a healing modality seems clear.

Embodied Minds and Mindful Bodies

Interesting questions arise as to how stress is experienced both in the mind *and* the body and how manipulation of soft tissue can change someone's emotional and intellectual state. What explains how the kneading of muscle and skin helps alleviate the mental tension of a bad day at the office or a difficult home life? How does relaxing the muscles calm the mind? These questions are related to anthropological discussions of somatization, dualism, and embodiment. The only reasonable answer to them is that there is a profound interaction between what we know in the United States as the mind *and* the body.

The cross-cultural study of somatization, or the expression of psychological or emotional problems through physical experiences, raises legitimate questions about what should be considered the "real" event in certain illnesses (Helman 1994; Obeyesekere 1985; Katon 1982). Is depression a state of hopelessness and sadness or is it an experience of sleeplessness, heaviness in the chest, and profound fatigue? Is depression maladaptive thought patterns or excessive, unconscious muscle tension leading to dull constant pain and exhaustion? Is it coming from the mind or is the body informing the mind that it is depressed through stomach tightening or heart palpitations or excessive sleep? While not a question that can be answered here, how do we privilege one over the other as "real"?

It turns out that the West is the unusual case for wanting to "psychologize" many problems that other cultures would describe in physical terms and seek tangible, mechanical therapies for such as acupuncture or herbs (Katon 1982). Asian cultures often scorn the idea of "talk therapies" in general and expect a medical appointment to end in physical treatment. If emotional and intellectual states are understood and experienced as ultimately grounded in the physical body, it would then make sense that altering the body somehow could actually change emotions, thought cycles, or other aspects of experience. This is the embedded message from many great body thinkers like Rolf and Alexander, and is also reflected in recent studies that show regular cardiovascular exercise to be as effective an antidepressant as leading prescription drugs (Blumenthal 1999). Jackson touches on this when he writes: "Altered patterns of body use may induce new experiences and provoke new ideas, as when a regulation and steadying of the breath induces tranquility of mind and a balanced pose bodies forth a sense of equanimity. Likewise, emotional and mental turmoil may induce corresponding changes in bodily attitude, as when depression registers in a slumped posture or grief is manifest in an absolute loss of muscle tonus" (1989:129).

However, the idea that physical changes induced by manual therapy may effect change on multiple levels of personal experience is simply not a part of the mainstream biomedical perspective. And though that profound interaction may be a part of our genetic inheritance and happening with every breath, we do not yet have the vocabulary to describe it, anyway. We remain suspended in a world of slashes and hyphens when discussing mind–body connections. People may find certain ailments disappear with changed circumstances, realize that their body seizes up in some situations or notice that they physically recoil from people they intellectually want to love, but these remain vague, amorphous anecdotes. Americans would seem to need a word like the Balinese *mekeneh* or "feel-think," which refers to what Balinese see as an inextricable relationship between thinking and physically feeling, as a way to reach true insights (Wikan 1991:285). While not part of our language or normal frame of reference, the absent body that Leder (1990) discusses is the ignored but ever present body of daily life. It is the inescapable agent of all corporeal activity as well as the constant witness, prisoner, and celebrant of the myriad ways we navigate the world.

On a deep, basic level, all mental and emotional events are inscribed on tissues every second of the day and neuroscience is slowly starting to unravel the mysteries of the cognitive and emotional brain (Pert 1997). Acknowledging this connection between mind and body is a recurring theme throughout world history and is not the new, radical concept some people suggest. Indeed, it is counterintuitive and contrary to experience to say there is no connection between mind and body, as anyone who has been intoxicated, had adrenalin injected into a vein, or had an orgasm can attest to. Diverse Western thinkers who rejected dualism include many of the ancient Greeks, Friedrich Nietzsche, Karl Marx, William James, and John Dewey. The American pragmatist Dewey was also an early practitioner of the movement therapy called the "Alexander technique" and once commented: "In ultimate analysis the mystery that a mind should use a body, or that a body should have a mind, is like the mystery that a man cultivating plants should use the soil; or that the soil which grows plants at all should grow those adapted to its own physico-chemical properties and relations" (1925:277).

While these mind–body connections remain difficult to articulate, this anthropological topic addresses a primordial reality of being human.

Conclusion

There is something fundamental and profound about the power of and need for the human touch (Montagu 1971; Harlow and Zimmerman 1958). Massage is an ancient, low-technology, physically intensive manual art that is unlikely to ever completely disappear. It is making its periodic return to mainstream medicine in a populace again emboldened by distrust of mainstream physicians and invasive treatments. Seemingly due to an intrinsic disbelief that physical manipulation of the body could affect its functioning, biomedicine still largely retains a blind spot for contemporary massage and other manual therapies. Yet when patients are trying to heal themselves on different existential levels, the physical comfort and human connection that massage offers helps fill a specific void left by highly technological, impersonal modern medicine. It may seem that massage's effects are only temporary, but then so are the effects of drugs. What is more, massage does not have a lengthy list of side effects.

Discussions about mind-body dualism reflect a separation that has been artificially introduced. While the title of this article seems to support a basic mind-body dualism, such a separation would be like separating plants from soil or lungs from a person. We can make the intellectual leap, but the structures are no longer alive as they were meant to be. A living human creature is composed of mind *and* body and perhaps spirit in ceaseless enmeshment. Endlessly trying to disentangle layers of mind or body degrades the majesty of the interconnection created by millions of years of evolution; it is an academic exercise divorced from reality. Over a hundred years ago, Nietzsche criticized the scientists and philosophers of his day as slandering the natural preconditions of life and materiality. He warned that the idea of "pure spirit" is "a piece of pure stupidity: take away the nervous system and the senses, the so-called 'mortal shell' and *the rest is miscalculation*—that is all!" (Nietzsche 1999[1895]:14). More recently, Juhan has written how the "skin is no more separated from the brain than the surface of a lake is separate from its depths. . . . The brain is a single functional unit, from cortex to fingertips to toes. To touch the surface is to stir the depths" (1987:43). An old Buddhist expression suggests the soul needs a body.

The experience of receiving massage demonstrates this unity of mind and body. In disuniting the whole to suggest that massaging the body can affect the mind and emotions, I hope to highlight their intimate connection and restore some reverence for this complex, dynamic system and the nature of its two-way conversations. This chapter may seem to have strayed from its aims of exploring the cultural context of massage therapy in the United States, but a thorough understanding of massage therapy must begin in acknowledging the basic power of being touched as an embodied being.

Notes

I would like to acknowledge the help and support of Lesley Sharp and Herve Varenne in the completion of this manuscript.

1. I am completing a Ph.D. in applied anthropology at Columbia University, have taught anatomy and physiology, medical anthropology, and anthropology of the body at the New School University, Marymount Manhattan College and the Swedish Institute of Massage Therapy. I have been a licensed New York State Massage Therapist since 1994.

2. Matthias Alexander (1869–1955) developed a system of manually and verbally guided exercises for reeducating the body and mind to facilitate good posture, ease of movement and body awareness. Ida Rolf, Ph.D. (1896–1979) developed a series of ten intense manual manipulation sessions that address the myofascial structure of the human body, change long-standing postural and movement habits and seek to create an efficient individual relationship with gravity. Joseph Pilates (1880–1967) developed a still innovative sequence of movements that stretch and strengthen the body while elongating it, by focusing on core abdominal muscles. Moshe Feldenkrais, D.Sc. (1904–1984) developed methods of movement education that emphasized graceful mind–body connections. Janet Travell, M.D. (1901–1996) helped develop the theory of pain caused by myofascial trigger points and wrote two influential and beautifully illustrated books on the subject. Leon Chaitow, D.O., N.D. is a senior lecturer at the University of Westminster, a prolific author on books about palpation, manual therapies, and health, and an articulate, contemporary spokesperson for the medical application of touch. Milton Trager, M.D. (1908–1997) developed a unique manual technique of gentle rocking, shaking, and self-exercise, which sought to reduce holding patterns and reeducate the body.

3. This became highly interesting to me as a medical anthropologist and eventually led me to write a masters thesis on stress (Walkley 1999), although it did not involve massage directly.

References

Ackerknecht, E.
  1982   *A Short History of Medicine.* Baltimore, Md.: John Hopkins University Press. American Massage Therapy Association
  2001   Massage Therapy Consumer Survey Fact Sheet. Opinion Research Corporation International.
Anderson, R.
  1996   *Magic, Science and Health: The Aims and Achievements of Medical Anthropology.* New York: Harcourt Brace.
Astin, J.
  1998   Why Patients Use Alternative Medicine: Results of a National Survey. *Journal of the American Medical Society* 279:1548–53.
Baer, H.
  1989   The American Dominative Medical System as a Reflection of Social Relations in the Larger Society. *Social Science and Medicine* 28:1103–12.
  2001   *Biomedicine and Alternative Healing Systems in America: Issues of Class, Race, Ethnicity, and Gender.* Madison: University of Wisconsin Press.

Birch, S., and I. Junko.
   1998 *Japanese Acupuncture: A Clinical Guide.* Brookline: Paradigm.
Blumenthal, J., M. Babyak, K. Moore, S. Craighead, S. Herman, and P. Khatri
   1999 Effects of Exercise Training on Older Patients with Major Depression. *Archives of Internal Medicine* 159:2349–56.
Boas, F.
   1936 The Relations between Physical and Social Anthropology. Pp. 15–17 in R. Lowie, ed. *Essays in Anthropology: Presented to A. L. Kroeber.* Berkeley: University of California Press.
Bonica, J.
   1990 *Management of Pain in Clinical Practice.* Philadelphia: Lea and Febiger.
Bourdieu, P.
   1980 *The Logic of Practice.* Stanford, Calif.: Stanford University Press.
Calvert, N.
   2002 *The History of Massage: An Illustrated Survey from around the World.* Rochester, Vt.: Healing Arts Press.
Cherkin, D., D. Eisenberg, K. Sherman, W. Barlow, T. Kaptchuk, J. Street, and R. Deyo
   2001 Randomized Trial Comparing Traditional Chinese Medical Acupuncture, Therapeutic Massage, and Self-Care Education for Chronic Low Back Pain. *Archives of Internal Medicine* 161(8):1081–88.
Conrad, P.
   1992 Medicalization and Social Control. *Annual Review of Sociology* 18:104–129.
   1994 Wellness as Virtue: Morality and the Pursuit of Health. *Culture, Medicine and Psychiatry* 18:385–401.
Csordas, T.
   1990 Embodiment as a Paradigm for Anthropology. *Ethos* 18:5–47.
Damasio, A.
   1994 *Descartes' Error: Emotion, Reason and the Human Brain.* New York: Putnam.
Davis, D., and P. Guarnaccia
   1989 Health, Culture, and the Nature of Nervios: Introduction. *Medical Anthropology* 11:1–13.
Dewey, J.
   1925 *Experience and Nature.* London: Open Court.
Doi, T.
   1973 *The Anatomy of Dependence.* New York: Kodansha.
Eisenberg, D., R. Davis, S. Ettner, S. Appel, S. Wilkey, M. Rompay, and R. Kessler
   1998 Trends in Alternative Medicine Use in the United States, 1990–1997. *Journal of the American Medical Association* 280:1569–75.
Eisenberg, D., R. Kessler, C. Foster, F. Norlock, D. Calkins, and T. Delbanco
   1993 Unconventional Medicine in the United States–Prevalence, Costs, and Patterns of Use. *The New England Journal of Medicine* 328:246–52.
Fabrega, H.
   1997 *Evolution of Sickness and Healing.* Berkeley: University of California Press.

Finkler, K.

1994   Sacred Healing and Biomedicine Compared. *Medical Anthropology Quarterly* 6:178–97.

Field, T.

2000   *Touch Therapy.* New York: Churchill Livingston.

Fritz, S.

2000   *Mosby's Fundamentals of Massage Therapy.* St. Louis, Mo.: Mosby.

Graham, D.

1890   *Manual Therapeutics.* Philadelphia, Pa.: J. B. Lippincott.

1902   *Manual Therapeutics, a Treatise on Massage: Its History, Mode of Application and Effects.* Philadelphia, Pa.: J. B. Lippincott.

Greenman, P.

1996   *Principles of Manual Medicine.* New York: Lippincott Williams and Wilkins.

Groopman, J.

2002   Annals of Medicine; A Knife in the Back: Is Surgery the Best Approach to Chronic Back Pain? *The New Yorker,* April 8.

Hahn, R., and A. Kleinman

1983   Belief as Pathogen, Belief as Medicine: "Voodoo Death" and the "Placebo Phenomenon." *Medical Anthropology Quarterly* 14:3–19.

Harlow, H., and R. Zimmerman

1958   The Development of Affectional Responses in Infant Monkeys. *Proceedings, American Philosophical Society* 102:501–509.

Helman, C.

1994   *Culture, Health and Illness.* Woburn, Mass.: Butterworth-Heinemann.

Hinojosa, S. Z.

2002   "The Hands Know": Bodily Engagement and Medical Impasse in Highland Maya Bonesetting. *Medical Anthropology Quarterly* 16:22–40.

Jackson, M.

1989   *Paths towards a Clearing: Radical Empiricism and Ethnographic Inquiry.* Indianapolis: Indiana University Press.

Jordan, B.

1993   *Birth in Four Cultures.* Long Grove, Ill.: Waveland Press.

Juhan, D.

1987   *Job's Body.* Barrytown, N.Y.: Station Hill Press.

Kahn, J.

2001   Massage Research: Direction for Future Research Projects. *Massage Therapy Journal* (Fall):105–114.

Kaptchuk, T.

1998   Persuasive Appeal of Alternative Medicine. *Annals of Internal Medicine* 129:1061.

Katon, W., A. Kleinman, and G. Rosen

1982   Depression and Somatization: A Review. *American Journal of Medicine* 72:127–35, 241–47.

Kellogg, J. H.

1895   *The Art of Massage: Its Physiological Effects and Therapeutic Applications.* Battle Creek, Mich.: Modern Medicine.

Kleinman, A.
1980 *Patients and Healers in the Context of Culture*. Berkeley: University of California Press.
Konner, M.
1976 Maternal Care, Infant Behavior, and Development among the !Kung. Pp. 218–45 in R. Lee and I. DeVore, eds. *Kalahari-Hunter*. Cambridge, Mass.: Harvard University Press.
Kostuik, J.
2002 Why Is Back Pain So Common? P. 19 in S. Margolis and J. Kostuik, eds. *The Johns Hopkins White Papers: Low Back Pain and Osteoarthritis*. Baltimore, Md.: Johns Hopkins University.
Leder, D.
1990 *The Absent Body*. Chicago: University of Chicago Press.
Lindsay, S.
1996 Hand Drumming: An Essay in Practical Knowledge. Pp. 196–212 in M. Jackson, ed. *Things as They Are*. Indiana: Indiana University Press.
Maretzki, T.
1989 Cultural Variation in Biomedicine: The Kur in West Germany. *Medical Anthropology Quarterly* 3:335–89.
Mead, M.
1935 *Sex and Temperament in Three Societies*. New York: William and Morrow.
Mitchell, S. W.
1877 *Fat and Blood and How to Make Them*. Philadelphia, Pa.: J. B. Lippincott.
Montagu, A.
1971 *Touching: The Human Significance of the Skin*. New York: Harper and Row.
Nichter, M.
1981 Idioms of Distress: Alternatives of Psychosocial Distress: A Case Study from South India. *Culture, Medicine, and Psychiatry* 5:399–408.
1991 Ethnomedicine: Diverse Trends, Common Linkages. *Medical Anthropology* 13:137–71.
Nietzsche, F.
1999[1895] The Anti-Christ. Tucson, Ariz.: Sharp Press.
Obeyesekere, G.
1985 Depression, Buddhism, and the Work of Culture in Sri Lanka. Pp. 134–52 in A. Kleinman and B. Good, eds. *Culture and Depression*. Berkeley: University of California Press.
Pernick, M.
1985 *A Calculus of Suffering*. New York: Columbia University Press.
Pert, C.
1997 *Molecules of Emotion: The Science behind Mind–Body Medicine*. New York: Simon and Schuster.
Rattray, F., and Ludwig, L.
2000 *Clinical Massage Therapy*. Toronto: Talus.
Rubel, A.
1977 The Epidemiology of a Folk Illness: Susto in Hispanic America. Pp. 119–28 in D. Landy, ed. *Culture, Disease, and Healing*. New York: Macmillan.

Sapir, E.

1968 [1929] The Status of Linguistics as a Science. Pp. 160–67 in D. Mandelbaum, ed. *Selected Writings of Edward Sapir in Language, Culture, and Personality*, 5th ed. Berkeley: University of California Press.

Scheper-Hughes, N.

1992 Hungry Bodies, Medicine, and the State: Toward a Critical Psychological Anthropology. Pp. 221–47 in T. Schwartz, G. White, and C. Lutz, eds. *New Directions in Psychological Anthropology*. Cambridge, England: Cambridge University Press.

Scheper-Hughes, N., and M. Lock.

1987 The Mindful Body: A Prolegomenon to Future Work in Medical Anthropology. *Medical Anthropological Quarterly* 1:6–41.

Taussig, M.

1992 *The Nervous System.* New York: Routledge.

Taylor, G.

1860 *An Exposition of the Swedish Movement-Cure.* New York: Fowler and Wells.

Tortora, G., and S. Grabowski

1993 *Principles of Anatomy and Physiology.* New York: Harper Collins.

Walkley, S.

1999 A Modern Affliction: Stress in the Contemporary United States. Master's thesis. Department of Applied Anthropology, Teachers College, Columbia University.

Wikan, U.

1991 Toward an Experience-Near Anthropology. *Cultural Anthropology* 6:285–305.

Wolf, E.

1997 *Europe and the People without History.* Berkeley: University of California Press.

Xinnong, C.

1987 *Chinese Acupuncture and Moxibustion.* Beijing: Foreign Language Press.

Competing Views of Chiropractic: Health Services Research versus Ethnographic Observation

3

IAN COULTER

CHIROPRACTIC, AN INDIGENOUS NORTH AMERICAN FORM of bonesetting, is the most extensively used complementary and alternative medicine (CAM) in the United States. It is also one of the most widely studied CAMs, drawing the attention of social scientists and increasingly of health service researchers. The latter, using data on the epidemiology of chiropractic and of health services utilization, efficacy, effectiveness, costs, appropriateness, quality of care, and outcomes, present an overall picture of chiropractic as a limited specialty. Chiropractic is seen as focusing on neuromusculoskeletal conditions and using predominantly spinal manipulative therapy. Such studies show patients in the study presenting a very limited number of health problems to be treated.

The view from anthropology and sociology, on the other hand, is entirely different. In this literature chiropractic is seen as a broad based, distinct alternative health paradigm, with its own metaphysic, philosophy, language, therapies, and health practices—and as one providing a unique health encounter. Numerous names have been used to describe this paradigm (patient centered, holistic, a wellness paradigm) but it suggests that chiropractic cannot be reduced simply to the manipulation of the spine and other joints. This chapter presents these two different views of chiropractic and then explores the basis of the differences.

The Health Services Research View

Overview

Recent studies have established that 30 to 40 percent of biomedical patients in North America utilize alternative health care and that the most common of these alternatives is chiropractic (Eisenberg et al. 1993, 1998). Chiropractic accounted for 31 percent of the total estimated number of visits for sixteen alternative therapies. Of the alternative medical systems, chiropractic represents one of the most firmly entrenched in North America. Approximately two-thirds of all outpatient visits for back pain are made to chiropractors (Shekelle et al. 1995a). The mean number of patient visits per week per chiropractor in 1994 was reported as 109 (American Chiropractic Association 1995). It is estimated that 7 percent of the total medical patient population used chiropractic in 1993 (Eisenberg et al. 1993). It has also been reported that 30 percent of people with low back injuries will directly seek chiropractic care (Carey et al. 1995).

A growing body of literature on chiropractic is in the area of health services research. Major areas of interest have included workman's compensation care (Nyiendo and Lamm 1991; Stano 1993), comparison of biomedical and chiropractic care (Cherkin et al. 1988; Cherkin 1992; Cherkin et al. 1989; Curtis and Bove 1992; Hurwitz 1994), evaluation by patients (Cherkin et al. 1989; Coulter et al. 1994), and testing of various hypotheses about chiropractic utilization using empirical data (Cleary 1982; Schmitt 1978; Yesalis et al. 1980). Health services have also included studies on the efficacy of chiropractic in clinical trials (Coulter 1998; Kane et al. 1974; Meade et al. 1990; Meade et al. 1995; Meeker and Haldeman 2002), metanalyses of studies on chiropractic care (Shekelle et al. 1992), appropriateness of spinal manipulation (Coulter et al. 1996; Shekelle et al. 1991; Shekelle et al. 1998), and economic costs of chiropractic (Jarvis et al. 1991; Stano 1993; Stano and Smith 1996; Shekelle et al. 1995a; Shekelle et al. 1995b). In trying to ascertain the role of the chiropractor in the current health care system, I draw on the studies of utilization.

Studies of Chiropractic Services Utilization

The data from utilization of chiropractic services suggest that chiropractors provide 18 to 38 million cervical manipulations per year for neck pain and headaches (Shekelle and Brook 1991). Both regional (New Haven Health Care 1976; Prima Health Systems 1976; Yesalis et al. 1980; Phillips and Butler 1982) and national (Schmitt 1978; Kelner et al. 1980; Coulter 1985; Von Kuster 1980; Mugge 1986; Hurwitz 1998; Coulter et al. 2002) studies of chiropractic utilization have shown that chiropractic users are more likely to be middle-aged, employed, and high school educated than the general population. With some exceptions, no gender or income differences have been seen. Low back pain is the most common symptom for those seeking care, and spinal manipulation accounts for the vast majority of services provided. Neck pain and headache combined constitute the next largest category of presenting complaints of chiropractic patients. Several studies have shown greater use by whites. Regional differences in rate of use have been seen, but no consistent pattern has emerged. The proportion of the U.S. population that uses chiropractic and the number of chiropractic visits per capita appears to have doubled in the past fifteen to twenty years (Von Kuster 1980; Shekelle and Brook 1991).

When chiropractic is examined epidemiologically, it is clear that the overwhelming majority of patients present for a narrow scope of conditions. Three conditions account for about 58 percent of the conditions presented: general back/spine, neck/shoulder, and lower back. All other categories are reported by less than 5 percent of patients (Coulter et al. 2002). National surveys by the National Board of Chiropractic Examiners (1993) also indicate that spinal subluxation/joint dysfunction and headaches are the conditions routinely seen. In addition, conditions listed as "often seen" are overwhelmingly neuromusculoskeletal in origin. Furthermore, as mentioned earlier, manipulation is the most frequently billed service by chiropractors (Shekelle and Brook 1991). The problem with such an approach, however, is that it gives no indication about the nature of the health encounter or the type of care that is delivered.

National expenditures on alternative care, which encompass chiropractic, provide revealing data of the place of chiropractic in health care. Eisenberg et al. (1993) estimate that expenditures on alternative care are at $11.7 billion in the United States. Similar estimates have been derived for the use of alternative services in Australia where 15 percent of the providers seen were chiropractors (MacLennan et al. 1996). Chiropractors in the United States are responsible for the largest amount of billed services for manipulation covered by insurance (94 percent), and the estimated annual expenditures for chiropractic services was $2.4 billion by 1988 (Shekelle 1994).

Care must be taken with accepting many of the studies at face value. Many of the studies on utilization of chiropractic services have had inadequate sampling designs, suffered from an inappropriately low response rate, are out-of-date, or exhibit some combination of these factors. Although all of the above work has contributed to our knowledge of chiropractic, much of it is limited in its usefulness for descriptive purposes either because it is based on data limited to a single state (Gesler 1988), to areas within a state (e.g., rural; Lavsky-Shulman et al. 1985), or relies on data from outside the United States (Kelner et al. 1980; Shapiro 1983; MacLennan et al. 1996). Even where U.S. community-based data has been used (Shekelle and Brook 1991), the analysis is based on data that is now dated. More recently, studies have been done through an established chiropractic practice network (Hawk et al. 2000; Hawk et al. 2001) but these are convenience samples and are therefore more constrained in terms of generalizations. The only current national data are from two recent publications from a single study (Hurwitz et al. 1998; Coulter et al. 2002) that used randomly selected practices and patients in a cluster sample in North America. But even here, the cluster sites were not chosen randomly, so generalizations from this study are also restricted. Most of the studies cited, however, suffer from a response rate low enough that their results cannot be generalized to the population as a whole. This makes much of the work invalid for describing chiropractic care in the twenty-first century.

There is, however, an increasing body of data on the epidemiology of chiropractic and the utilization of chiropractic (Hurwitz et al. 1998), and a growing body of health services research (Mootz et al. 1997). The picture presented of chiropractic is that of a limited specialty focusing on neuromusculoskeletal conditions (Shekelle 1998) and using predominantly spinal manipulative therapy (Christensen and Morgan 1993). Studies show patients presenting with a very limited number of health problems (Barlett 2001). The overall sense of these studies is that chiropractic is limited in scope both in terms of the therapies used and the type of health condition brought to chiropractors by patients. This has led some commentators to argue that chiropractic is akin to a subspecialty within medicine and not a broad-based alternative to traditional biomedicine (Nelson 1994; Bartlett 2001; Shekelle 1998).

Studies also suggest, nonetheless, that chiropractic health care is not used exclusive of biomedical care but in addition to it (Yesalis et al. 1980; Cleary 1982; Shapiro 1983; Gesler 1988). They provide little data, though, about how patients combine mainstream and chiropractic care and virtually no outcome data looking at the results of combining different providers. Some writers such as Eisenberg and his colleagues (1993) have postulated that unconventional therapy may be used for nonserious biomedical conditions, health promotion, or disease prevention.

Much more research is needed that examines outcomes of chiropractic, including research based on more than simply the clinical outcomes from spinal manipulation. Comparatively speaking, there now exists an extensive body of controlled trials on manipulation (Meeker and Haldeman 2002), the findings of which indicate that manipulation is an efficacious therapy for nonchronic low back pain (Shekelle et al. 1992; Coulter 1998) and for some cervical vertebral problems (Coulter et al. 1996). However, none of these studies address the question of effectiveness—that is, outcomes from its use on patients in average and real clinical settings, as opposed to trials in ideal settings, which can only address efficacy. The work to date deals with efficacy not effectiveness.

Efficacy is established through random controlled trials, double blinded if possible, conducted under ideal conditions. By their nature, they do not provide evidence for how a given procedure or therapy will work in an average practice, with an average practitioner, and with an average patient. Effectiveness is established through studies conducted in real practices under normal conditions. While it is unlikely that a therapy with no efficacy could have any effectiveness, it is possible that something with efficacy could be low in effectiveness. This could arise from the difficulty of providing the therapy in practice, the difficulty in getting patient compliance with a difficult regimen, or the variation in the clinical skills of the provider of the therapy. It might also be the case that a therapy that has efficacy, such as manipulation, varies widely in effectiveness because of the nature of the health encounter itself. While allopathic doctors might manipulate, they may have less effectiveness than chiropractors.

The View from Anthropology and Sociology

Early Writings and the Labeling of Chiropractic

From the early 1950s until the mid-1970s, writings in anthropology and sociology often reflected the same cultural bias against chiropractic as found in society at large. The early focus of this work was on the assumed marginality of chiropractic, its cultism, its professionalism or lack of it, and its deviant theory of disease (Coulter 1983a). By labeling chiropractic as a marginal profession, alternative profession, and pseudoprofession, they adversely influenced the legitimacy of the profession. Anthropologists and sociologists labeled few groups as negatively as they did chiropractic. Coulter (1991a) has termed this early work an exercise in ideological hegemony because it contributed to the process of biomedical hegemony vis-à-vis chiropractic.

The conceptualization of chiropractic as a marginal profession was widely adopted by sociologists (and other social scientists) for some thirty years. Wardwell (1952) introduced the concept of marginality to describe the status of chiropractic. By using this concept, he conveyed the fact that the chiropractor's role was not as institutionalized as that of the biomedical physician. Wardwell (1955) also examined the psychological reactions of chiropractors to the tension and frustration that result from a marginal role. Marginality became one of the accepted and self-evident features about the chiropractic role. Subsequent investigations were therefore not aimed at examining marginality as a hypothesis, but at illustrating some of its consequences for chiropractors.

This perspective led to a series of studies on the professionalization of chiropractic (Leis 1972; Lin 1972; Sternberg 1969; Evans 1973a, b; Rootman and Mills 1974; White and Skipper 1971). Chiropractic was usually portrayed as an interesting hybrid, one with some of the features of a profession but also stigmatized. Professionalism and stigma are normally thought to be incompatible (Sternberg 1969). Much of this work was also focused on how the profession and chiropractic students cope with this dilemma (Leis 1972; Lin 1972). These studies saw chiropractic not as a profession that had already arrived, but as one struggling for legitimacy through the process of professionalization.

Scholars focusing on the practice of chiropractic gave prominence to the marginality thesis. McCorkle (1961), in an anthropological account of the growth of chiropractic in Iowa, conceded that chiropractic was the most "influential" of the alternative health care systems, but nevertheless titled his paper "Chiropractic: A Deviant Theory of Disease and Treatment in Contemporary Western Culture." Roebuck and Hunter (1972), who focused on health care quackery, and Cowie and Roebuck (1975), also presented chiropractic as deviant. The latter subtitled their ethnographic study "Definitions of a Deviant Situation." Both studies purported to establish that important labeling groups in the United States saw chiropractic as deviant or marginal; both therefore concluded that chiropractic had a deviant or marginal role in health care. Their position, of course, did not accord with that of chiropractors or their patients. Cowie and Roebuck recognized that they might even be contributing to this labeling when they stated, "It is ironic that even Roebuck and Hunter, who have delineated the labeling bodies in this section, have contributed to the deviant image of chiropractic by publishing an article which designates it as such to a scientific reading public" (1975:4). The irony of the statement seems to have been lost on the authors.

Some writers reinforced this position by challenging the scientific basis of chiropractic theory despite their lack of competence to do so. Cobb, using an anthropological perspective, noted, "Writers of every persuasion are unanimous in their contention that the chiropractic theory of disease causation has no scientific validity" (1977:2), and that, "Chiropractic has, over the years, taken on a variety of apparent professional trappings" (1977:13). To explain how such a group could obtain legitimacy, Cobb argued that a new era of pluralism provided the coattail on which chiropractic was riding. Reading Cobb's article, the implication that chiropractors were doing something illegitimate is difficult to avoid.

Wardwell (1972, 1976, 1979, 1980a, b, c, 1981) continued to publish on chiropractic in this early period (1960s to the 1970s), but his later writings (1976, 1978) explored, for the most part, changes in the status of the profession (from a marginal to a limited biomedical profession, as opposed to a parallel profession [1979, 1980a]) and postulated the possible future directions of chiropractic (1980b, c). In his more recent writings, he sees chiropractic as a challenge to biomedical dominance (1981, 1992). While he still uses the term "marginal" (Wardwell 1994), chiropractors are no longer considered part of this group and have evolved into limited medical practitioners.

Surveying this early work by social scientists, we find the following array of terms used to describe chiropractic: marginal, deviant, stigmatized, and heterodox (Hewitt and Wood 1975; Baer 1984). Other terms of note include caste and outcaste (Anderson 1981; Weisner 1983). In spite of its productive vocabulary, the early literature on chiropractic in the social sciences gives very little factual information about chiropractic. It is focused on the conceptualization of the role of the profession in society and on theorizing either about the causes or the effects of that role. Whatever the term actually used by social scientists, they were interested in investigating chiropractic as a hybrid and an oddity within the health care system of North America. Their work reinforced the impression that chiropractic was either not a profession, or that it was a quasi profession or a group en route to becoming a profession (Rosenthal 1981; Coulter 1991b).

A New Era in the Social Sciences

A new era in social science writings was signaled by the publication of an issue of *Sociological Symposium* (Skipper 1978) focused on chiropractic. Most of the articles began to acknowledge that the earlier conceptualizations were not based on empirical data. In the symposium, theories about chiropractic were examined in relation to utilization data (Schmitt 1978); and, for the first time, the idea that the focus on marginality was no longer appropriate, and that it was in all likelihood a politically created marginality, was put forward (Wild 1978). At the same time, the idea that chiropractic might be a distinct health paradigm and legitimate in its own right was suggested (Nofz 1978).

The same change in perspective could also be seen in the new empirical studies being done on chiropractic. In their work, Kelner et al. (1980) dispensed entirely with earlier conceptualizations and used random samples, extensive surveys, and observation to evaluate the evidence for considering chiropractic as an alternative paradigm of health care. They provided a rich database combining qualitative and quantitative data for examining the chiropractic curriculum (Coulter 1981), the chiropractic model of education (Coulter 1983b), the chiropractic patient (Coulter 1985), and the chiropractor's role (Coulter 1992b). Caplan (1984, 1988) further advanced the alternative paradigm argument by maintaining that if chiropractors became the musculoskeletal experts that biomedicine was increasingly willing to accept, they would, in fact, lose their distinctive health paradigm.

A second defining event in the literature was the publication by the *Journal of Manipulative and Physiological Therapeutics* of a special edition titled "The Sociology of Chiropractic" (Lawrence 1991). Its contributing researchers departed significantly from the earlier perspectives. Their work had come to consider the political basis of marginality, linking it to the sociological thesis of biomedical dominance (Willis 1983, 1991). The work also avoided labeling chiropractic and focused on the political attempts by biomedicine (including its use of labels) to exclude chiropractic. This new perspective had been used in work by Coulter (1991a), which focused on biomedical ideology and hegemony, and by Coburn and Biggs (1986),

Biggs (1991), and Coburn (1991, 1993), which examined various aspects of chiropractic legitimacy and the state.

Nowhere is this change in the perspective of social sciences more clearly manifested than in the more recent ethnographic and observational studies of chiropractic. Several authors (Kleynhans and Cahill 1991; Coulter 1993b; Jamison 1994) have suggested that the traditional positivist/empiricist/quantitative research paradigm is incapable of capturing a grounded understanding of chiropractic practice and must be supplemented with qualitative studies. This can only be done via observation-based studies of chiropractic practice, focusing on the chiropractic health encounter. To date, few such studies exist. The remainder of the chapter examines four such studies. Although the four studies were conducted quite independently and in different sites (one in Canada, two in the United States, and one in Australia) their findings are extremely consistent.

The Canadian study by Kelner et al. (1980) involved a random sample of 1 in 5 of 349 Canadian chiropractors, from which seventy practices were chosen for in-depth interviews with the chiropractors. A rapid ethnographic observation study of the clinics over a single day was conducted and interviews were held with 10 randomly chosen of 658 patients. Out of these multiple sources, the researchers constructed a model of the healing encounter. The study showed that despite what appears to be a very limited epidemiological scope in the practice, the chiropractor has constructed a broad-based health paradigm around these apparent limitations. The chiropractor "is also involved, with the patient's cooperation, in preventing occurrences of health problems, either through continuing chiropractic treatment or by effecting changes in the patient's behavior" (1980:169). In sum, the authors found that chiropractic offers the patient care that is holistic, conservative, available, immediate, personal, intelligible, and cooperative.

In another observational study, Coulehan (1985), a biomedical physician and epidemiologist, interviewed and observed ten chiropractors and describes a health encounter very similar to the one documented by Kelner et al. (1980). The chiropractor, according to Coulehan (1985), brings to the encounter a belief system with not only a positive regard for the patient and "genuineness" (the ability to be oneself in the relationship without hiding behind a role or facade [1985:387]), but also with a positive view that what they do helps the patient. Where the biomedical practitioner sees back problems as difficult and uncertain, the chiropractor sees them as solvable. Coulehan calls this the faith that heals (1985:387). According to the study, chiropractors use mechanical and holistic explanations that are understandable to the patient. The former concepts are acceptable in a rationalistic society and the latter appeal to the patient's sense that the person is not subtracted from the encounter. Chiropractic also stresses a positive dynamic and a drug-free view of health. As Coulehan puts it, "The net effect is a logical set of beliefs which appeal to common sense, use scientific terminology, yet promote a natural, non-invasive, holistic approach rather than a biomedical approach" (1985:388).

The chiropractors do something to the patient, rather than simply talk or write prescriptions, according to Coulehan (1985). This also involves extensive laying on of hands that attends to bodily pain and touching. The encounter is a plan "that requires patient commitment and cooperation" (1985:388). This may include a program of exercise, nutritional counseling, stress management techniques, and behavioral change. Coulehan (1985:388) concludes, "Chiropractic care, as opposed to spinal adjustment as an isolated treatment, must be viewed as a process or interaction."

In the third study, Jamison (1993) observed thirty Australian clinics, interviewed practitioners, and viewed patient files. The chiropractic care involved manual, emotional, and psychosocial contact. It was cooperative; focused on the well-being of the patient; used a low level of technology; focused on objective, subjective, and effective data; was directed at understanding the whole person; and was personalized. She concluded that the chiropractors were providing holistic care. Her study also identified three ideal chiropractic types, two or sometimes three of which operate simultaneously within the doctor–patient relationship. The types (paradigms) she identified were biomechanical, conventional holism, and alternate holism. The first stresses the body as a machine, the second stresses the multifactorial nature of health care, and the last focuses on a vitalistic version of holism. Like Coulehan (1985), Jamison found that at the level of explanations to the patients the chiropractors tend to use rationalistic, reductionist concepts of biomechanics. However, if the focus is on the chiropractors' understandings and expectations—the cognitive commitment—then the concepts used when chiropractors talk about themselves to patients clearly is holistic. The objective for the chiropractor is the total well-being of the patient, even if the initial focus is manipulation of a specific lesion. At the level of the presenting symptoms and during the application of therapy, the encounter may resemble that of a reductionist, nonholistic practitioner. This however, overlooks how the therapy is actually delivered within a much broader paradigm.

The last observation study is that of Oths (1994). In analyzing communication in a chiropractic clinic, she also stresses that chiropractic explanations are simple and understandable and harmonize very well with the way individuals conceptualize things in an industrialized society. She further notes that there is a high degree of congruence between the explanations the patients give of their illness and those of the chiropractor. Her conclusion is that patients internalize the chiropractic model of disease to a high degree. In her study, the communication was reinforced by pamphlets, charts, diagrams, and models in all the rooms in the clinic, and with videos. As did Coulehan (1985), Oths found the chiropractor made extensive use of analogies and constantly translated biomedical jargon into lay terms the patient can understand. For her, this demystified medicine as well as the patient's health problem.

These studies collectively show that scholars increasingly agree that chiropractic care in general, and care focused on low back pain in particular, is and will be characterized by a holistic regard for the patient.

Lessons from the Social Sciences

Despite more than fifty years of anthropological and sociological publications on chiropractic, only a modest amount of good research is available. Considering that chiropractic is the most used CAM therapy and is the third largest primary contact profession in the United States after biomedicine and dentistry, this paucity of data is surprising. However, the literature does provide evidence of one major change. From the late 1940s, when some chiropractors were prosecuted and jailed for practicing medicine without a license, to the 1990s, a radical transformation occurred in the way chiropractic was perceived. Social scientists have become increasingly willing to view chiropractic as an alternative form of health care, or as a specialty within the health care system, rather than as a deviant theory of disease in Western society. It is therefore increasingly difficult to portray chiropractic as a marginal profession playing a marginal role in health care.

Whatever the status of chiropractic in the past, by the late 1980s it had established a secure niche within the health care system. Whereas the survival of chiropractic had once been problematic because of their attributed marginality, the question of chiropractic's future role within the health care system has now been foregrounded.

Many terms have been used by anthropologists and sociologists over the years to describe chiropractic. As noted above, not all of them have been very flattering. These terms have attempted to both capture its essence and position it within the health care system. On the more positive side, anthropologists and sociologists have termed it: complementary medicine (Mills 1989–1990), chiropractic medicine (Salmon 1984), holistic health care (Caplan 1988), wellness care (Coulter 1990b; Hawk 2000), and primary health care (Coulter 1992a). All of these signal conceptions of a paradigm broader than that of simply manipulative therapy for neuromusculoskeletal problems.

The Health Services Approach versus the Social Science Approach

Why the Different Approaches

As outlined above, social scientists and health services researchers have adopted different approaches to the study of chiropractic. On the one hand, epidemiology and health services research has focused on such matters as the presenting condition, the diagnosis, the distribution of conditions among the patients, utilization patterns, cost of the care, objectively measured outcomes and satisfaction with the care, and efficacy of the care, which usually means the efficacy of manipulation (Mootz et al. 1997). On the other hand, sociologists and anthropologists have been more likely to focus on the total health encounter and the effectiveness of the care. They tend to consider all elements making up the social/cultural/psychological aspects of the care. In this sense they are more concerned with care than are health services researchers who are more concerned with treatment.

The use of different research methods and types of data collected has also been a distinguishing feature between epidemiologists and health services researchers and social scientists. Epidemiologists and health services researchers have tended to collect quantitative data derived from patient files (Shekelle et al. 1998), surveys (Hawk et al. 1998), billing records (Stano and Smith 1996), clinical assessment instruments (Christensen and Nilsson 1998), validated health status instruments (Vernon and Mior 1991), and validated satisfaction instruments (Coulter et al. 1994; Coulter et al. 2000). Anthropologists and sociologists, however, have been much more likely to use observation techniques and collect qualitative data (Anderson 1998). They are also more interested in discovering the meaning of the care to the patient, which is more likely to be predicated on the use of a qualitative research methodology. There are exceptions where both methods are used by social scientists (e.g., Oths 1994; Kelner et al. 1980).

A third difference in approach between the two groups of researchers derives from their different research objectives. In anthropology and sociology, much more emphasis is placed on discovery, at least in areas where the body of knowledge is sparse, than on justification of therapy. The dominant concern of much of health services research, however, as evidenced in the elevation to supremacy of random controlled trials and the use of systematic literature reviews and met-analysis, is for determining "legitimacy" of a therapy by efficacy studies. Herein can be seen the difference between a focus on effectiveness and one on efficacy. In studies on effectiveness by social scientists, the outcome of the therapy is measured within the context of the whole health encounter as it occurs in real practice and not just for manipulation in a controlled trial. Here legitimacy includes both patient assessment of outcomes and sociocultural legitimacy. By contrast, in efficacy studies, patient assessment of outcomes is thought to be suspect because of the placebo effect, and emphasis is not placed on the whole encounter.

The Future Role of Chiropractors

The two distinct approaches for evaluating chiropractic outlined above point to at least two distinct futures for chiropractic. At the risk of oversimplifying these futures, one of these situates chiropractors within the role of health care specialists. The other future, meanwhile, envisions chiropractors as providing broad-based alternative health care. It is the second possibility I wish to explore here.

Coulter (1991b) has argued that chiropractic is a broad health paradigm and that the concept of a sub-biomedical specialist is inappropriate. In view of this, the term *holistic* captures well the characterization of the chiropractic role, and has historically been favored by many in the profession. It was initially used by Coulter to describe chiropractic (1990a). However, since then, Coulter has argued that "to the extent that chiropractic focuses on the whole individual as opposed to the etiology of illness it could be claimed that it moved further in the direction of holism. However if holism implies considering the individual in the full context of their spiritual, psychological, social and biological well-being, chiropractic has proceeded on a very 'truncated individual'" (1993a: 158).

Chiropractic makes a claim for treating the whole person, something that neither the education nor practice of chiropractic can substantiate (Coulter 1999). This position does not deny that chiropractors could choose to be holistic. But such a claim has remained more at the level of rhetoric than reality. This begins to problematize some of the claims of chiropractic, to challenge some of the rhetoric. The end result might be a view of the chiropractic role that is broader than that of a specialist but not as broad as a full alternative health care system. While the dominant focus of the care is on neuromusculoskeletal problems brought to the chiropractor and the dominant therapy is adjustments, it is broader in several ways. First, while treating the neuromusculoskeletal problems, their treatment expands into problem areas that were not brought initially to the chiropractor for care. As this occurs, and if the care is successful, the patient expands the number and nature of problems they bring for treatment. Second, the chiropractor also provides lifestyle counseling (about weight, posture, stress, exercise, sleeping habits, work environment, etc.). This places the adjustments in a broader paradigm. Third, the care expands to include a whole range of other therapies (herbs, heat, massage, acupuncture, electrical, etc.), unless the chiropractor is a "straight" (uses hands only and adjusts only the spine). The end result is that the majority of the practice is broader than that portrayed by health services research and narrower than that often claimed by chiropractors and sometimes portrayed by social scientists.

One question posed by the analysis presented here is whether the changed view of chiropractic as presented by social scientists reflects changes in chiropractic over time or changes in the social scientists' way of seeing this profession. Coburn (1993) has suggested that under the drive to legitimate themselves, chiropractors have changed their claims and their practice. His thesis is that this has lead to a narrowing of the scope of practice. But the observational studies of chiropractic would suggest that the practice is still very broad. It may be that at the level of political rhetoric, chiropractors have found it expedient to limit the scope of practice they claim, while at the level of practice they are doing what they have always done.

With regard to the writings by social scientists, it must be acknowledged that these are also linked to broader social trends. The original work on chiropractic in both sociology and anthropology predated the emergence of the work on biomedical dominance. As biomedicine was increasingly challenged by such political movements as feminism, the antipsychiatry movement, the gay movement, and the consumer movement, intellectually social scientists moved from seeing biomedicine as the exemplar for what constitutes a fully developed profession to seeing professions generally as a way of protecting the interests of professions at the expense of the public. As professions such as medicine and law started to lose their cache and the trust placed in them by the public, "marginalized professions" such as chiropractic found it increasingly possible to challenge biomedical dominance. In chiropractic in the United States, this culminated in their successful antitrust suit against the American Medical Association in the 1976 Wilkes et al. case. In conclusion, the changes in the perspective on chiropractic need to be situated in the social context of their times, although this task is beyond the purpose of this chapter.

References

American Chiropractic Association
   1995   Summary of the 1994 ACA Annual Statistical Study. *Journal of American Chiropractic Association* (Jan.):57–63.
Anderson, R. T.
   1981   Medicine, Chiropractic and Caste. *Anthropology Quarterly* 54:157–65.
   1998   Strong and Weak Measures of Efficacy: A Comparison of Chiropractic with Biomedicine in the Management of Back Pain. *Journal of Manipulative and Physiological Therapeutics* 21(6):402–409.
Baer, H. A.
   1984   A Comparative View of a Heterodox Health System: Chiropractic in America and Britain. *Medical Anthropology* 8:151–68.
Bartlett, E. E.
   2001   Benchmarking in the Clinical and Financial Characteristics of Chiropractic Offices. *Topics of Clinical Chiropractic* 8(2):13–19.
Biggs, L.
   1991   Chiropractic Education: A Struggle for Survival. *Journal of Manipulative and Physiological Therapeutics* 14(1):22–28.
Caplan, R. L.
   1984   Chiropractic. Pp. 86–87 in J. Salmon, ed. *Alternative Medicines: Popular and Policy Perspectives.* New York: Tavistock.

1988   Holistic Healers in the United States and the Changing Health Care Environment. *Holistic Medicine* 3(1):167–74.

Carey, T. S., J. Garrett, A. Jackman, et al.

1995   The Outcomes and Costs for Care for Acute Low Back Pain among Patients Seen by Primary Care Practitioners, Chiropractors, and Orthopaedic Surgeons. *New England Journal of Medicine* 333(14):913–17.

Cherkin, D. C.

1992   Family Physicians and Chiropractors: What's Best for the Patient? *Journal of Family Practice* 35(5):505–506.

Cherkin, D. C., F. A. MacCornack, and A. O. Berg

1988   The Management of Low Back Pain: A Comparison of the Beliefs and Behaviors of Family Physicians and Chiropractors. *Western Journal of Medicine* 149(4):475–80.

1989   Family Physicians' Views of Chiropractors: Hostile or Hospitable? *American Journal of Public Health* 79(5):636–37.

Cherkin, D. C., and F. A. MacCornack

1989   Patient Evaluations of Low Back Pain Care from Family Physicians and Chiropractors. *Western Journal of Medicine* 150(3):351–55.

Christensen, M., and D. Morgan, eds.

1993   Job Analysis of Chiropractic. A Project Report of the Practice of Chiropractic within the United States. Greely, Colo.: National Board of Chiropractic Examiners.

Christensen, H. W., and N. Nilsson

1998   The Reliability of Measuring Active and Passive Cervical Range of Motion: An Observer-Blinded and Randomized Repeat-Measures Design. *Journal of Manipulative and Physiological Therapeutics* 21:341–47.

Cleary, P. D.

1982   Chiropractic Use: A Test of Several Hypotheses. *American Journal of Public Health* 72(7):727–29.

Cobb, A. K.

1977   Pluralistic Legitimation of an Alternative Therapy System: The Case of Chiropractic. *Medical Anthropology* 1:1–23.

Coburn, D.

1991   Legitimacy at the Expense of Narrowing of Scope of Practice: Chiropractic in Canada. *Journal of Manipulative and Physiological Therapeutics* 14(10):14–21.

1993   State Authority, Medical Dominance, and Trends in the Regulation of the Health Professions: The Ontario Case. *Social Science and Medicine* 37(7):841–50.

Coburn, D., and C. L. Biggs

1986   Limits to Medical Dominance. *Social Science and Medicine* 22(10):1035–46.

Coulehan, J. L.

1985   Chiropractic and the Clinical Art. *Social Science and Medicine* 21:383–90.

Coulter, I. D.

1981   The Chiropractic Curriculum: A Problem of Integration. *Journal of Manipulative and Physiological Therapeutics* 4:143–54.

1983a   Chiropractic Observed: Thirty Years of Changing Sociological Perspective. *Chiropractic History* 3:43–47.

1983b   Chiropractic and Medical Education: A Contrast in Models of Health and Education. *Journal of Canadian Chiropractic Association* 27:151–58.

1985   The Chiropractic Patient: A Social Profile. *Journal of Canadian Chiropractic Association* 29:25–28.

1990a   The Chiropractic Paradigm. *Journal of Manipulative and Physiological Therapeutics* 13(5):279–87.

1990b   The Patient, the Practitioner, and Wellness: Paradigm Lost, Paradigm Gained. *Journal of Manipulative and Physiological Therapeutics* 13(2):107–110.

1991a   Sociological Studies of the Role of the Chiropractor: An Exercise in Ideological Hegemony? *Journal of Manipulative and Physiological Therapeutics* 14(1):51–58.

1991b   The Sociology of Chiropractic: Future Options and Directions. Pp. 53–59 in S. Haldeman, ed. *Principles and Practice of Chiropractic.* Norwalk, Conn: Appleton and Lange.

1992a   Is Chiropractic Care Primary Care? *Journal of Canadian Chiropractic Association* 36:96–101.

1992b   The Chiropractic Role: Marginal, Supplemental, or Alternative Health Care? In D. Coburn and L. Torrance, eds. *Health and Canadian Society.* Toronto: Fitzhenry & Whitesides.

1993a   The Physician, The Patient, and the Person: The Humanistic Challenge. *Journal of Chiropractic Humanities* 1:9–20.

1993b   Alternative Philosophical and Investigatory Paradigms for Chiropractic. *Journal of Manipulative and Physiological Therapeutics* 16(6):419–25.

1998   Efficacy and Risks of Chiropractic Manipulation: What Does the Evidence Suggest? *Integrative Medicine* 1(1):61–66.

1999   *Chiropractic: A Philosophy for Alternative Health Care.* Oxford: Butterworth-Heinemann.

Coulter I. D., R. D. Hays, and C. D. Danielson

1994   The Chiropractic Satisfaction Questionnaire. *Topics of Clinical Chiropractic* 1(4):40–43.

Coulter I. D., E. L. Hurwitz, A. H. Adams, B. J. Genovese, R. Hays, and P. G. Shekelle

2002   Patients Using Chiropractors in North America: Who Are They and Why Are They in Chiropractic Care? *Spine* 27(3):291–98.

Coulter I. D., E. L. Hurwitz, A. H. Adams, W. C. Meeker, D. T. Hansen, R. D. Mootz, P. D. Aker, B. J. Genovese, and P. G. Shekelle

1996   The Appropriateness of Manipulation and Mobilization of the Cervical Spine. RAND, Santa Monica, MR-781-CCR.

Coulter I. D., E. L. Hurwitz, K. Spitzer, B. J. Genovese, and R. D. Hays

2000   A Chiropractic Supplemental Item Set for the Consumer Assessment of Health Plan Study. *Topics in Clinical Chiropractic* 7(4):50–56.

Cowie, J. B., and J. B. Roebuck

1975   *An Ethnography of a Chiropractic Clinic: Definitions of a Deviant Situation.* New York: Free Press.

Curtis, P., and G. Bove
  1992   Family Physicians, Chiropractors, and Back Pain. *Journal of Family Practice* 35(5):551–55.

Eisenberg, D. M., R. B. Davis, S. L. Ettner, S. Appel, S. Wilkey, M. Van Rompay, and R. C. Kessler
  1998   Trends in Alternative Medicine Use in the United States, 1990–1997: Results of a Follow-up National Survey. *Journal of the American Medical Association* 280(18):1569–75.

Eisenberg, D. M., R. C. Kessler, C. Foster, F. E. Norlock, D. R. Calkins, and T. L. Delbanco
  1993   Unconventional Medicine in the United States. *New England Journal of Medicine* 328(4):246–52.

Evans, G. D.
  1973a   Treatment Technologies and Publics. Their Relevance to Achieving Professional Status. *Journal of the Canadian Chiropractic Association* 21:11–15.
  1973b   A Sociology of Chiropractic. *Journal of the Canadian Chiropractic Association* 21:6–18.

Gesler, W. M.
  1988   The Place of Chiropractors in Health Care Delivery: A Case Study of North Carolina. *Social Science and Medicine* 26(8):785–92.

Hawk, C.
  2000   Should Chiropractic Be a "Wellness" Profession. *Topics of Clinical Chiropractics* 7(1):23–26.

Hawk, C., C. R. Long, and K. T. Boulanger
  1998   Development of a Practice-Based Research Program. *Journal of Manipulative and Physiological Therapeutics* 21(3):149–56.
  2001   Patient Satisfaction with the Chiropractic Clinical Encounter: Report from a Practice-Based Research Program. *Journal of Neuromusculoskeletal System* 9(4):109–117.

Hawk, C., C. R. Long, K. T. Boulanger, E. Morschhauser, and A. W. Fuhr
  2000   Chiropractic Care for Patients Aged 55 Years and Older: Report from a Practice Based Research Program. *Journal of American Geriatric Society* 48(5):534–45.

Hewitt, D., and P. H. N. Wood
  1975   Heterodox Practitioners and the Availability of Specialist Advice. *Rheumatology Rehabilitation* 14:191.

Hurwitz, E. L.
  1994   The Relative Impact of Chiropractic versus Medical Management of Low-Back Pain on Health Status in a Multispecialty Group Practice. *Journal of Manipulative and Physiological Therapeutics* 17:74–82.

Hurwitz, E. L., I. D. Coulter, A. H. Adams, B. J. Genovese, and P. G. Shekelle
  1998   Use of Chiropractic Services from 1985 through 1991 in the United States and Canada. *American Journal of Public Health* 88(5):771–75.

Jamison, J. R.
  1993   Chiropractic Holism: Interactively Becoming in a Reductionist Health Care System. *Chiropractic Journal of Australia* 23(3):98–105.

1994   Clinical Communication: The Essence of Chiropractic. *Journal of Chiropractic Humanities* 4:26–35.

Jarvis, K. B., R. B. Phillips, and E. K. Moris

1991   Cost per Case Comparison of Back Injury Claims of Chiropractic versus Medical Management for Conditions with Identical Diagnostic Codes. *Journal of Occupational Medicine* 33:847–52.

Kane, R. L., C. Leymaster, D. Olsen, and F. R. Woolley

1974   Manipulating the Patient: A Comparison of Physician and Chiropractic Care. *Lancet* 1:3333–36.

Kelner, M., O. Hall, and I. Coulter

1980   *Chiropractors: Do They Help?* Toronto: Fitzhenry & Whiteside.

Kleynhans, A. M., and D. N. Cahill

1991   Paradigms for Chiropractic Research. *Chiropractic Journal of Australia* 21:102–107.

Lavsky-Shulman, M., R. B. Wallace, and F. J. Kohout

1985   Prevalence and Functional Correlates of Low Back Pain in the Elderly: The Iowa 65+ Rural Health Study. *Journal of American Geriatric Society* 33:23–28.

Lawrence, D., ed.

1991   The Sociology of Chiropractic (special issue): *Journal of Manipulative and Physiological Therapeutics* 14, 1.

Leis, G. L.

1972   The Professionalization of Chiropractic. PhD thesis. State University of New York.

Lin, P. L.

1972   The Chiropractor, Chiropractic, and Process: A Study of the Sociology of an Occupation. PhD thesis. University of Missouri.

MacLennan, A. H., D. H. Wilson, and A. W. Taylor

1996   Prevalence and Cost of Alternative Medicine in Australia. *Lancet* 347:569–73.

McCorkle, T.

1961   Chiropractic: A Deviant Theory of Disease and Treatment in Contemporary Western Culture. *Human Organization* 20:20–23.

Meade, T. W., S. Dyer, W. Browne, and A. O. Frank

1995   Randomized Comparison of Chiropractic and Hospital Outpatient Management for Low Back Pain: Results from an Extended Follow-Up. *British Medical Journal* 311:349–51.

Meade, T. W., S. Dyer, W. Browne, J. Townsend, and A. O. Frank

1990   Low Back Pain of Mechanical Origin: A Randomized Comparison of Chiropractic and Hospital Outpatient Treatment. *British Medical Journal* 300:1431–37.

Meeker, W. C., and S. Haldeman

2002   Chiropractic: A Profession at the Crossroads of Mainstream and Alternative Medicine. *Annals of Internal Medicine* 136:216–27.

Mills, S.

1989–90 Inside the Academy. The Center for Complementary Health Studies Opens at Britain's Exeter University—A Landmark Event for Complementary Medicine. *Journal of Traditional Acupuncture* (Winter):28–33.

Mootz, R. D., I. D. Coulter, and D. T. Hansen
  1997   Health Services Research Related to Chiropractic: Review and Recommenda-
         tions for Research Prioritization by the Chiropractic Profession. *Journal of Ma-
         nipulative and Physiological Therapeutics* 20:201–17.
Mugge, R. H.
  1986   Utilization of Chiropractic Services in the United States. Paper presented at
         the Meetings of the American Public Health Association in Las Vegas, Nevada,
         on October 1.
National Board of Chiropractic Examiners: Job Analysis of Chiropractic
  1993   A Project Report, Survey Analysis, and Summary of the Practice of Chiro-
         practic within the United States. Greely, Colo.: NBCE.
Nelson, C. F.
  1994   Chiropractic and Wellness Care. *Journal of Chiropractic Humanities* 4(1):319. New
         Haven Health Care, Inc., National Chiropractic Center for Health Planning,
         Connecticut Chiropractic Association, Inc.
  1976   Ambulatory Chiropractic Practice in Connecticut. Final report, Contract No.
         HSM 110-72-377. Washington, D.C.: Health Services and Mental Health Ad-
         ministration, Department of Health, Education, and Welfare.
Nofz, M.
  1978   Paradigm Identification and Organizational Structure: An Overview of the
         Chiropractic Health Care Profession. *Sociological Symposium* 22:18–32.
Nyiendo, J., and L. Lamm
  1991   Disabling Low Back Oregon Worker's Compensation Claims. Part I: Method-
         ology and Clinical Categorization of Chiropractic and Medical Cases. *Journal of
         Manipulative and Physiological Therapeutics* 14(3):177–84.
Oths, K.
  1994   Communication in a Chiropractic Clinic: How a D.C. Treats His Patients. *Cul-
         ture, Medicine, and Psychiatry* 18(1):83–113.
Phillips, R. B., and R. Butler
  1982   Survey of Chiropractic in Dade County, Florida. *Journal of Manipulative and Phys-
         iological Therapeutics* 5(2):83–89.
Prima Health Systems, Inc.
  1976   Ambulatory Care Survey. Final Report Prepared for the American Chiroprac-
         tic Association, November.
Roebuck, J. B., and B. Hunter
  1972   The Awareness of Health Care Quackery as Deviant Behavior. *Journal of Health
         and Human Behavior* 15:3–10.
Rootman, I., and D. L. Mills
  1974   Professional Behavior of American and Canadian Chiropractors. *Journal of
         Health and Human Behavior* 15:3–12.
Rosenthal, F.
  1981   Marginal or Mainstream: Two Studies of Contemporary Chiropractic. *Social Fo-
         cus* 14:271–85.

Salmon, J. W., ed.
  1984   *Alternative Medicines: Popular and Policy Perspectives*. New York: Tavistock.
Schmitt, N. I.
  1978   The Utilization of Chiropractors. *Sociological Symposium* 22:55–71.
Shapiro, E.
  1983   The Physician Visit Patterns of Chiropractic Users: Health-Seeking Behavior of the Elderly in Manitoba, Canada. *American Journal of Public Health* 73:553–57.
Shekelle, P. G.
  1994   Spinal Manipulation. *Spine* 19(2):858–61.
  1998   What Role for Chiropractic in Health Care? *New England Journal of Medicine* 339(15):1074–75.
Shekelle, P. G., A. H. Adams, and M. R. Chassin
  1991   The Appropriateness of Spinal Manipulation for Low-Back Pain: Project Overview and Literature Review. Santa Monica, Calif.: The RAND Corporation, R-4025/1 CCR/FCER.
Shekelle, P. G., A. Adams, M. R. Chassin, E. L. Hurwitz, and R. H. Brook
  1992   Spinal Manipulation for Low-Back Pain. *Annals of Internal Medicine* 117:590–98.
Shekelle, P. G., and R. H. Brook
  1991   A Community-Based Study of the Use of Chiropractic Services. *American Journal of Public Health* 81(4):439–42.
Shekelle, P. G., D. Coulter, E. L. Hurwitz, B. Genovese, A. H. Adams, S. A. Miro, and R. H. Brook
  1998   Congruence between Decisions to Initiate Chiropractic Spinal Manipulation for Low Back Pain and Appropriateness Criteria in North America. *Annals of Internal Medicine* 129(1):9–17.
Shekelle, P. G., M. Markovich, and R. Louie
  1995a   Factors Associated with Choosing a Chiropractor for Episodes of Back Pain Care. *Medical Care* 33(8):842–50.
  1995b   Comparing the Costs between Provider Types of Episodes of Back Care Pain. *Spine* 20(2):221–27.
Skipper, J. K., ed.
  1978   Sociological Symposium. *The Sociology of Chiropractors and Chiropractic* 22.
Stano, M.
  1993   A Comparison of Health Care Costs for Chiropractic and Medical Patients. *Journal of Manipulative and Physiological Therapeutics* 16(5):291–99.
Stano, M., and M. Smith
  1996   Chiropractic and Medical Costs of Low Back Pain Care. *Medical Care* 34:191–204.
Sternberg, D.
  1969   Boys in Plight. A Case Study of Chiropractic Students Confronting a Medically Oriented Society. PhD thesis. New York University.

Vernon, H., and S. Mior

    1991   The Neck Disability Index: A Study of Reliability and Validity. *Journal of Manipulative and Physiological Therapeutics* 14:409–15.

Von Kuster, T., Jr.

    1980   Chiropractic Health Care: A National Study of Cost of Education, Service, Utilization, Number of Practicing Doctors of Chiropractic, and Other Key Policy Issues. Washington, D.C.: The Foundation for the Advancement of Chiropractic Tenets and Science.

Wardwell, W.

    1952   A Marginal Professional Role: The Chiropractor. *Social Forces* 30:339–46.

    1955   The Reduction of Strain in a Marginal Role. *American Journal of Sociology* 61:16–26.

    1972   Orthodoxy and Heterodoxy in Medical Practice. *Social Science and Medicine* 6:759–63.

    1976   Whither Chiropractic. *Digest of Chiropractic Economics* 18(5):87–89.

    1978   Social Factors in the Survival of Chiropractic: A Comparative View. *Sociological Symposium* 22:6–15.

    1979   Limited and Marginal Practitioners. In Freedman H. E., Levine G., and Reeder L. S., eds. *Handbook of Medical Sociology.* 3rd ed. Englewood Cliffs, N.J.: Prentice Hall.

    1980a   The Present and Future Role of the Chiropractor. Pp. 25–41 in S. Haldeman, ed. *Modern Developments in the Principles and Practice of Chiropractic.* New York: Appleton-Century Croft.

    1980b   The Triumph of Chiropractic—And Then What? *Journal of Sociology and Social Welfare* 7(3):425–29.

    1980c   A Sounding Board—Future of Chiropractic. *New England Journal of Medicine* 302:688–90.

    1981   Chiropractors—Challengers of Medical Domination. *Research in the Sociology of Health Care* 2:207–250.

    1992   *Chiropractic: History and Evolution of a New Profession.* St. Louis, Mo.: Moseby Year Book.

    1994   Alternative Medicine in the United States. *Social Science and Medicine.* 38(8):1061–68.

Weisner, D.

    1983   A Caste and Outcaste System in Medicine. *Social Science and Medicine* 17:475.

White, M., and J. K. Skipper

    1971   The Chiropractic Physician: A Study of Career Contingencies. *Journal of Health and Social Behavior* 12:300–310.

Wild, P. B.

    1978   Social Origins and Ideology of Chiropractors: An Empirical Study of the Socialization of the Chiropractic Student. *Sociological Symposium* 22:33–54.

Willis, E.

    1983   *Medical Domination.* Sydney: George Allen & Unwin.

    1991   Chiropractic in Australia. *Journal of Manipulative and Physiological Therapeutics* 14(1):59–69.

Yesalis, C. E., R. B. Wallace, W. P. Fisher, and R. Tokheim

    1980   Does Chiropractic Utilization Substitute for Less Available Medical Services? *American Journal of Public Health* 70:415–17.

Divergences in the Evolution of Osteopathy in Four Anglophone Countries
The United States, Canada, Britain, and Australia

4

HANS A. BAER

WHEREAS MANY CROSS-CULTURAL STUDIES of biomedicine have been conducted, often as part of a rich literature on comparative health systems, relatively little attention has been paid to the cross-cultural study of alternative or heterodox medical systems. One exception is Roth's (1976) examination of "natural medicine" in the United States and West Germany. Another is Unshuld's (1980) demonstration that the status of homeopathy, anthroposophy, and botanical medicine in West Germany and East Germany, particularly with respect to their use of alternative drug therapy prior to the reunification of 1990, had been shaped by the larger sociopolitical systems in those countries. This chapter examines the divergent evolutionary trajectories of osteopathy in four Anglophone countries, namely the United States, Canada, Great Britain, and Australia, within the context of their larger national health care systems.

Andrew Taylor Still, an allopathic physician, developed osteopathy in the Midwest of the United States as a manual medical system in the late nineteenth century in response to what he considered to be the inadequacies of allopathic medicine. In the early part of the twentieth century, osteopathy diffused to various other Anglophone countries, particularly Canada, Britain, and Australia, where it has undergone distinct evolutionary trajectories shaped by the larger political economies of those countries.

The Emergence of Osteopathy in the United States

Andrew Taylor Still (1828–1917), the son of a Methodist minister and a dabbler in mesmerism and spiritualism, developed what he termed "osteopathy" in the 1860s (Trowbridge 1991). Although Still briefly studied at the Kansas City College of Physicians and Surgeons in 1860 (Booth 1924), he obtained his medical training as his father's apprentice. He became disenchanted with regular medicine when it failed to prevent the death of three of his children from meningitis. Based upon detailed anatomical investigations, Still asserted that many, if not all, diseases are caused by faulty articulations or "lesions" in various parts of the musculoskeletal system. Such dislocations produce disordered nerve connections that in turn impair the proper circulation of the blood and other body fluids. Still maintained that structure and function of the body are intricately intertwined and that disorders in one organ affect other parts of the body. In his private practice, Still began to rely more and more on osteopathic manipulation therapy (OMT) as a form of therapy, not only for musculoskeletal problems but also ailments in other organs. He argued that health could be best promoted by ensuring that the musculoskeletal system was in as perfect alignment as possible and obstructions to blood and lymph flow were minimized. Still strongly opposed the use of drugs, vaccines, serums, and modalities such as electrotherapy, radiology, and hydrotherapy. In essence, he synthesized some of the major components of magnetic healing and bonesetting into a unified heterodox medical system. His system also had a metaphysical component in that he viewed osteopathy as "God's law" and the body as a God-given machine.

After Baker University in Baldwin, Kansas—an institution that Still's father and brothers helped establish—denied him permission to present his ideas, he established a base of operations in Kirksville in northeast Missouri, where he applied his concepts in private practice from 1874 to 1892. Still reported that on June 22, 1874, he "flung to the breeze the banner of Osteopathy" (Still 1908). He presented himself as the "Lightening Bone Setter" and as an itinerant physician who spread the gospel of osteopathy from town to town in Missouri (McKone 2001:16–17).

Still established, along with William Smith, a Briton and graduate of the University of Edinburgh medical school, the American School of Osteopathy in Kirksville in September 1892. Smith served as the first lecturer in anatomy and provided the new institution with impeccable credentials and an aura of legitimacy. The early faculty of the American School included several other physicians with degrees from both regular and homeopathic colleges. In addition to anatomy and OMT, the curricula emphasized histology, physiology, and toxicology.

Osteopathy appealed to thousands of ordinary rural and small-town people, particularly those who were suffering from chronic spinal or joint ailments. The creation of an additional seventeen osteopathic schools between 1895 and 1900 offered many individuals of humble origins the hope of becoming medical practitioners (Albrecht and Levy 1982:74). Despite the fascination of some regular physicians with osteopathy as an adjunct to their practices, most regular physicians were hostile to the new manual medical system. Notwithstanding the opposition of these physicians, along with that of various homeopathic and eclectic physicians, osteopaths—with the support of satisfied patients, some of whom were state legislators, and patrons—quickly obtained at least limited practice rights in most states during the 1890s and the first decade of the twentieth century. Among those sympathetic to osteopathy was Mark Twain, who wrote in his *Notebook* around 1900: "To ask a doctor's opinion of osteopathy is equivalent to going to Satan for information about Christianity" (quoted in McKone 2001:20). He came in contact with it in Hannibal, Missouri, where Still had an office for several months in late 1889. Twain supported legislation for osteopathy before a New York assembly committee meeting in 1901.

The Evolution of Osteopathy into Osteopathic Medicine and Surgery in the United States

Despite Still's eschewal of drugs and surgery except in extreme circumstances, osteopathy began to incorporate more and more aspects of regular medicine or biomedicine. The early history of U.S. osteopathy entailed spirited debates between the "lesion osteopaths," who wished to closely adhere to the principles delineated by Still, and the "broad osteopaths," who favored incorporating elements from regular medicine as well as other medical systems such as naturopathy and electrotherapy (Gevitz 1982:61–66). At roughly the same time that regular medicine was evolving into biomedicine—a system based heavily on germ theory and controlled scientific research, osteopathy began to accommodate itself to its parent. Although Still objected to surgery except as a last resort, the Committee of Education of the American Osteopathic Association (AOA) relaxed this injunction in 1902 by stating: "Surgery is very closely related to osteopathy. . . . Osteopathic cases sometimes require a little surgery, while nearly all surgical operations would be profitably supplemented by osteopathic treatment" (American Osteopathic Association 1902). Gradually, osteopaths adopted other biomedical practices, including the administration of drugs, vaccines, and antibiotics.

By the 1930s, osteopathy in the United States had evolved into osteopathic medicine and surgery or a parallel medical system with an emphasis on primary care. DO's (doctors of osteopathy) referred to themselves as osteopathic physicians rather than osteopaths. The osteopathic profession began to create its own hospitals in the early 1930s and established the American Osteopathic Hospital Association in 1934. Today, few American osteopathic physicians specialize in osteopathic manipulation therapy, despite the centrality of this modality in the system that Still developed. Instead, the vast majority use it as an adjunct therapeutic modality or not at all. As the majority of biomedical physicians vacated primary care for various specialties, many osteopathic physicians found a niche as primary care providers. In contrasting themselves to biomedical practitioners, osteopathic physicians often assert that they treat the "person rather than the disease." In reality, this assertion has not been empirically demonstrated, but appears to serve as a rhetorical device by which U.S. osteopathic physicians can distinguish themselves from their biomedical counterparts. In a survey of a rural community in central Michigan, Riley (1980), a medical anthropologist who later went "native" by becoming an osteopathic physician, found that a substantial majority of his subjects did not perceive any difference between DOs, and MDs in terms of practice, although they tended to regard biomedicine more favorably than osteopathic medicine. Detailed ethnographic studies comparing and contrasting the "bedside manner" of biomedical and osteopathic physicians are long overdue.

A fair degree of tension persists between the AOA and the American Academy of Osteopathy, a body that serves as a quasi-certifying board for those DOs who specialize in OMT. Within the culture of U.S. osteopathic medicine, whereas most practitioners are referred to as "three-fingered osteopaths," in that they regularly administer injections, members of the academy are referred to as "ten-fingered osteopaths" because they use all of their fingers to manipulate patients. The 2001 AOA fact sheet indicates that only 430, or 1 percent, of 41,574 active DOs in the United States specialize in OMT (AOA 2002). Conversely, the overwhelming majority of chiropractors in the United States and other countries around the world specialize in the manipulative or manual medicine underlying their field from its inception.

Despite the efforts of biomedicine to legally contain osteopathy in the United States (Baer 2001:55–57), the latter managed to obtain full practice rights in about three quarters of states by 1960. As a result, biomedicine shifted its policy to co-option. The climax of this strategy occurred in 1961 when the California Medical Association and California Osteopathic Association merged. Consequent to this merger, 86 percent of the DOs in California (about two thousand) became MDs, the California College of Osteopathic Physicians and Surgeons in Los Angeles became the University of California College of Medicine–Irvine, and most of the osteopathic hospitals in the state were converted into biomedical ones. Those practitioners who chose to retain their DO degrees were reorganized as the Osteopathic Physicians and Surgeons of California.

Regardless of how rank-and-file members of the osteopathic profession may have viewed the California merger, the general reaction of its leadership in the AOA was one of strong disapproval and alarm. Despite some other attempts at mergers, such as those in Pennsylvania and Washington, the osteopathic profession successfully prevented the loss of other state societies to organized medicine. Because most DOs in California became MDs, the leadership of the osteopathic profession fell on a Michigan association that responded by establishing a private school in Pontiac. When the osteopathic profession in Michigan realized that it could not financially support a college on its own, it turned to support from the state legislature. In large part because DOs, particularly since World War II, had provided much of the primary care in Michigan, the state legislature approved the annexation in 1969 of the osteopathic college to Michigan State University. This measure prompted legislatures in six other states—namely Texas, Oklahoma, West Virginia, Ohio, New Jersey, and New York—to fund osteopathic medical colleges. Since 1976, an additional eight private osteopathic colleges have been established in the United States, bringing the total number of schools to nineteen, in contrast to a low of five osteopathic colleges in the country in the wake of the demise of the California Osteopathic Association in 1961. The Harvey Peters Foundation has plans to open a new osteopathic medical school in Virginia (Lareau 2001:2).

The number of practicing DOs in the United States increased from 8,410 in 1932 to 13,708 in 1960; it then fell slightly to 13,454 in 1970. The number rose again to 18,820 in 1980, to 25,429 in 1986, and to 41,574 in 2001 (from AOA, 2002 Fact Sheets). In essence, the U.S. osteopathic profession has undergone an organizational rejuvenation over the course of the past three decades or so. By the early 1970s, the osteopathic profession had achieved full practice rights in all fifty states and the District of Columbia.

Although U.S. osteopathy initially attracted regular physicians and other individuals who wanted to practice a heterodox form of therapy, eventually many if not most of those who entered the profession did not do so because they wanted to become osteopaths per se. They wanted to become physicians but found admission to biomedical schools closed to them for structural reasons, ranging from class bias favoring upper and upper-middle-class students over lower-middle and working-class students on admissions standards to quotas on the number of Jewish students once widespread in biomedical schools (New 1958; Sharma and Dressel 1975).

Various state legislatures opted to fund osteopathic schools due to the paucity of primary physicians in biomedicine. In 1967–1968 the national percentage of practitioners in general practice was 29 percent for biomedical physicians and 90 percent for osteopathic physicians; by 1978, the percentage had dropped significantly to 18 percent for biomedical physicians, but remained high at 88 percent for osteopathic physicians (Albrecht and Levy 1982:191). Ironically, an increasing number of osteopathic physicians have turned to the specialties in the past two decades or so. Conversely, as U.S. osteopathic medicine increasingly abandoned its therapeutic birthright, chiropractic emerged as the foremost promoter of manual therapy in the United States and has achieved status as a semilegitimate professional heterodox medical system whose practitioners now outnumber osteopathic physicians (Baer 2001). Despite its more or less complete legitimacy, American osteopathy continues to face an identity dilemma concerning whether or not it constitutes a distinct medical system with a need for separate organizational structures, such as professional associations, colleges, and hospitals (Miller 1998). Osteopathic physicians frequently practice in biomedical settings. Osteopathic hospitals, which tend to be smaller than their biomedical counterparts, are having difficulty filling their residencies. Young DOs face pressures to view themselves as less and less different from MDs.

Regardless of the views of individual DOs and their patients, the AOA has engaged in extensive public relations efforts to underscore that osteopathic physicians are authentic physicians and that osteopathic medicine constitutes a comprehensive and holistic form of health care. In an effort to differentiate itself from biomedicine, U.S. osteopathic medicine has been urging greater emphasis on OMT as a treatment, and has increased research on its efficacy. Nevertheless, it continues to suffer from what Norman Gevitz (2001:176), a sociologist at the Ohio University College of Osteopathic Medicine, terms an "osteopathic invisibility syndrome" in that the general public is generally unaware of the profession. He asserts that osteopathic schools need to encourage research more than they have in the past, including on OMT, so that the osteopathic profession can better differentiate itself from biomedicine.

Whereas U.S. osteopathy moved away from its roots as a manual medical system, its closely related rival, chiropractic, has evolved by and large in the United States into a musculoskeletal specialty. Daniel David Palmer, the founder of chiropractic, administered his first spinal adjustment in Davenport, Iowa, in September 1895, when he cured an African American janitor of a seventeen-year deafness. Chiropractic constitutes the most visible and successful alternative medical system in the United States, despite the fact that its history has been marked by considerable factionalism between the "straights"—those practitioners who rely primarily or exclusively on spinal adjustment, and the "mixers"—those practitioners who also rely on a wide array of other modalities, including physiotherapy, vitamin and nutritional therapy, and even acupuncture (Baer 2001:67–84).

Despite vigorous opposition from organized biomedicine, U.S. chiropractic has undergone considerable legitimization since the early 1970s. Governmental support for chiropractic has included (1) coverage for chiropractic care under Workers' Compensation in all fifty states and the District of Columbia, (2) the allowance of sick leave for federal civil service employees based on a statement from a chiropractor, (3) federal income tax deductions for chiropractic care, and (4) coverage for chiropractic in all or nearly all states under Medicaid or Medicare. In 1974, the United States Office of Education authorized the American Chiropractic Association's Council on Chiropractic Education to act as the official accrediting agency of chiropractic colleges. The CIC currently extends accreditation to fifteen chiropractic colleges. While statistics on the number of chiropractors in the United States fluctuate widely, chiropractic has undergone considerable growth and can be expected to do so for some time. The 1990 Official Directory of the Federation of Chiropractic Boards listed 44,904 "resident D.C.'s" in the United States (cited in Wardwell 1992:232).

The Canadian Scenario

Despite its geographical proximity to the United States, the osteopathic profession in Canada has always been small and has only had limited practice rights. The first osteopaths arrived in Canada before 1900 and others arrived shortly after (Mills 1966:219). The Ontario Osteopathic Association was established in 1901 with roughly eight members (Mills 1966:221). The first osteopaths set up practice in New Brunswick around 1903 and in British Columbia no later than 1909 (Mills 1966:223). The Canadian Osteopathic Association was organized under a federal charter in 1926 (Mills 1966:10).

By the end of the 1930s, Canada had only about two hundred practicing osteopaths (Mills 1966). This number declined to 124 in 1954 and 105 in 1962 (Gray 1981). Most osteopaths in Canada obtained their training at U.S. osteopathic colleges, and many belonged to the American Osteopathic Association. Despite efforts to obtain full practice rights and hospital privileges like their American counterparts, Canadian osteopaths had been forced to work under limited practice legislation for decades (Mills 1966:49). Osteopaths had special osteopathic licensing boards in Ontario, Manitoba, and Saskatchewan, but practiced under other provisions in other provinces (Mills 1966:235). Osteopathy has been a much smaller profession than chiropractic in Canada, despite the fact that both essentially function as manual medical systems. Whereas there were reportedly 1,073 chiropractors in Canada in 1961, there were only 105 osteopaths (Mills 1966:17).

Although some provinces began to grant full practice rights to graduates of U.S. osteopathic medical schools in the 1960s, few of them chose to take advantage of these provisions. Svoboda reports that "[b]y 1999, the number of DOs had dwindled to 29, and within that remnant, many are retired or semi-retired" (2000:57).

Osteopathy has started to make a modest comeback in Canada with the creation in 1981 of the Collège d'Etudes Ostepathiques de Montreal. This Canadian College of Osteopathy has branches in Quebec, Toronto, Halifax, and Vancouver (Canadian College of Osteopathy 2003). Still unaccredited, the institution offers weekend courses in osteopathy and offers a "Doctorate in Osteopathic Manual Practice" for students who opt to write a thesis in addition to their clinical training. While the Canadian College of Osteopathy holds out the promise of the rejuvenation of osteopathy as a manual medical system in Canada, Charles E. Findlay, the president of the Canadian Osteopathic Association and a family practitioner in Calgary, Alberta, asserted that the physician shortage in Canada has created a climate in which "the five Canadian provinces and two territories that have not yet granted DOs full practice rights seem ready to do so, with the exception of Ontario" (Svoboda 2000:57). He contended that the "achievements of U.S. DOs at home and abroad is helping to raise the status of the osteopathic medical profession in Canada" (Svoboda 2000:58). If indeed more provinces eventually grant full practice rights to DOs, there is the possibility that Canadian osteopathic medicine will evolve into a medical system parallel to biomedicine, as it has in the United States.

Although osteopathy experienced decline, at least until recently, in Canada, chiropractic has enjoyed increasing growth and legitimatization (Coburn and Biggs 1986). The number of chiropractors in Canada grew rapidly after World War II when the Canadian Memorial Chiropractic College was established in Toronto in 1945. Canada has some five thousand practicing chiropractors, almost half of whom are in Ontario (Clarke 2000:357). Chiropractors are licensed in all provinces except for Newfoundland. Canada's national health insurance or Medicare provides coverage for general chiropractic and x-ray examinations for a limited number of visits per year in every province where they are licensed, except in Saskatchewan, which does not restrict the number of visits. Only time will tell to what extent graduates of the various branches of the Canadian College of Osteopathy will come to compete with chiropractors who have achieved considerably more legitimization.

The British Scenario

The most important figure linking osteopathy between the two sides of the Atlantic was John Martin Littlejohn (1865–1947), a native of Glasgow, Scotland. After having served as the president of Amity College in College Springs, Iowa, his poor health forced him to resign his position, but led him to visit Still in Kirksville for several treatments. After being cured, Littlejohn enrolled as a student at the American School of Osteopathy and, shortly thereafter, was appointed its dean of faculty and professor of physiology. After receiving his DO in 1900, he founded, with his brothers, the American College of Osteopathic Medicine and Surgery, the forerunner of the Chicago College of Osteopathic Medicine. In 1898, Littlejohn introduced osteopathy to Britain by reading a paper on it before the Society of Science and Arts in London (Hall and Wernham 1974:8). F. J. Horn was the first person to practice osteopathy in Britain when he opened an office in London in 1902. By the 1920s, practitioners trained in U.S. schools, and others trained in osteopathy as apprentices or by self-instruction, were practicing in Britain. In contrast to the United States, where state licensing laws made heterodox practitioners marginal, the British government withheld statutory recognition and the creation of a state-sanctioned register, at least up until recently in the cases of osteopathy and chiropractic. According to Falder and Munro (1981:4), the "practice of alternative forms of therapy is a customary right in the UK and is part of Common Law. There are no legal restrictions under the law of any kind of treatment, although there are certain restrictions relating to certain diseases, appellations, and remedies."

A group of twelve osteopaths convened in 1910 or 1911 in Manchester to establish a society, which became the British Osteopathic Association (BOA) (Baer 1984). This is the premier association of British osteopathy and the only one recognized by the American Osteopathic Association. Most osteopaths in the first few decades of the twentieth century in Britain received their training in England rather than U.S. osteopathic schools. With the assistance of Horn, Littlejohn established the British School of Osteopathy in London in 1917. Various osteopathic schools and associations were formed in Britain during the 1920s and 1930s—a period described by the "old osteopaths" as the heyday of British osteopathy (Baer 1984). The Osteopathic Association of Great Britain came to fruition during this period and evolved until recently primarily as the alumni association of the British School of Osteopathy (BSO).

The British osteopathic profession went into a holding pattern during World War II, and after the war the British Osteopathic Association founded a postgraduate institution called the British College of Osteopathy. The school ceased operations in 1975 and was reestablished in 1978 as the London College of Osteopathic Medicine (Baer 1984). Admission to the college was available only to biomedical physicians, and this widened the already existing rift between the association and the BSO graduates.

As naturopathy, or nature cure, lost some of its appeal due to the advent of "wonder drugs," some naturopaths turned to osteopathy (Baer 1984). In 1961, the British Naturopathic Association was renamed the British Naturopathic and Osteopathic Association, and its associated training institution, the British College of Naturopathy, was renamed the British College of Naturopathy and Osteopathy. The Society of Osteopaths and the European College of Osteopathy emerged in the early 1970s as a result of a schism in the College of Naturopathy and Osteopathy. The society thereafter attracted disgruntled osteopaths affiliated with the OAGB and the BNOA. Also, since its beginnings, British osteopathy has had freelance practitioners who have not been eligible for membership in the major osteopathic associations (Baer 1984). These osteopaths have over the years formed a number of small associations of their own, many of which are affiliated with part-time schools offering courses in osteopathy and other natural therapies.

Since its diffusion to Britain in the early twentieth century, osteopathy has achieved a substantial degree of legitimacy there (Baer 1984). Sharma (1992:180) notes it constitutes the one "form of non-orthodox medicine which is best understood by and most acceptable to orthodox doctors." Many biomedical general practitioners have contracted with osteopaths to provide OMT for their National Health Service patients (General Osteopathic Council 2000:1). Some NHS hospitals employ osteopaths within their physiotherapy departments, and some NHS community trusts employ osteopaths to work at community health centers. At any rate, in many ways osteopathy in Britain today resembles osteopathy as it existed in the United States eighty or more years ago. Unless they have obtained training as regular medical practitioners, osteopaths in Britain are restricted from engaging in various biomedical procedures, such as prescribing legally defined dangerous drugs and performing surgery. Although British osteopaths (other than those who received biomedical training at the London College of Osteopathic Medicine) may employ various naturopathic techniques in their scope of treatment, by and large they function as musculoskeletal specialists, much in the same way that chiropractors in Britain and other countries do.

As we have seen, British osteopathy has undergone several lines of development, resulting in a hierarchy of organizations. While each of the osteopathic bodies continued to retain organizational independence, they achieved partial unity for a period of time under a voluntary registry called the General Council and Register of Osteopaths. The Osteopathic Association of Great Britain and the British Naturopathic and Osteopathic Association merged in spring 1992. During the course of the 1990s, the British School of Osteopathy, the British College of Naturopathy and Osteopathy, and the European School of Osteopathy became affiliated with various polytechnic colleges, enabling them to award BSc degrees approved by the Council for National Academic Awards.

In 1993, Parliament passed the Osteopaths Act, which finally provided the British Osteopathic profession with the statutory recognition it had long sought (Baer 1984). Practitioners trained in four-year osteopathic colleges in Britain as well as the London College of Osteopathic Medicine must register with the General Osteopathic Council (GOC). In contrast to the General Medical Council that has little power to sanction a biomedical physician for alleged incompetence, the GOC Council can rule that certain members have engaged in "unacceptable professional behavior" (Vincent and Furnham 1997:74). Britain's Faculty of Homeopathy constitutes the only statutory heterodox medical body in Europe with historical precedence over the GOC (Vincent and Furnham 1997:76). In the wake of the creation of statutory

recognition, the British Osteopathic Association proposed a merger that re-
sulted in a new BOA that incorporated the former Osteopathic Association of
Great Britain, the British Naturopathic and Osteopathic Association, and the
Society for Osteopaths (British Osteopathy Organization 2002).

Other than osteopathy, chiropractic is the only other heterodox medical
system in Britain that is regulated. Chiropractors achieved statutory recognition under the Chiropractors Act of 1994 and must register with the General
Chiropractic Council. Furthermore, the Anglo-European College of Chiropractic in Bournemouth offers a Council for National Academic Awards–
approved degree. British graduates of this institution, which also trains a large
number of practitioners from other countries, are eligible for membership in
the British Chiropractic Association. Graduates of two smaller chiropractic
schools can join the Institute of Pure Chiropractic or the British Association
of Chiropractic. Compared to the United States, British chiropractic remains
a tiny enterprise. According to one in-house source, "Osteopathy is better
known in the UK than Chiropractic. Britain is the only country where Osteopaths outnumber Chiropractors" (British Chiropractors' Association
n.d.:11). In 1999, Britain had 2,325 registered osteopaths and 1,118 registered
chiropractors (Zollman 1999).

The Australian Scenario

In contrast to the other three Anglophone countries under consideration, the development of osteopathy has been closely intertwined with that of chiropractic
in Australia. Many osteopaths transformed themselves into chiropractors with
the creation of the United Chiropractors' Association in 1961 (Hawkins and
O'Neill 1990: 27). Fredrick George Roberts established the Chiropractic and
Osteopathic College of Australasia in 1959 (Chiropractic and Osteopathic College of Australia 2001). In the mid-1960s, this institution dropped the designation "osteopathic" from its name. The college transferred its operations in 1981
to the Preston Institute of Technology which is now the Royal Melbourne Institute of Technology. The Australian Chiropractors' Association and the Australian
Osteopathic Association discussed the establishment of a joint organization in
the 1960s but have remained separate organizations (Hawkins and O'Neill
1990:35). The government-sponsored Webb Report (1977) grouped osteopaths
and chiropractors together. Indeed, some Australian practitioners have attempted
to institutionalize a merger of chiropractic and osteopathy as evidenced by the
names of two professional bodies, namely the Australian Chiropractors, Osteopaths, and Naturopathic Physicians Association and a group called Chiropractic and Osteopathic Incorporated (Webb Report 1977:261).

Willis provides the following overview of the sociopolitical status of osteopathy in Australia in the late 1980s:

> There were estimated to be between 250 and 300 osteopaths in Australia in 1986, with statutory registration in all states and territories except Western Australia and Tasmania, often conjointly with chiropractic. To a considerable extent, osteopathy has ridden on the coat-tails of chiropractic, and owes much of its success to that relationship. The 1983 *Health Survey* found quite low levels of utilization of osteopathic services; demand was only 10 percent of that for chiropractic and 40 percent of that for natural therapies. (Willis 1989:264)

As a point of comparison, there were 1,475 chiropractors in Australia in 1984 (Willis 1989:263).

Practitioners who attended regular clinical meetings at the Ringwood Clinic in Melbourne formed the Chiropractors and Osteopaths Musculo-Skeletal Interest Group (COMSIG) in 1990 (Chiropractic and Osteopathic College of Australia 2001). Under the banner of the Chiropractic and Osteopathic College of Australia, COMSIG functions as the leading provider of seminars and conferences for chiropractors and osteopaths in Australia. Both chiropractic and osteopathic programs are offered in state-supported institutions in Australia. The Philip Institute of Technology in Melbourne began granting a Diploma in Chiropractic in 1981 and the Diploma in Osteopathy in 1984. Osteopathy is presently taught at the baccalaureate level in three Australian institutions of higher education—the Royal Melbourne Institute of Technology, the Victoria University of Technology, and the University of West Sydney–MacArthur (Chiropractic and Osteopathic College of Australia 2002). Students at the latter two institutions may also obtain a master's degree in osteopathy. Since 1991, the Australian Osteopathic Association, which was formed in 1955 in Victoria, has regarded itself as a federal body representing osteopaths in all states.[1]

Social Forces Accounting for the Divergent Evolution of Osteopathy in Four Anglophone Countries

Biomedicine constitutes the predominant medical subsystem in all plural medical systems in the modern world, including the United States, Canada, Britain, and Australia. As a result, I refer to this structural arrangement as the dominative medical system, one which consists of a rank hierarchy with (1) biomedicine at the apex; (2) certain specific parallel medical systems (such as osteopathic medicine within the U.S. context and homeopathy within the Britain context); (3) various professionalized heterodox medical systems (such as chiropractic and naturopathy in the United States or osteopathy, chiropractic, and naturopathy in Canada, Britain, and Australia); (4) various partially professionalized heterodox medical systems (such as massage therapy, Rolfing, herbalism); (5) religious healing systems (such as Christian Science or Pentecostalism), and (6) a wide array of folk medical systems prevalent among ethnic minorities and indigenous people situated in complex societies (Baer, Singer, and Susser 1997; Baer 2001).

Ultimately, the ability of biomedicine to achieve dominance depends on support from what Freidson (1970:72-73) terms "strategic elites." These strategic elites include members of the corporate class interested in health issues, their political allies in the state sector, and health policy makers in the government, private foundations, and think tanks. However, biomedicine's dominance over rival medical systems that it achieved around the world in the beginning of the twentieth century has never been absolute. The state, which primarily serves the interests of the corporate class, must periodically make concessions to subordinate social groups in order to maintain social order. As a result, certain heterodox practitioners, with the support of influential patrons, have been able to obtain legitimization in the form of full practice rights (e.g., osteopathic physicians in the United States and homeopathic physicians in Britain) or limited practice rights (e.g., chiropractors and naturopaths in the United States and osteopaths, chiropractors, and naturopaths in Canada, Britain, and Australia).

Osteopathy in the United States has evolved away from its initial emphasis on manipulative therapy and essentially functions as a parallel medical system to biomedicine. Only a small number of "ten-fingered" osteopaths associated with the American Academy of Osteopathy specialize in osteopathic manipulation therapy. In contrast, osteopathy continues to function primarily as a manual medical system in Canada, Britain, and Australia. However, as noted earlier, a few Canadian provinces have granted full practice rights to graduates of U.S. osteopathic colleges. In Britain, biomedical physicians who have studied at the London College of Osteopathic Medicine function as specialists in OMT. Elsewhere in Europe, Germany recently became the first country to offer full licensure to graduates of U.S. osteopathic schools (Glassman 1998:596). Furthermore, the German Society of Manual Medicine—an affiliate of the German Medical Association—offers a 480-hour OMT/manual medicine training program to biomedical physicians.

While it has obtained statutory or parliamentary recognition in Commonwealth countries, osteopathy functions, by and large, as does chiropractic, as a heterodox musculoskeletal specialty. Some osteopaths in these settings broaden their scope of practice by employing various naturopathic techniques. To a large extent, the full legitimization of osteopathy in the United States occurred because it helped address the paucity of primary care physicians associated with a largely privatized, capital-intensive political economy of health care. In contrast, the nationalized health care systems of Canada, Britain, and Australia have resulted in a roughly 50-50 split between generalists and specialists and a lack of the pressures that have prompted health policy makers in the United States to seek alternate sources for primary care providers. However, this situation appears to be changing in Canada. Ironically, whereas in the United States insurance companies and Medicare and Medicaid cover services provided by osteopathic physicians, the governments of Canada, Britain, and Australia provide some financial reimbursement for osteopathic services. In contrast to the United States where osteopathy and chiropractic have evolved in quite different directions, osteopathy shares roughly the same niche as chiropractic in the medical marketplaces of Canada, Britain, and Australia.

Osteopathy can be considered, on the whole, politically stronger than chiropractic in Britain, but it has come to play second fiddle to chiropractic in Canada and Australia. As tenuous as osteopathy's future in Canada appears to be, its status in Britain and Australia bears some resemblance to Coburn's observations about chiropractic in Canada—observations that in large part apply to chiropractic in much of the world today. He argues:

> Chiropractic, however, from being a complete alternative to medicine, has been partly tamed and "medicalized." Its education now consists to a great deal of traditional "medical" basic science. In order to be able to deal with patients directly rather than having to have a medical referral chiropractic has had to teach "general diagnosis" in a manner little different from medical schools. Many of the original claims to being a complete alternative to medicine have been downplayed as chiropractic has sought to distance itself from anything faintly disreputable. (Coburn 1993:846)

Ironically, osteopathy clearly no longer functions as a heterodox medical system in the United States where it is barely distinguishable from biomedicine. Although osteopathy in Canada, Britain, and Australia tends to resemble what osteopathy looked like 60 or 70 years ago in the United States, it also has, like chiropractic, been partially medicalized in these settings as it has embarked upon a path of professionalization and legitimization.

Notes

An earlier version of this essay was presented at the combined meeting of the Society for Applied Anthropology and the Society for Medical Anthropology in Merida, Yucatan, Mexico, March 28–April 1, 2001.

1. Osteopaths in New Zealand in the past have obtained their training in Britain, Australia, and possibly elsewhere and belong to the New Zealand Register of Osteopaths. The first master's degree program in osteopathy entailing five years of study was established in February 2002 in Auckland. The Department of Orthopaedic Surgery and Musculoskeletal Medicine at the Christchurch School of Medicine offers a postgraduate certifi-

cate in Musculoskeletal Medicine that includes training in osteopathy and chiropractic (University of Otago 2002).

References

Albrecht, Gary L., and Judith A. Levy
  1982 The Professionalization of Osteopathy: Adaptation in the Medical Marketplace. Pp. 161–206 in Julius A. Roth, ed. *Research in the Sociology of Health Care: Changing Structure of Health Service Occupations.* vol. 3. Greenwich, Conn.: JAI Press.
American Osteopathic Association
  1902 Report of the Committee for Education. *Journal of the American Osteopathic Association* 2:10–19.
  2002 Information. Available at www.aoa-net.org (accessed April 19, 2002).
Australian Osteopathic Association.
  2002 Osteopathic Undergraduate Degree Courses. Available at www.osteopathic.com .au/education.htm (accessed April 19, 2002).
Baer, Hans A.
  1984 The Drive for Professionalization in British Osteopathy. *Social Science and Medicine* 19:717–24.
  2001 *Biomedicine and Alternative Healing Systems in America: Issues of Class, Race, Ethnicity, and Gender.* Madison: University of Wisconsin Press.
Baer, Hans A., Merrill Singer, and Ida Susser
  1997 *Medical Anthropology and the World System: A Critical Perspective.* Westport, Conn.: Bergin & Garvey.
Booth, E. R.
  1924 *History of Osteopathy and Twentieth-Century Medical Practice.* Cincinnati, Oh.: Caxton.
British Chiropractors' Association
  n.d.   *The British Chiropractic Handbook.* Chelmsford, Essex.
British Osteopathic Association
  2002 History of the Association. Available at www.osteopathy.org/n_history.htm (accessed April 19, 2002).
Canadian College of Osteopathy.
  2003 Available at www.osteopathy-canada.com/academicprogram.htm (accessed June 26, 2003).
Chiropractic and Osteopathic College of Australasia
  2001 The History of the Chiropractic and Osteopathic College of Australasia. Available at www.com.au/history.htm (accessed January 1, 2001).
Clarke, Juane Nancarrow
  2000 *Health, Illness, and Medicine in Canada.* Don Mills, Ontario: Oxford University Press.
Coburn, David
  1993 State Authority, Medical Dominance, and Trends in the Regulation of the Health Professions: The Ontario Case. *Social Science and Medicine* 37:841–50.
Coburn, David, and Lesley Biggs
  1986 The Limits to Medical Dominance: The Case of Chiropractic. *Social Science and Medicine* 22:1035–46.

Falder, S., and R. Munro

    1981 *The Status of Complementary Medicine in the United Kingdom.* London: Threshold Foundation.

Freidson, Elliott

    1970 *Profession of Medicine: A Study of the Sociology of Applied Knowledge.* New York: Dodd, Mead

General Osteopathic Council

    2000 Osteopath and Medicine: Working with the NHS. Available at www.osteopathy
        .org.uk/goc/medicine/working.shtml (accessed May 3, 2004).

Gevitz, Norman

    1982 *The D.Os: Osteopathic Medicine in the Americas.* Baltimore: Johns Hopkins University Press.

    2001 Researched and Demonstrated: Inquiry and Infrastructure at Osteopathic Insti-
        tutions. *Journal of the American Osteopathic Association* 101(3):174–79.

Glassman, J.

    1998 International Recognition of Osteopathic Medicine. *Journal of the American Osteo-
        pathic Association* 98:596.

Gray, Charlotte

    1981 Osteopathy: Is There a Place in Canadian Medicine? *Canadian Medical Association
        Journal* 125 (July 1):108-111.

Hall, T., and J. Wernham

    1974 *The Contribution of John Martin Littlejohn to Osteopathy.* Maidstone, Kent, England:
        Maidstone Osteopathic Clinic.

Hawkins, Peter, and Arthur O'Neill

    1990 *Osteopathy in Australia.* Bundoora, Australia: Philip Institute of Technology Press.

Lareau, Chris

    2001 Osteopathy Officially Recognized as a Complete Equal School of Medicine.
        The D.O. Health Network, April 11–18. Available at www.dohealthnet.com (see
        article 1171) (accessed May 3, 2004).

McKone, W. Llewellyn

    2001 *Osteopathic Medicine: Philosophy, Principles & Practice.* Oxford: Blackwell Science.

Mills, D. L.

    1966 *Study of Chiropractors, Osteopaths, and Naturopaths in Canada.* Royal Commission on
        Health Services. Ottawa: Queen's Printer.

Miller, Katherine

    1998 The Evolution of Professional Identity: The Case of Osteopathic Medicine. *So-
        cial Science and Medicine* 47:1739–48.

New, Peter Kong-Ming

    1958 The Osteopathic Students: A Study in Dilemma. Pp. 413–421 in E. Gartley
        Jaco, ed. *Patients, Physicians, and Illness.* Glencoe, Ill.: Free Press.

Riley, James Nelson

    1980 Client Choices among Osteopaths and Ordinary Physicians in a Michigan Com-
        munity. *Social Science and Medicine* 14B:111-20.

Roth, Julius A.

    1976 *Health Purifiers and Their Enemies.* New York: Prodist.

Sharma, S., and P. Dressel
1975 Interim Report of an Exploratory Study of Michigan State University of Osteopathic Medicine Training Programs. East Lansing: Office of Institutional Research, Michigan State University.

Sharma, Ursula
1992 Complementary Medicine Today: Practitioners and Patients. New York: Routledge.

Still, Andrew T.
1908 Autobiography of Andrew T. Still, with a History of the Discovery and Development of the Science of Osteopathy. Kirksville, Mo.: Andrew T. Still.

Svoboda, Jill
2000 Come on, Take Your Medicine—Global. The DO (December):56–58.

Trowbridge, Carol
1991 Andrew Taylor Still, 1828–1917. Kirksville, Mo.: Thomas Jefferson State University Press.

University of Otago
2002 Musculoskeletal Medicine. Available at otago.ac.nz/subjects/msme.html (accessed April 19, 2002).

Unshuld, Paul L.
1980 The Issue of Structured Coexistence of Scientific and Alternative Medical Systems: A Comparsion of East and West German Legislation. Social Science and Medicine 143:15–42.

Wardwell, Walter I.
1992 Chiropractic: History and Evolution of a New Practice. St. Louis, Mo.: Mosby.

Webb Report
1977 Report of the Committee of Inquiry into Chiropractic, Osteopathy, Homeopathy and Naturopathy. Canberra: AGPS.

Vincent, Charles, and Adrian Furnham
1997 Complementary Medicine: A Research Perspective. Chichester, England: John Wiley & Sons.

Willis, Evan
1989 Complementary Healers. Pp. 259–79 in Gillian M. Lupton and Jake M. Najman, eds. Sociology of Health and Illness: Australian Readings. Melbourne, Australia: Macmillan.

Zollman, Catherine
1999 Users and Practitioners of Complementary Medicine. British Medical Journal 319 (7213): 836–83.

Achy-Breaky Art
The Historical Development and Contemporary Practice of Tuina

5

JENNIFER MINOR, MIRANDA WARBURTON, AND H. VINCENT BLACK

TRADITIONAL CHINESE MEDICINE (TCM) has experienced a surge in popularity in the United States in recent years. In this chapter, the authors examine the historical development of Chinese culture, TCM, and, more specifically, Tuina (Chinese manual therapy) to illustrate that: TCM is a complete and independent medical system shaped by complex cultural and social processes and environmental influences over several millennia, TCM functions as an intricate system of related modalities, and Tuina is an integral component of TCM and a successful mode of treatment. The goal of this exploration of TCM and Tuina is to further understand the structure and function of TCM, preserve the cultural elements of TCM education and practice, and contribute to the dialogue on TCM practice and research in the United States.

The Role of Culture in the Development of Medical Systems

Traditional Chinese Medicine is frequently equated with acupuncture. A glance at any of a number of TCM classics easily leads to this misapprehension; while these works focus on fundamental theory, acupuncture (*zhenjiu*) is often used as the primary application. Students and patients of Traditional Chinese Medicine quickly learn, however, that TCM is not based on one therapeutic mode. Rather, TCM is a complex system of treatment modalities designed to prevent or treat a myriad of illnesses. Chinese herbs (*zhongyao*), Chinese massage (*Tuina*), and acupuncture form the three pillars of TCM and comprise a holistic system of medicine. The three pillars are connected by shared theoretical and philosophical principles, so a TCM practitioner may use each component independently or in concert to boost treatment efficacy. Thus, TCM constitutes what Topley (1978:111) refers to as a system, or a set of phenomena connected to form a complex unit.

Leslie (1978:236) and Kleinman (1978:86) assert that all medical systems are by nature cultural systems, a concept valuable to the study of TCM. Conceptualizing TCM as a system allows social scientists to study its cultural and social roots, structure, and organization, which can provide a more developed understanding of the mechanisms of care and the level of potential for TCM to prevent or treat illness, including those illnesses currently deemed "untreatable" in other medical systems. Cultural beliefs about health, disease, and treatment guide the formation of an autonomous medical system. A social system of medicine evolves concomitantly and creates an intricate social structure of interrelated roles, such as practitioners and patients, medical establishments, and teaching institutions (Janzen 2002).

As is the case with many medical systems, the components of TCM developed at different stages in the evolution of Chinese society and culture; however, all three components developed within the same Chinese cultural milieu. Thus, Tuina can be best understood, appreciated, and practiced by professionals, students, and researchers alike, if one first understands the social and cultural environment in which Tuina arose.

A Historical Perspective of Traditional Chinese Medicine

The roots of Traditional Chinese Medicine extend back to the beginnings of Chinese civilization. Manipulation of bone and tissue is in many ways the most obvious precursor to both TCM and biomedicine. Since time immemorial, humans have suffered from fractures, bruises, sore muscles and joints, and torn ligaments, tendons, and muscles. The principles of Tuina developed early in tribal China, and until relatively recently Tuina practice was the medical domain of rural farmers, nomads, and poorer urban dwellers, people whose medical skills were handed down from generation to generation within family or clan lines. Unfortunately, Chinese archaeological remains and historical documents primarily provide insights into medical practices of Chinese elite rather than average citizens, who out of economic necessity relied on herbalists and bonesetters within their extended families. Using available archaeological and historical documents, we trace the development of TCM and its central theoretical constructs to delineate the role of Tuina within that historical and cultural development.

The ancestors of Chinese civilization are recognizable in Yang-shao period villages, which date as early as 5000 BC. During this time, the area known today as China was settled by numerous heterogeneous tribal groups of nomads and farmers (Wenke 1984). In the transition from the Yang-shao period to the succeeding

Lung-shan period (ca. 2300–1850 BC), the shift to larger and more settled villages with a concomitant greater reliance on agriculture represented significant changes in social structure (Wenke 1984:326–27). TCM scholars note that inhabitants of these early towns "suffered diseases and traumatic injuries in their fight against poisonous snakes or wild beasts, and in their labor and wars, so they kept exploring and searching for various ways of conquering nature and relieving the suffering of diseases" (Zhang 1996:1).

Perhaps the extreme suffering from disease and trauma during this period served as the catalyst that transformed early TCM from an integral part of life to a more conscious, externalized, and more formalized means of learning. The beginning of a written system allowed medical practitioners to summarize medical theory and practical experience, like massage and herbal poultices, into a form that could be passed on and further developed. Stone and bone needles recovered archaeologically from this time point to the early practice of acupuncture in the region as well (Zhang and Rose 1999:151).

Three legendary Emperor Gods, Fu Xi, Shen Nong, and Huang Di, are attributed with creating the essential elements of the subsequent florescence of Chinese civilization during the latter Yang-shao and early Lung-shan periods. Legend clearly predominates over fact in discussions of contributions by these Emperor Gods; nonetheless, they are significant in the development of Chinese civilization and influential in the development of TCM (Zhang and Rose 1999:149).

Fu Xi (ca. 2900 BC) is credited with greatly influencing social and economic life; some credit him with teaching his people the practices of hunting, fishing, and animal husbandry (Cleary 1986:3). Most importantly for TCM, Fu Xi is considered the creator of the signs of the *I Ching*, the eight trigrams (figure 5.1). Chinese medical practice is inextricably intertwined with Chinese philosophy, especially Daoism, a system wherein culture and nature are one and change is constant. The core of this philosophy is The Dao, or The Way, which is conceptualized as the powerful flow of the universe.

Shen Nong (ca. 2800 BC), the second Emperor God, is renowned for his role in the development of herbal medicines. Living in a time of natural calamities and disasters, which led to rampant disease, Shen Nong is said to have sampled hundreds of plants, examining their properties, tastes, and medicinal qualities to discover what was safe to eat and effective in treating illness. His research is considered the foundation of contemporary herbal medicine.

The legendary Huang Di (ca. 2700 BC) is considered the author of the oldest extant medical text, the *Huang Di Nei Jing*, also referred to as the *Yellow Emperor's Canon of Internal Medicine*. Of its two sections, the *Ling Shu* and the *Su Wen*, the latter is most firmly associated with Huang Di, and is considered to be derived from older, more foundational principles, such as the *I Ching*.

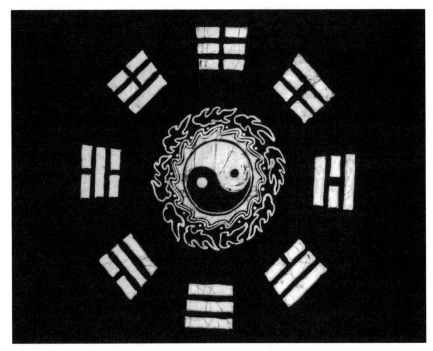

Figure 5.1.   Depiction of the Eight Trigrams of the *I Ching* attributed to Fu Xi. (Photo by David Stickles.)

The *Huang Di Nei Jing* is a significant work that provides insight into the historical development of Chinese cultural beliefs and TCM, and many TCM scholars and practitioners have studied the *Huang Di Nei Jing* in the years since its creation. Its primary appeal is that the text reflects the position of medicine as integral to philosophy and religion, and emphasizes human oneness with nature (Veith 1972:10). Additionally, the text covers basic theoretical underpinnings of TCM, including Yin and Yang and the Five Elements.

The first recorded discussion of anmo, the predecessor of Tuina, also appears in the *Yellow Emperor's Canon*. A section of the *Su Wen*, entitled *The Different Methods of Treatment and the Appropriate Prescriptions*, refers to medical treatment with "breathing exercises, massage of skin and flesh, and exercises of hands and feet" (Qi Gong and Tuina) (in Veith 1972:147–48). In another section of the *Yellow Emperor's Canon*, when Huang Di requests that his minister Qi Bo describe therapeutic bodywork and massage, The Divine Healer replied: "In the spring and summer, when food is plentiful and humans tend to become lazy and slothful, finger pressure is used to increase digestive fire and restore vigor" (Dubitsky in Sun 1993:xiii). This statement indicates the early development of the foundational principles of Tuina, specifically the use of massage within Five Element Theory. In keeping with the holistic ideology presented in *The Yellow Emperor's Canon*, a contemporary Tuina practitioner will often use the Five Element Theory in conjunction with the Yin-Yang Theory to diagnose and treat patients. Together these two theories form the foundation of Traditional Chinese Medical thought and practice (Maciocia 1989:15).

Yin-Yang Theory

The concepts of balance and the nature–culture relationship, as discussed in the *Huang Di Nei Jing*, are reflected in the dualistic principle of Yin and Yang. The Chinese characters for Yin and Yang refer to the "dark side of the hill" and the "sunny side of the hill" respectively, and these concepts lay the groundwork for classifying all phenomena in the natural world and the human body (Maciocia 1989:2; Veith 1972:13). Although the characters represent opposite phenomena, Yin and Yang refer to continuous and infinitely divisible phenomenological cycles in the universe, like day and night, that are opposite and yet complementary.

Because all phenomena in the universe are Yin or Yang in nature, a TCM physician can categorize every symptom, physiological function, existing pathogenic factors, and the patient's overall physical, mental, and emotional constitution into Yin or Yang categories and devise a treatment protocol to return the patient to a balanced state of health.

Five Element Theory

The *Yellow Emperor's Canon* also references five elements and provides an explanation of the relationships between humans, health, and the environment in relation to those elements, although it is not systematized and formally presented as a theoretical underpinning of TCM until the Song Dynasty (ca. AD 1000) (Zhang and Rose 1999:160).

The core principles of Five Element Theory are evident in its Chinese translation and in the principle correspondences between the elements and the organs of the body. In Mandarin, Five Elements Theory is referred to as *wu xing*, where *wu* is "five" and *xing* translates to "movement" or "conduct, behaviour" (Maciocia 1989:15). In medical application, the Five Elements Theory explains the self-regulating relationships of the internal organs, the energetic (Qi) connections between the organs, and the physiological relationships between the organs and the other parts of the human body. Each element corresponds with a set of paired organs, one Yin and one Yang organ (table 5.1), and all other phenomena in the universe—ranging from the symptoms of disease to links with the environment. Tuina practitioners use the correspondences in conjunction with other diagnostic

Table 5.1.   **Five Element Correspondences**

Element	Yin Organ	Yang Organ
Metal	lungs	large intestine
Water	kidneys	urinary bladder
Wood	liver	gall bladder
Fire	heart	small intestine
Earth	spleen	stomach

tools of TCM, such as Yin-Yang, to effectively diagnose and treat patients (Maciocia 1989:22).

Qi

The concept of Qi is central to the Chinese worldview as well as TCM, and it is clearly rooted in the philosophies of the *I Ching* and the *Huang Di Nei Jing*. Huai Nan Zi (c. 122 BC) delineates the central role of Qi in relation to the Dao and the development of Yin and Yang: "Dao originated from Emptiness and Emptiness produced the universe. The universe produced Qi. . . . That which was clear and light drifted up to become heaven [Yang], and that which was heavy and turbid solidified to form earth [Yin]" (in Maciocia 1989:36). Thus, Qi is the origin of all phenomena in the universe (nature) and the human body, a principle that led Chinese philosophers to understand Qi as the root of human existence and the basis of human health and disease.

Qi manifests in many forms and carries out many important functions, chief of which is that it circulates through a system of meridians and collaterals to support and stimulate the Blood and internal organs of the body to protect and maintain health (Cheng 1987:47; Maciocia 1989:36; Ni 1996:1). Blood has a different, more comprehensive sense in Chinese medicine than in Western medicine. Although it carries nutrients throughout the body, it is inseparable from Qi. "Qi infuses life into Blood; without Qi, Blood would be an inert fluid" (Maciocia 1989:48). Qi and Blood together form the material basis for the body's functional activities. When Qi is in balance and moving freely throughout the system, the body is healthy; when Qi becomes stagnant or deficient due to internal or external environmental factors, disease may occur. It is then the goal of a TCM practitioner to help the system return to a balanced state; this is similar to the principle of homeostasis in biomedicine. In this capacity, practitioners are especially successful in using Tuina techniques, herbs, and/or acupressure to influence the flow of Qi and restore balance.

The meridian and collateral system, *Jingluo*, functions as a network of vessels that carry materials, mainly Qi and Blood, from one location to another (figure 5.2). This intricately networked system of meridians allows TCM practitioners to

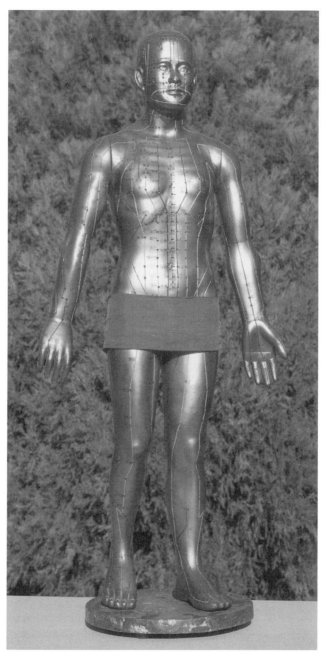

Figure 5.2.   Bronze figure depicting meridians on the human body, developed by Wang Wei Yi during the Song Dynasty. (Photo by David Stickles.)

affect deep, internal illness as well as superficial injuries without invasive techniques. To correct a disharmony, practitioners stimulate superficial acupoints using acupuncture (the insertion of needles into specific points along meridians) and/or Tuina techniques (bonesetting and massage along the meridians and at specific points) to increase or decrease the flow of Qi and Blood in different locations of the body (Deadman 1998:13).

Traditional Chinese Medicine and the Rise of Cultural Complexity

Lung-shan culture is replaced by Early Bronze Age China and the Shang Dynasty (1850 BC to 1112 BC); it is during this time that we see increased cultural complexity as well as the spread of traits that are the hallmarks of China, including widespread use of writing, architecture, art, and ideology (Wenke 1984:328). The shift in cultural complexity was profoundly influential in elite society, but for the average farmer or village dweller life during this period was not much different than it had been for thousands of years. Only the elite members of society possessed craft specialization or specialization of services, including medical practitioners and associated medical paraphernalia, such as bronze needles. It is likely, therefore, that there was a parallel development of elite and folk medical disciplines, which while united under the same philosophical precepts of the Dao and Yin and Yang, remained divided by social and economic status. Anmo and *Moshou*, or what we would today consider Tuina and bonesetting, likely continued to be practiced widely among nonelites to treat a variety of ailments during this time.

Traditional Chinese Medicine, Confucianism, and Daoism in Imperial China

Chinese civilization flourished from approximately 1027 BC to AD 220. The former sociopolitical structure of relatively autonomous warlords gave way to a structure with a king and noble elite at the apex and a base consisting of the nation's millions of peasants. More humanistic philosophy and religion began to permeate intellectual thought and manifested in an emphasis on studying and developing medical theories and techniques (Zhang and Rose 1999:151).

Confucius, one of the greatest influencers of Chinese civilization, was born in the state of Lu in 551 BC. His conservative vision called for the acceptance of social hierarchies and, consequently, social responsibility to those being ruled (Allen and Phillips 1999:15). The Taoist philosophy of the prophet Laozi (b. 604 BC) arose simultaneously and competed with Confucianism in influencing Chinese thought. In the *Dao Te Jing*, Laozi emphasized natural order and solitude, promoting the natural order of the Dao, Yin and Yang, and the Five Elements as the foundation of Chinese life and TCM. These concepts became the basis of Taoist philosophy and denoted a stark contrast with Confucianism.

During the Qin Dynasty (ca. AD 220) under Huang Di, the first emperor, the first text devoted to the practice of anmo, *Huang Di Qi Bo An Mo Jing Shi Juan*, was produced. Unfortunately, this volume was lost in a great fire, but the knowledge from this comprehensive, foundational work continues to be passed on from teachers to students through oral tradition (Xu 1994:6). Under imperial proclamation, many libraries were burned and many important medical texts lost during Huang Di's reign, leaving practitioners and students to once again rely solely on oral history and experience. In 1973, the Tombs of Ma Wang Dui, sealed since AD 168, were opened and copies of many historically and clinically significant texts were recovered. This is a pivotal event in TCM history; among the texts recovered were the *Yellow Emperor's Canon of Internal Medicine* (Zhang and Rose 1999:103) and the *Fifty-two Medical Formulas* and *Illustrated Health Exercises*, which illustrated and referenced particular anmo hand and bonesetting techniques.

One of the most famous of all Chinese doctors was Bian Que, who lived during Huang Di's reign. Bian Que was renowned as a great diagnostician, acupuncturist, and pediatrician. He is also credited with being the author of the *Nan Jing*, a text exemplifying the systematic approach to TCM promoted by Confucianist practitioners. Bian Que's research is notable because of his theoretical presentation of difficult pathological and physiological problems (Porkert 1990:247).

Hua Tuo (ca. AD 140–203), another early and famous practitioner, is noted for his contributions to the practice of anmo. He is credited with developing a system of calisthenics based on the movements of animals, strength training, and QI building movements that may be the precursor to Taiji and other Chinese Internal Martial Arts (Porkert 1990:25). He also established the method of *Gaomo*, which involves the use of herbal poultices and liniments to reduce fever and purge superficial pathogens, techniques that are still used as adjunct therapy in Tuina practice today (Xu 1994:7).

The Three Pillar System Arises in Traditional Chinese Medicine (AD 265–present)

Zhang and Rose (1999:156) characterize the period from AD 265 to 960 as "the full development of Chinese medicine." During the Tang Dynasty, Chinese culture prospered, providing an infrastructure for the development of science and learning that lead to the systematization of TCM (Zhang and Rose 1999:156). Sun Simo (AD 582–682), the last in a procession of great practitioners in the esoteric medical tradition, lived as a hermit sage in a remote mountain pass and spent his years working on a synthesis of all medical knowledge. This work, entitled *Qianjin Yaofang* or *Vital Prescriptions Worth a Thousand Gold Pieces*, includes information on all aspects of TCM, from therapeutic principles, to ethics, diagnosis, and even career recommendations (Porkert 1990:254–55; Zhang and Rose 1999:158; Zhang 1996:3).

By the Song Dynasty (AD 960–1279), the practice of all arts and sciences fell under the dominion of the state and its imperial bureaucracy. The Great Medical Authority *Taiyiju* sponsored a medical school and a university medical press, which carefully reviewed and edited the classics as well as more recent works. Although the initial effect of this institution was stimulating, its longest lasting effect was to create a rift between academic intellectual research on TCM and the practical application of medicine (Porkert 1990:256–57; Zhang and Rose 1999:158).

Essentially the greatest scholars of TCM were confined to this one institution and interacted only with one another, eventually leading to intellectual stagnation and the unfortunate result that "medicine became a branch of literature and bibliography rather than an applied science" (Porkert 1990:257). A by-product of this development was that individuals involved in the applied practice of medicine developed a folk medicine education that returned to a form of master–apprentice training, which was beyond official court control and thus perpetuated the rift between court and folk medicines (Zhang and Rose 1999:158).

Officials in the Institute of the Imperial Physician, the state medical school, established a Department of Anmo by the beginning of the Song Dynasty; an act that signified the official adoption of Anmo, Moshou, and Gaomo into the system of TCM and supported applied medical practice (Xu 1994:8). Tuina had achieved increased prominence, and numerous texts on the subject of traumatology and orthopedics were published reflecting "the precious and rich theories and experience of the Chinese working people accumulated in their long struggle against traumatic injuries and bone and joint disease" (Zhang 1996:6–7). It is at this point that the term "Tuina" enters the lexicon to denote manual therapy (Xu 1994:11).

By the mid-1800s, Western civilization, and especially biomedical and scientific methods, began to supplant TCM practice. In 1925, the National Government refused to include TCM in medical school curricula. The coup de grace, however, occurred in 1929 when the National Committee on Public Health resolved to abolish TCM (Zhang and Rose 1999:167).

Following the Communist takeover in 1949, Mao and his government supported reestablishment of TCM because the nationalists had taken such a strong stance against it, and it provided an inexpensive way to bring medical attention to the populace (Zhang and Rose 1999:167). Since the 1950s, TCM in China has witnessed a great resurgence with establishment of many universities and colleges of TCM. Many volumes specific to Tuina, including bonesetting, traumatology, massage, and Tuina hand techniques, have been published in the late twentieth century (Cheng 1987; Sun Chengnan 1993; Sun Shuchun 1989; Wu Xianlin 1997; Xu Xiangcai 1994, 2002; Zhang Zhigang 1996). And today, millions of Chinese still rely on the whole system of TCM for their primary health care needs.

Contemporary Practice of Tuina

The preceding historical discussion is intended to demonstrate that Traditional Chinese Medicine is a viable system of medicine shaped over millennia by cultural values. It is also intended to illustrate how Tuina and bonesetting developed into an integral part of the larger system of TCM and were often used in combination with acupuncture and herbs to treat disease. Contemporary practice of TCM should not be isolated from those foundational values. Yet today, particularly in the United States, we often see acupuncture, herbs, and Tuina used independently.

In the remainder of this chapter, we examine the contemporary practice of Tuina through a discussion of the structure and function of the Tuina system, diagnosis, a selection of more common techniques, education protocols, and a case study demonstrating the process and efficacy of Tuina. The intent is to illustrate that from a practical or clinical perspective, as well as a historical and cultural perspective, Tuina, like acupuncture and herbs, is an integral component of TCM and a successful mode of treatment. It is through principles shared with acupuncture and herbs, and by frequently combining techniques from the other pillars of TCM, that Tuina is able to restore physiological balance to the body and reduce physical pain.

Tuina Techniques

A technique is defined as the way in which a practitioner executes a standard technical maneuver on a joint, following a meridian, or on a specific area of the body for medical purposes (Xu 2002:57). As discussed earlier, ancient TCM philosophers and practitioners developed manual manipulation techniques through observation, scientific experimentation, and practical experience. They often retained the most efficacious techniques for their own practice, handing them down to descendants within their family or school lineage (Zhang 1996; Xu 1994).

Contemporary Tuina texts commonly classify techniques into one of two categories: soft-tissue or bonesetting manipulations (Mercati 1997; Sun 1989). The categories are broad and the techniques generally classified based on their standardized functions. Consistent with the I-Ching principle of constant change, however, the specific function of a manipulation will change each time the practitioner applies it. The practitioner's intention, force, angle, and the area of application are adjusted with each application to account for the factors impacting the treatment.

In part, the practitioner ascertains the many factors that determine a treatment protocol and the specifics of each technique at the beginning of a treatment through an extensive interview and diagnostic process known as differential diagnosis. In this phase of the treatment, the TCM practitioner observes face color and pallor, demeanor, posture, and the body to detect physical and energetic restrictions and gauge the level and balance of Qi, Blood, and Spirit, or "Shen." For example, a patient with black under the eyes, pain in the knees and low back, edema in the legs, and no vitality in the face could be diagnosed with deficient Kidney Qi and treated with a series of Tuina techniques, and perhaps an herb poultice, to increase the Qi and Blood of the Kidney. This is not to say that the physical organ of the kidney is damaged; rather, this is an indication that the energetic level of the Qi, Blood, Shen, and/or Water Element is out of balance and may need regulating. A few of the additional diagnostic techniques that the practitioner will employ to hone in on a diagnosis are palpating the pulse and injured areas of the body; observing the color, body, and coat of the tongue; listening to the quality of the voice and the breath; and inquiring about the patient's symptoms, bodily functions, feelings, emotions, and even the patient's family, community, and home environment. The differential and contextual diagnostic process allows the practitioner to tailor the protocol to the individual's specific condition. With this information, the practitioner may also modify the standardized Tuina techniques, tailoring them to the specific energetic imbalance and physiological restriction(s), possibly even using a combination of manipulations simultaneously to treat energetic and structural imbalances that induce physical pain.

Structurally, Tuina techniques release restrictions in joints and soft tissues to promote Qi and Blood flow, which will result in the reduction of pain. Energetically, Tuina manipulations (1) restore balance to Blood and Qi (Yin and Yang Theory), (2) harmonize the Qi of the viscera (Five Elements Theory), (3) promote and regulate the flow of Qi in the meridians (Meridian Theory), and (4) release external pernicious influences (Mercati 1997; Xu 2002). In accordance with the *I Ching*, *The Dao*, and the *Huang Di Nei Jing* as discussed earlier, the effects of Tuina manipulations on the body clearly reflect the underpinnings of the cultural beliefs of holism, balance, and the connection to the natural environment that guided the development of the medical system, its diagnostic and treatment procedures, and even how students learn the system.

Whether a practitioner wants to learn Tuina first or the combination of Tuina, acupuncture, and herbs simultaneously, the training is the same—everyone must learn foundational TCM theory, pathology, and diagnosis. Historically, students learned Tuina through apprenticeship training. As time progressed, the continually changing political forces and competing schools of thought dictated changes in levels of formalization and standardization of TCM teaching and practice (Unschuld 1985). In present-day China and the United States, TCM education and practice is highly formalized.

In the United States, TCM schools and clinics are segregated from the hegemonic biomedical community of medical schools, hospitals, and clinics. This trend is changing as the public demand for TCM continues to increase and biomedical researchers and practitioners focus more of their research efforts on TCM efficacy and safety (Eisenberg et al. 1998; World Health Organization 2002).

Conversely, in modern China the intrinsic understanding of TCM theory and practice, combined with several millennia of efficacy research, laid the groundwork for a more collaborative environment. While some biomedical and TCM schools share research facilities and classes, the vast majority of TCM schools are still segregated from biomedical schools (Dr. Gong Shuhua, personal communication, April 16, 2001). Nevertheless, in China's larger cities citizens may choose to visit the acupuncture, Tuina, and herb clinics or the biomedical doctor for medical services. During several trips to Beijing, the authors observed the collaborative nature of the biomedicine–TCM relationship firsthand in numerous area hospitals. Chinese biomedical doctors commonly refer walk-in patients to TCM clinics and frequently prescribe repeated TCM treatments for hospital inpatients. TCM practitioners reciprocate, referring patients to biomedical doctors if the patient's condition would be better served by biomedical treatment or a combination of treatment modalities. TCM practitioners in biomedical hospitals may also prescribe diagnostic tests, such as x-rays, and they are trained to read and interpret the results.

Despite differing degrees of acceptance and collaboration between TCM and biomedicine practitioners in China and the United States, a TCM practitioner's education in either country is rigorous and extensive. TCM schools educate practitioners using a complex arrangement of didactic, clinical, and mentored education. Tuina students take courses and acquire clinical experience in TCM observation, diagnosis, and pathogenesis, as well as biomedical anatomy, physiology, pathology, and diagnosis (Xu 1994).

In spite of the technological age in which we live, much of the study and practice of TCM retains its traditional philosophical orientation. A student of Tuina devotes untold hours of study to the classic theoretical texts of diagnostics, therapeutics, orthopedics, and traumatology, some written over a millennium ago. The practice of Tuina is mentally and physically demanding for the student and practitioner. Therefore, students must cultivate strength and endurance and develop a comprehensive familiarity with the physical, mental, and emotional body in order to properly perform the techniques for the duration of the treatment (Xu 2002). Students build these skills through a variety of means; however, a more traditional education stresses the importance of training in Chinese internal martial arts in conjunction with training in TCM.

Chinese Internal Martial Arts include Taiji Chuan, Xingyi Chuan, Bagua Zhang, and numerous other styles of Qi Gong. Li Zi Ming (1993:xii), Master of Liang Zhen Pu Bagua Zhang and the teacher of one the authors of this chapter (Black), once said that practicing martial arts "can develop the practitioner's physical health to restore essence, tonify the brain, dispel illness, prolong life, and maintain optimum vitality." The martial arts also provide the practitioner with a greater sensitivity to detect and move Qi, and a deeper knowledge of the anatomic structure and physiologic functioning of the human body. Thus, studying Chinese internal martial arts furnishes the physical, mental, and emotional strength and stability necessary for Tuina practitioners to build and maintain their own health and effectively heal patients. To illustrate the physical demands placed on the practitioner and the patient, and demonstrate the efficacy of Tuina, we next introduce three commonly used techniques, *Gun Fa*, *Na Fa*, and *Ban Fa*, and provide a case study that uses all three.

Gun Fa (rolling). Gun Fa is a technique used extensively as a preventative measure and to treat a wide range of conditions. The most common instrument used to perform Gun Fa is the dorsal (back) surface of the hand, from the medial edge of the fifth metacarpal to the lateral edge of the first metacarpal; although, it can also be performed using the belly of the thumb, the dorsal surface of all four fingers, and the forearm, depending on the location where the practitioner applies the technique. For most situations, the practitioner rolls the back of his hand across the affected area at a pace of 140 to 160 times per minute with deep, even, constant, and smooth strokes, taking care to avoid sliding across the body surface and working to maintain a proper body posture, ensuring proper depth of force, speed, and angle of application (Mercati 1997:64; Xu 2002:67). The movement is challenging and, at first, quite exhausting; however, when performed by experienced practitioners, the technique often feels smooth and round—so much so that patients often equate it with the feel of a rolling pin or ball rolling across the treated area.

The appeal of Gun Fa lies in its safety and applicability to large areas of the body, with the exception of the craniofacial, anterior-cervical, and thoracico-abdominal regions (Xu 2002:67). Practitioners use Gun Fa to relax the muscles, tendons, ligaments, and vessels; lubricate the joints; warm and activate the meridians; encourage Blood circulation; and relieve spasms and stop pain. From a TCM perspective, practitioners use Gun Fa when the external pernicious influences (EPIs) of wind, damp, and/or cold invade the body and cause energetic imbalance and deleterious structural changes. In biomedical terms, this manipulation is effective in treating disorders of the motor and nervous systems (Xu 2002:68).

At the beginning of a treatment, it is not uncommon for a practitioner to perform Gun Fa along the patient's back, legs, the sides of the body, and portions of the front of the body. On the physical level, this achieves all of the expected therapeutic functions and generally relaxes the patient. On the social level, this introduces a break from the patient's everyday life, sets up a quiet and relaxed environment for the treatment, and allows the patient and practitioner time to interact before the practitioner digs into her work, sometimes literally!

Na Fa (grasping). Unlike Gun Fa, Na Fa does not have the added effect of immediately relaxing the patient; in fact, it can actually be somewhat uncomfortable. It is a powerful stimulus that practitioners apply to the tight, cordlike soft tissue in the neck, shoulders, back, and limbs to release the exterior (body surface) by encouraging perspiration and expel the EPIs of wind and cold from the body. Much like Gun Fa, it relaxes the muscles and tendons, promotes Blood circulation, and relieves muscle spasms and pain (Mercati 1997:56; Xu 2002:60). In extreme cases, practitioners may also use Na Fa to resuscitate a patient.

To determine whether Na Fa is the appropriate manipulation to use, the practitioner first observes the patient to sense the flow (or stagnation) of Qi, and palpates to locate the muscle(s) where the energy is most excessive or most deficient, which may also be the area of greatest pain. To perform Na Fa, the practitioner places his thumb and fingers on opposite sides of the muscle and then squeezes the proximal surface of the fingers and thumb together to create a slight lift in the tissues. Once the practitioner has a secure hold on the muscle, she applies force to further lift the tissue, keeping the force symmetrical and perpendicular to the body surface until the muscles relax and the Qi is again flowing smoothly (Xu 2002:60). To minimize the level of discomfort and still achieve the maximum therapeutic result, the practitioner must introduce the technique with slow, light movements and repeat it numerous times, increasing the strength of the squeeze with each application.

Ban Fa (pulling). Practitioners use Ban Fa in many forms and throughout the entire body. Basically, it is used to pull a joint in two opposite directions in order to remove energetic and physical restrictions and to restore the flow of Qi along the meridians. To apply this technique effectively, safely, and without effort requires extensive understanding of human anatomy and the angles, direction of motion, range of motion, and the axis of each joint (Xu 2002:79). This technique serves different purposes, depending on the strength of its execution. Implementing this technique lightly allows practitioners to gently draw energy along the meridians in the affected area while stretching the joint. Diligent practice of Ban Fa with light force cultivates the skill and power to set the joints and correct joint malalignments, dislocations, and bone breaks. Less experienced physicians often practice Ban Fa gently for many years to build up their practical understanding of the joints and correct posture and position for the patient and physician, which in turn creates the foundation for performing actual joint manipulations safely and effectively.

Ban Fa can be used throughout the entire body. In its more gentle form, practitioners frequently use it on the fingers or toes at the end of a treatment involving any of the limbs, or in any situation where the practitioner intends to move stagnant energy from the center of the body out to the ends of the limbs. Following Xu (2002:89) and Sun (1993:67), to perform Ban Fa on the fingers, the practitioner grasps the patient's finger firmly between her first and second phalanges and takes the patient's wrist with the other hand. The practitioner stabilizes the wrist, tractions back slightly, and applies pressure to retain the grip, starting at the proximal end of the patient's finger. The practitioner then pulls distally and with a slight upward lift to traction the joint in a direction that follows the curve of the finger. Overall, this technique, whether performed gently or with more force, spreads or separates the tendons and removes physical restrictions, lubricates the soft tissue and joints, increases Blood circulation, increases the flow of Qi, dredges the meridians, sets the bones, and relieves pain (Sun 1993:68).

A Case Study in Tuina—Beijing, China

In April 2001, one of the authors (Minor) spent ten days at the China, Beijing International Acupuncture Training Center to augment her apprenticeship training in TCM in the United States. Minor participated as a student at the Center. She spent each morning working in a clinic that focused on either Tuina or acupuncture, and each afternoon attending lectures on Tuina, acupuncture, and herbs. For the first five days, Minor observed and performed clinical work in a Tuina clinic. Minor worked closely with lead TCM doctors in the clinic and recorded extensive participant observation notes on breaks, in the evenings, and during clinic practice whenever possible.

The coalescence of biomedicine and TCM in the hospitals of Beijing proved an interesting phenomenon guided by what the authors observed as an unequal reciprocity. The Chinese biomedical establishment instituted specialization among TCM practitioners and confined the practitioners and TCM clinics to a supporting role in patient care. TCM practitioners alleviated some pressures from the biomedical practitioners in regard to the mass of outpatients visiting the hospital on a daily basis.

TCM practitioner specialization was created along perceived margins between the three pillars of TCM (Tuina, herbs, and acupuncture) by dividing the three into entirely separate clinics within the hospital setting and by limiting the physicians' medical practices to their assigned modalities (Dr. Fan, personal communication, April 12, 2001). The supporting role of TCM practitioners and the responsibility of the TCM practitioners to treat large numbers of patients are indicated in the standard hospital procedures. Patients are commonly seen by a biomedical doctor for their initial visits and are then referred to an in-house TCM physician once any acute symptoms are alleviated, or if the visit is for a chronic condition that TCM may treat more effectively.

Two of the authors (Minor and Warburton) have visited and/or assisted in hospitals and TCM clinics in Beijing in recent years; Black accumulated several years of Chinese Medical practice in hospitals and clinics in Beijing, Shanghai, and Taiwan in the 1970s and 1990s. During the authors' visits to the hospitals, it was common to see anywhere from two to twenty patients waiting for treatment in the various TCM clinics. Many of the patients in both the Tuina and acupuncture clinics suffered from facial paralysis, frozen shoulders, stiff necks, or stroke—all syndromes that may be induced by the invasion of the external pernicious influence of wind.

In the Tuina clinic at the Center, Minor and several other students worked with two TCM physicians, Dr. Fan and Dr. Feng. Fan, as the lead practitioner, diagnosed patients, dictated treatment protocols, and supervised the apprentices. Early on the morning of the second day, a patient, obviously in extreme pain, entered the clinic. Fan quickly assessed her condition as she walked across the room, observing how she moved and what did not move freely when she walked, how she sat down in the chair, how she spoke, and the color and pallor of her skin. Fan followed up his observations with additional standard TCM diagnostic techniques, including palpating her pulses and observing the appearance of her tongue. Fan then directed Minor to start with Gun Fa (rolling) on her left shoulder. Fan and Minor worked simultaneously on the patient's arms as he questioned her about her injury, which turned out to be a severe stiff neck and frozen shoulder that developed the evening before, after many hours riding her bike in the wind.

Fan and Minor used the Gun Fa technique along her shoulders and up and down both arms until the skin started to turn red and she started to relax. Fan followed this with several minutes of Na Fa (grasping) on the patient's neck and then her shoulders, focusing on the meridians with the most stagnant Qi—in this case, the Gall Bladder and San Jiao meridians. Like most experienced TCM practitioners, Fan was able to detect the areas with the greatest Qi stagnation and Qi deficiency through observation, palpation, and clinical experience. TCM practitioners hone the ability to detect Qi flow through continued clinical practice, where they gain skill with each patient that they treat, and through martial arts/Qi Gong training, where they cultivate the ability to feel and control the flow of Qi in their own bodies. The pain in the patient's neck was so extreme, and the muscles in such spasm, that Fan began with very gentle manipulation, followed by more work on the shoulders by both practitioners. Within minutes her shoulders relaxed and Fan and Minor applied the technique more firmly along the shoulders, while Fan still gently worked her neck. As the muscles in the patient's neck finally began to relax, the stagnant Qi and Blood began to be released. In keeping with the fundamental principle to restore the natural flow of Qi to the body, the practitioners continued with Na Fa, moving slowly down the patient's arms and periodically returning to the neck and shoulders to work out any remaining stagnation.

The treatment continued with Fan and Minor performing Na Fa along the major muscles of her arms, particularly in the areas where the meridians run from the posterior portion of the neck and superior portion of the shoulders, through the lateral and posterior portions of the arms and to the fingertips. Within twenty minutes the patient was relaxed and sleeping despite continued Na Fa manipulations along her arms. When Fan and Minor reached the wrists with the Na Fa technique, they rotated the wrist and finger joints through their ranges of motion, using a technique called *Yao Fa* (rotating). Rotating the wrists and fingers further released the joints and opened the flow of Blood and Qi all of the way to the fingers. To completely remove the Qi and Blood stagnation that was drawn out of the patient's neck and shoulders and down her arms, Fan and Minor finished the treatment with Ban Fa on her fingers—this also served to gently wake the patient. Fan then directed the patient through a series of range-of-motion tests for her neck and arms. The patient was able to move her head and shoulders through the full ranges of motion and reported no pain in her neck, upper back, or arms. Her pallor and color were now bright and normal and her demeanor more energetic.

Not every patient and every syndrome can be cured in one session and not everything can be cured with Tuina alone, hence the need for the three pillars of TCM. This treatment, however, is an example of Tuina as a simple, effective, expedient, and noninvasive method of treatment.

Conclusion

This case study reflects the fundamental concepts of Tuina and elucidates its unique design and capacity for quickly and effectively treating common ailments. Tuina is an art as well as a treatment modality, and the demands it makes on its students shape them into effective practitioners with practical skills to address a multiplicity of chronic and acute conditions.

Learning and practicing Tuina requires diligence and focus; knowledge of human anatomy, biomechanics, physiology, thought, and emotion; awareness and sensitivity to one's physical surroundings and circumstances; knowledge of more esoteric concepts like Qi and Yin-Yang; and physical strength. Sustaining the diligence and focus necessary to successfully learn and practice Tuina requires a profound understanding of the role of Tuina in the larger system and practice of

TCM and a comprehensive knowledge of Chinese cultural development, particularly related to scientific thought and medical practice.

TCM cannot be effectively understood apart from its cultural history—an interplay of political, economic, religious, and social forces that has molded it into its present form. This is becoming more of an issue as societies worldwide become increasingly interested in and receptive to the practice of TCM. Possible reasons for this increased interest in TCM include: a comprehensive, holistic nature; the ability to treat chronic and acute conditions effectively, inexpensively, and noninvasively; the physician–patient relationship; the reassuring hands-on techniques to treat the patient, which allows the practitioner to connect with the patient on a personal and physical level; and, the emphasis on preventive medicine, which can bring about fundamental constitutional changes resulting in increased Qi and balanced Yin and Yang for a healthier life.

TCM can be effectively employed in other cultural contexts, provided that its practitioners recognize that it is a complete, complex, and independent medical system that holds the potential to cure diseases and heal patients differently from biomedicine or in situations where biomedicine cannot. To explore these differences and build a true collaboration, it is imperative to approach TCM learning and practice not from the mechanistic perspective of the hegemonic biomedical system, but from the holistic perspective inherent to the history and culture to which the medical tradition was born. Hence, the purpose of this exploration into the historical and practical aspects of TCM was to further understand the synergistic forces connecting the structure and function of TCM, preserve the practice of TCM as it continues to spread across national borders, and contribute to the dialogue on creating more appropriate and effective means of practice and research of TCM in the United States.

Note

Jennifer Minor wishes to thank her family for their support in this ever changing journey; Miranda Warburton, Gail Derin-Kellogg, and Vince and Kim Black for their guidance, encouragement, and generosity; and all of the teachers before them who have contributed to the collective knowledge and traditions of Chinese Medicine and martial arts. Miranda Warburton would like to thank her mother, Margarett Vernon, for introducing her to alternative medicine when Miranda was very young. She also wishes to acknowledge David Nicoletti, the late Kris Greening, and especially Gail Derin-Kellogg for presenting the fundamentals of Traditional Chinese Medicine in such a way that its beauty, complexity, and practicality were enticing, and above all, Kim and Vince Black, whose unconditional support and vast stores of knowledge and experience have been an inspiration and life-changing force. Vince Black wishes to thank Hsu Hong Chi, Mah Gong Wong, Liao Wu Chang, Jiang Jia Bao, and all the others for their knowledge, guidance, and compassion.

References

Allen, Tony, and Charles Phillips
   1999   *Land of the Dragon: Chinese Myth.* London: Duncan Baird Publishers.
Cheng Xinnong
   1987   *Chinese Acupuncture and Moxibustion.* Beijing: Foreign Languages Press.
Cleary, Thomas, trans.
   1986   *The Taoist I Ching.* Boston: Shambhala.
Deadman, Paul, and Mazin Al-Khafaji with Kevin Baker
   1998   *Manual of Acupuncture.* Sussex: Journal of Chinese Medicine Publications.
Eisenberg, David M., R. B. Davis, S. L. Ettner, S. Appel, S. Wilkey, M. Van Rompay, and
   R. C. Kessler
   1998   Trends in Alternative Medicine Use in the United States, 1990–1997: Re-
      sults of a Follow-up National Survey. *Journal of the American Medical Association*
      280(18):1569–75.
Janzen, John
   2002   *Social Fabric of Health.* Boston: University of Kansas Press.
Kleinman, Arthur
   1978   Concepts and a Model for the Comparison of Medical Systems as Cultural Sys-
      tems. *Social Science and Medicine.* 12:85–93.
Leslie, Charles
   1978   Pluralism and Integration in the Indian and Chinese Medical Systems.
      Pp. 111–41 in A. Kleinman, P. Kunstadter, E. R. Alexander, and J. L. Gate, eds.
      Culture and Healing in Asian Societies: Anthropological, Psychiatric, and Public Health Studies.
      Cambridge, Mass.: Schenkman Publishing Company.
Li Zi Ming
   1993   *Liang Zhen Pu Eight Diagram Palm.* H. Vincent Black ed., Huang Guo Qi, trans. Pa-
      cific Grove, Calif.: High View Publications.
Maciocia, Giovanni
   1989   *The Foundations of Chinese Medicine: A Comprehensive Text for Acupuncturists and Herbalists.*
      New York: Churchill Livingstone.
Mercati, Maria
   1997   *Handbook of Chinese Massage: Tui Na Techniques to Awaken Body and Mind.* Vermont: Heal-
      ing Arts Press.
Ni, Yitian, with Richard L. Rosenbaum
   1996   *Navigating the Channels of Traditional Chinese Medicine.* San Diego, Calif.: Oriental Med-
      icine Center.
Porkert, Manfred
   1990   [1982] *Chinese Medicine as a Scientific System: Its History, Philosophy, and Practice, and How
      It Fits with the Medicine of the West.* New York: Henry Holt and Company.
Sun Chengnan, ed.
   1993   *Chinese Bodywork: A Complete Manual of Chinese Therapeutic Massage.* Berkeley, Calif.: Pa-
      cific View Press.

Sun Shuchun, ed.

1989   *Atlas of Therapeutic Motion for Treatment and Health: A Guide to Traditional Chinese Massage and Exercise Therapy.* Beijing: Foreign Language Press.

Topley, Marjorie

1978   Chinese and Western Medicine in Hong Kong: Some Social and Cultural Determinants of Variation, Interaction, and Change. Pp. 111–41 in A. Kleinman, P. Kunstadter, E. R. Alexander, and J. L. Gate, eds. *Culture and Healing in Asian Societies: Anthropological, Psychiatric, and Public Health Studies.* Cambridge, Mass. Schenkman Publishing Company.

Unschuld, Paul U.

1985   *Medicine in China: A History of Ideas.* Berkeley: University of California Press.

1998   *Chinese Medicine.* Brookline, Mass.: Paradigm Publications.

Veith, Ilza, trans.

1972   [1949]   *Yellow Emperor's Classic of Internal Medicine.* Berkeley: University of California Press.

Wenke, Robert J.

1984   *Patterns in Prehistory: Humankind's First Three Million Years.* 2nd edition. New York: Oxford University Press.

World Health Organization

2002   Traditional Medicine: Growing Needs and Potential. WHO Policy Perspectives on Medicines, May 2:1–6.

Wu Xianlin, ed.

1997   *Sun Zi's Art of War and Health Care: Military Science and Medical Science.* Beijing: New World Press.

Xu Xiangcai, ed.

1994   *The English-Chinese Encyclopedia of Practical Traditional Chinese Medicine.* Beijing: Higher Education Press.

Xu Xiangcai

2002   *Chinese Tui Na Massage: The Essential Guide to Treating Injuries, Improving Health, and Balancing Qi.* Boston, Mass.: YMAA Publication Center.

Zhang Yu Huan, and Ken Rose

1999   *Who Can Ride the Dragon? An Exploration of the Cultural Roots of Traditional Chinese Medicine.* Brookline, Mass.: Paradigm Publications.

Zhang Zhigang

1996   *Bone-Setting Skills in Traditional Chinese Medicine.* Beijing: Shangdong Science and Technology Press.

EXPERIENCE AND EMBODIMENT IN PRACTITIONER–PATIENT ENCOUNTERS

II

IN THIS PART OF THE BOOK, we shift from the broad historical sweep of bone-setting practice to a close scrutiny of actual clinical interactions between healer and client, with some intriguing permutations of this dyadic relationship. These accounts include those of two practitioners from distinct cultural backgrounds and training negotiating the same client (O'Malley), and two healer-clients assessing the same healer by submitting their own bodies to therapeutic participant observation (Anderson and Klein). In two cases, supernatural elements enter into healing (sacred divinatory objects in Guatemala, magic and shrine offerings in Bali), while in the other two the practice is strictly naturalistic (Filipino bonesetting and Rolfing). Curiously, two chapters view the manipulative skills of musculoskeletal healers of all types as similar and competent (O'Malley and Jacobson), while in another coauthors disagree over the competence of one specific healer (Anderson and Klein).

All chapters foreground the phenomenological aspects of manipulating with, and being manipulated by, human hands in a "somatic mode of attention" (Csordas 1994), which allows bodies to attend other suffering bodies on a nonconscious level (Hinojosa). O'Malley's and Jacobson's theoretically informed ethnographic clinical accounts take us deep into this realm. Somehow, the healers' hands "know how," which stands in relationship to but is not the same as "know that," or theoretical knowledge (O'Malley). "Know how" derives from an embodied experience of action within the context of specific knowledge.

If we pay closer attention to the actual practice and experience of bodywork, we might better appreciate "the body's role as an agent in healing, as well as its role as an instrument of healing," as suggests Hinojosa. Notable across the contributions is the acquisition by bonesetters, whether through apprenticeship, formal training, observation, divine inspiration, years of hands-on experience, or some combination of the above, of an embodied hand-based knowledge. These skilled musculoskeletal therapists seem to simply follow their body's lead as they search out and correct adhesions, blocked *uat* or *ugat*, spasms, and breaks. As the touch-mediated knowledge is preconscious, healers have only partial success articulating what they are doing and how, signaled by their preference for demonstrating their procedures to the learner rather than talking about them.

Each author endeavors to demonstrate the inseparable link between a people's cultural beliefs and values and the agreed-upon ethnopathophysiological explanation for the origin of a musculoskeletal problem and the proper way to relieve it. Following Heidegger, O'Malley contends that one's "way-of-being-in-the-world" affects touch-perception and is a prerequisite to understanding a healing art.

In chapter 6, Servando Z. Hinojosa informs us that the experience of Maya bonesetters with biomedical physicians has been fraught with tension, with most doctors refusing to acknowledge the skill of bonesetters and some discrediting bonesetting as a rogue activity. Yet, while still placing primacy on the hands in diagnosis and healing, bonesetters in Guatemala have managed to incorporate into their practice some accoutrements of biomedicine, such as pharmaceuticals and x-rays, in ways that enhance rather than threaten their authority on musculoskeletal matters. They find x-rays primarily useful as a confirmatory rather than diagnostic tool; by itself, the appearance of being conversant with the technology further legitimates their healing role by reassuring a clientele that has come to have a degree of faith in and respect for biomedicine.

The bonesetter's clinical protocol consists of first relaxing the patient, especially given that with broken bones one can anticipate the treatment to be less than pleasant. Next, the healer carries out a medical history and physical exam, and finally treatment is given using skin lubricants while palpating, massaging, mobilizing, prodding, and pulling. Their practice is an "eminently manual craft, one underwritten by the hands' ability to probe and access bodily information." Finally, the set joint or bone is immobilized with a removable cast. Analgesics, anti-inflammatory drugs, and topical ointments may be prescribed as well.

How practitioners of two radically different traditions acquire and embody manipulative skills is the subject of John O'Malley's work (chapter 7). The end result is that while their etiological rationales for treatment are dissonant—the Filipino bonesetter (*hilot*) is certain that blood flow blocked by *lamig* (cold substance) is the problem, whereas chiropractors see the world in terms of aberrant joint movement and spasming muscles—they operate in a nearly identical fashion in terms of manual techniques. "The key element they have in common is skill, and skill is the corollary of experience" contends O'Malley.

In sharp relief from the interdisciplinary conflict seen in other chapters, O'Malley, a chiropractor, spent over a year collaborating with indigenous *hilots*. O'Malley poses the provocative notion that the scientific explanation for why Western musculoskeletal healers proceed as they do is really epiphenomenal to the experiential knowledge gained by long-term work with ailing bodies. The body is the teacher. Nonetheless, he finds that for both traditions, clinical models do serve a purpose: They provide a starting point for action, and ultimately influence the embodiment of technical skill by orienting the placement of hands, the direction of massage, the thrust vector and timing, the area of contact, and so on. Going even further, O'Malley suggests that the empirical results are largely the same across all manual medicine traditions, despite a thematic knowledge that reflects local concepts of etiology and, by its partial nature, distorts manipulative practice to some extent.

One of the essential requirements of the social scientific endeavor is the replication of research findings, without which the accumulation of knowledge is hampered. Yet rarely in anthropology do two researchers study the same locale, much less the same issue with the same informant. In chapter 8, Robert Anderson and Norman Klein, both dually trained in anthropology and chiropractic, report radically different experiences in their self-reflexive encounters with the same Bali bonesetter (*balian*). Their friendship and scholarly maturity allowed them to critically examine their starkly contrasting conclusions and offer possible explanations.

On the one hand, Klein depicted two healing encounters that he witnessed, as well as the therapy he received personally, as successful. He highlighted the sacred elements of *balian* practice, and contended that they survive in competition with many other health care specialists—traditional, modern, and alternative—because of their attention to the spiritual dimension of illness. On the other hand, Anderson focused on the secular and structural aspects of *balian* practice, contending that treatment is almost entirely naturalistic, not supernatural. He was unsatisfied with the treatment received and had to conclude that the three *balian*s he studied were not competent, caused gratuitous pain, and might indeed potentially do harm. That they took no medical history nor did any physical exam he found alarming. In exploring their difference of opinion, Anderson and Klein came to realize that the *balians*' presentation of self was a response to what they perceived as the expectations of each researcher. Klein, more of a cultural relativist, accepted Balinese culture on its own terms without question, whereas Anderson, as a cultural critic, sought to evaluate *balians* based on Western standards of medical evidence. These two authors together have pushed the boundaries of discovery beyond that which one of them acting in isolation could ever pretend to achieve.

In chapter 9, "Getting Rolfed," Eric Jacobson weds his years of practical healing experience with his honed skill in observational research to arrive at a truly unique vantage point from which to gain insight into the genesis of much of the seemingly idiopathic musculoskeletal disorder distinctive of North Americans. Myofascia, the connective tissue that wraps all muscles, are, as Ida Rolf contended, the "organs of structure." Jacobson demonstrates how the body is made rigid by injury and strain as well as by past episodes of bodily discipline regarding comportment. The imbalances created make the body compete against rather than be enabled by gravity. Not only do deep-tissue Rolfing techniques restore relaxation, flexibility, and grace of movement by biomechanically releasing the myofascial adhesions that hold bodies in unhealthful poses, they can also release buried affect, induce personal maturity, and restore confidence in the self. As a Rolfer, Jacobson is keen to discern the visible, embodied traces of disciplinary tactics about which local culture is silent—that is, gender-proscribed movements ("Stand up like a man!"), or more consequentially, physical and sexual abuse, tactics that impact the posture and movement of people of every class, ethnicity, and age. Posture is "a continuous, dynamic aspect of all behavior" and Jacobson's goal as a healer is not the unattainable one "of fully delivering each client to [Rolfing] ideals, but rather of progressively approximating them." He notes that Rolfing's recognition of the intimate relationship between biomechanics, the self, and social relations is a trait shared across many other forms of structural bodywork.

Hinojosa predicts that the future of manual medicine, and the direction of its changes, will hinge on the dialogue between the distinct and self-validating domains of the various healers with differential access to power. These chapters document the collaboration between differently situated healers or researchers, from traditional bonesetters and physicians in Guatemala to a chiropractor and his *hilot* instructor-informant in the Philippines. This new direction in medical anthropological research provides a model to be emulated.

Reference
Csordas, Thomas, ed.
   1994 *Embodiment and Experience: The Existential Ground of Culture and Self*. Cambridge, England: Cambridge University Press.

The Hands, the Sacred, and the Context of Change in Maya Bonesetting

6

SERVANDO Z. HINOJOSA

ALTHOUGH AN EMPIRICAL FIELD, Maya bonesetting takes shape in different ways in the hands of different practitioners. In this chapter, I discuss how Maya bonesetters of two highland Guatemala towns, San Juan Comalapa and San Pedro la Laguna, experience their work, perform their work, and respond to a changing technological and professional environment. To do this, I first situate manual medicine in historical and regional perspective, paying particular attention to the Maya area of Middle America. Then, turning to the communities, I underline how different vocational tendencies are found in Maya bonesetting today. These tendencies are each predicated on a hand-based knowledge that makes bonesetting possible.

The chapter next reviews the contemporary environment of Maya bonesetting. A major aspect of this environment is the availability of resources such as pharmaceuticals and x-rays. Although fairly recent arrivals in the countryside, these products are making significant inroads into popular healing, not only supplementing time-honored methods of bonesetting, but likely adding a legitimating force to them. Following this discussion, I offer a critical look at how bonesetters and physicians relate to each other. Presenting the points of view of bonesetters and physicians, I highlight how each class of practitioner actively defines the other and the limits of the other's work. Barriers to cooperation become apparent in this situation, but a limited dialogue continues between popular and institutional healing specialists.

Bonesetting takes place in a context of tradition, changing resources, and professional tension. It continues in Guatemala because bonesetters are adapting to new realities. This chapter stresses that while recent decades have brought new challenges to highland Maya bonesetters, these persons are responding with cautious creativity to the challenges, thereby enabling their craft to continue.

Bonesetting in Global and Local Context

The bonesetting craft has been known to humans since before recorded time. It has deep roots among peoples of antiquity, notably among the Greeks and Egyptians (Filer 1996:86–90; Majno 1975:73–75; Nunn 1996:174–81). Later, beginning in the seventh century, Muslim medicine applied formal attention to bonesetting (Douglass 1994:181), anticipating its subsequent entry into Western medicine (Anderson 1983:14). Innumerable other world peoples have also developed systems for dealing with bodily injury, acknowledging the reality of traumatic injury everywhere (Peltier 1990).

In Middle America, Spanish chroniclers Sahagún (1961) and Ruiz de Alarcón (1984) provided valuable insight into sixteenth and seventeenth-century bonesetting among Nahuas, recording how they treated stiffness, swelling, and fractures with invocations, plants, and splints. Comparable information about pre-Columbian and Maya bonesetting is lacking, however. Aside from a few references to colonial practice (Orellana 1987:106), the existing documentation of Middle American bonesetting refers to the modern period. Contemporary manual medical practices and practitioners have been identified throughout the Maya region (Bricker 1973; Cosminsky 1972; Douglas 1969; Fabrega and Silver 1973; Holland 1962; Instituto Indigenista Nacional 1978; Paul 1976; Redfield and Villa Rojas 1962; Rodríguez Rouanet 1969; Tedlock 1992) and the Mexican cultural sphere (Anderson 1987; Huber and Anderson 1996).

Middle American peoples continue finding ways of dealing with musculoskeletal injury, approaching their work with the experience and skills needed to treat different kinds of physical problems. Most of these problems, understandably, derive from the rural, largely agricultural work in which many Middle Americans participate (Figueroa Ibarra 1980), but also include problems associated with an increasingly mechanized, urban world (Nash 1958). Maya bonesetters, especially, bring a range of backgrounds and experience into their work. Living in a land intersected by at least three national borders, Maya bonesetters of different language groups work among people like themselves, with little distinguishing them economically or socially from their neighbors. Their practical importance to the world of daily life, and its underlying symbolic matrix, accounts for their enduring place in many communities.

Although bonesetting is often mentioned in contemporary Maya and other regional accounts, its importance is downplayed, giving the impression that it is a field of limited complexity or value. So infrequently are bonesetters and massagers actually discussed, in fact, that it might seem Middle Americans have had little need of them. Recent works by Hinojosa (2002, In press), Huber and Anderson (1996), McMahon (1994), and Paul and McMahon (2001), though, have partly redressed this deficit. Working in Mexican and Guatemalan contexts, they show how Middle Americans respect and seek help from competent bonesetters, and suggest how the bonesetters' work deserves closer study.

Since the term "bonesetter" can mean different things in different places, I will first clarify what I mean by it. Bonesetters are persons who "[move] bones as a form of medical treatment," as Huber and Anderson (1996:31) put it. Such moving of bones may be limited to dislocation reduction, or may include fracture reduction. Persons who do this generally also perform massage, though not all persons who practice massage also move bones therapeutically. Middle American curers who do both are often called *hueseros, componehuesos, componedores de hueso, jaladores de hueso,* or simply, *sobadores.* The latter term is often applied only to individuals who limit their practice to bodily massage and who do not move bones. Highland Mayas resort heavily to these bonesetters, especially when their ailments involve non-Western understandings of the body. Such understandings are not uncommon among the Maya (Cosminsky 1982; Holland 1962; Villa Rojas 1980) and underwrite much manual medicine work. Via the different kinds of manual practitioners, Mayas avail themselves of healing options Western medicine does not provide.

Setting and Methods

The bonesetters covered in this chapter live in the towns of San Juan Comalapa and San Pedro la Laguna and its immediate vicinity, both located in the central Guatemalan highlands. In Comalapa, the bonesetters, whom I will call Armando, Bartolomé, Eduardo, Paulino, Tomás, Rómulo, and Lupito, are of Kaqchikel Maya background. Bonesetters of the San Pedro la Laguna area are Tz'utujiil Maya and I refer to them as Flavio, Victorino, Lázaro, Cipriano, Martín, and Imelda.[1] I initially met four bonesetters in Comalapa in 1992, spending three months visiting and interviewing them. In the years between 1998 and 2002, I resumed interaction with surviving bonesetters from the earlier period and met numerous new ones in each town, interacting with them and observing their work for a total of four months. Comalapa lies at 2,110 meters above sea level and has a population of about 28,380 (Asturias de Barrios 1994:193–94). The *municipio* of San Pedro la Laguna, in contrast, lies at 1,610 meters above sea level on the western shore of Lake Atitlán and numbers about 8,508 inhabitants (McMahon 1994:10). In each community, Mayas make up the overwhelming majority of inhabitants.

It might appear at first that, as the bonesetters do not work in clinics, there is no place for biomedical elements in their practices. While they may not actually work in clinics, biomedicine has nonetheless affected their practices. Bonesetters in each area evaluate and sometimes incorporate elements of Western traumatology into their work, but they do not do this in the same ways or degrees. Nor do they incorporate such elements to the point of obviating their manual techniques, the cornerstone of their craft. Despite the variations found in highland Maya bonesetting, it offers the kind of care favored by most Mayas I have spoken with. Maya bonesetting enjoys this preference despite how some elements of the medical establishment have tried discrediting bonesettting as a rogue activity. Physicians who take this position are motivated by the fact that Maya bonesetters possess healing modalities unavailable to, and structurally antithetical to, establishment medicine: modalities focused on the hand.

The Knowing Hands of the Craft

Oths (2002) contends that despite the recent anthropological interest in embodiment paradigms, little attention has been directed to the actual practice of bodywork by healers. Had closer attention been paid to actual bodywork, we might have appreciated the body's role as an agent in healing, as well as its role as an instrument of healing. More often, though, the body has been brought forward in its role as a surface to be acted upon, or as a medium upon and through which power is played out (Maines 1999; Martin 1992; Scarry 1985). The latter approach speaks particularly to how power structures are evident in medical practice and condition the legitimation of knowledge (Foucault 1994; Taussig 1987).

Western medicine has had delegitimating effects on traditional modes of healing in many parts of the world, including Guatemala (Annis 1981; Tedlock 1987). In many cases, the performance of healing modalities has had to change, as a result, or face extirpation. Nonetheless, Maya bonesetters have continued relying on their hands as their primary means of healing, something that has earned them the enmity of physicians and the patronage of other people. So close is the relationship between Maya bonesetters and their hands that the story of this craft centers repeatedly on the hands as the sine qua non of healing and as the lightning rod for medical criticism. A review of the hands' activities will clarify why this is.

When an injured person visits a Guatemalan bonesetter, the person knows that the bonesetter will deal with the injury with his or her hands, and that this will not be a painless procedure. The bonesetter begins the initial encounter, though, by getting the client to relax and explain how the injury happened. The persons, if any, who brought the injured person might contribute information, especially if a child has been injured. The bonesetter is most interested in the type and severity of the injury and when it occurred. Generally, the more recent the injury, the more readily can the bonesetter consider the case treatable. Visual signs on the body,

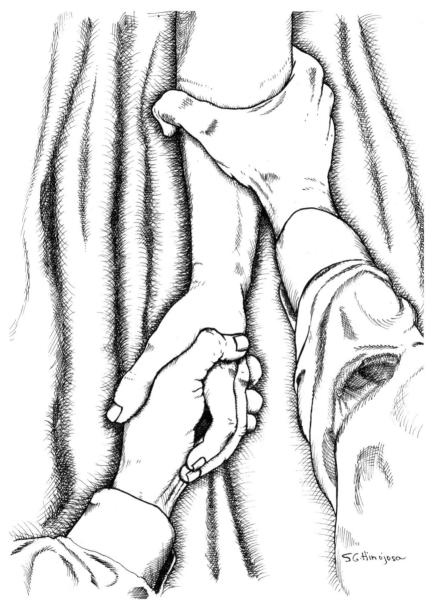

Figure 6.1.   A San Juan Comalapa bonesetter grasping a client's hand while massaging her injured forearm. (Drawing by Servando G. Hinojosa.)

such as deformity, reddening, edema, and bruising, suggest the type of injury and help the bonesetter locate it. The bonesetter also learns about the injury by checking the range of motion of the client's injured limb or torso, insofar as the client can move.

Typically, the bonesetter then applies a lubricating and/or warming agent to his hands and the client's body. Bonesetters of different communities might use beef fat or pig fat for this, or commercial products like cooking oil, rubbing alcohol, or pomades. The lubricant allows the healer's hands to move smoothly across the body, enabling more information about the injury to be accessed. The bonesetter moves his hands around the injury while pressing gently, watching for cues of discomfort and pain. As he palpates, his hands locate the trouble spots, detecting swelling, tenderness, and temperature irregularity. Together with what the client tells him, this information allows the bonesetter to assess the injury.

Most of the time, the bonesetter will diagnose either a relatively simple *golpe*, a deep soft tissue bruise, or a *safadura*, a strained, sprained, or disarticulated joint. In either case, if swelling is not excessive, the bonesetter can alleviate some of the pain and restore movement through steady but firm massage and limb mobilization. The client may be asked to return once or twice more for reexamination and continued treatments. If a fracture is detected, however, depending on its severity and on the bonesetter's abilities, hand-based reduction may take place. The Comalapan Rómulo explains that when a long bone is treated, "You've got to make a little effort, pull it a little, get to the end of the bone where it's broken, because you can't do it just with pressure, the point won't get to where it has to be, that would be impossible. You've got to give it a little pull, and give it the movement it needs until it arrives at the right spot, you know."

The bonesetter may ask others to help hold the client during treatment. Helpers, perhaps the injured person's relatives, might hold the seated client's torso while the bonesetter extends and pulls on his leg, or they might stabilize his shoulder while the healer treats the client's arm. An elderly bonesetter like Tonia of Comalapa might likewise ask for help, especially if her client is large or heavy.

Once the fracture has been realigned, as confirmed by palpation, it is immobilized using removable materials. Maya bonesetters seldom apply hard casting precisely because it is difficult to remove and would impede the critical reexamination of the injury site and/or the postalignment checks the bonesetter performs. During the first postalignment check, three to six days after the initial treatment, the bonesetter's hands check that the fracture has remained stable and aligned. Tomás, from Comalapa, relates that when a fracture follow-up is done, "Well, you have to feel it, you have to check if it's still protruding, it's, there's like, the bone forms a little step. Or it's, it's leveled, the bone, it's level, joined back together. If it has some steps, I have to lower these, flatten these, gently, gently, gently."

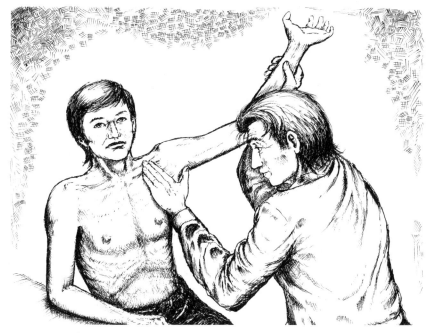

Figure 6.2.   A bonesetter from San Pedro la Laguna realigning a young client's fractured clavicle. (Drawing by Servando G. Hinojosa.)

His words strengthen the sense that Maya bonesetters practice an eminently manual craft, one underwritten by the hands' ability to probe and access bodily information. Bonesetters say their hands can directly detect problems in the body. They speak of how their hands simply "know" the body, both its surface and beneath, and that when they place their hands on a suffering body, their hands act of their own accord in locating the problem areas. They insist, furthermore, that they did not acquire this ability in any teaching setting (see Magan 1982; Paul and McMahon 2001). It is something that arose within them and that remains located within them. The bodily empathy revealed through the hands is of primary importance to Maya bonesetters, and most bonesetters rely on this alone to diagnose and treat suffering bodies. Their method evokes what Csordas (1993) describes as a somatic mode of attention, a capacity of the body to attend to other bodies, including suffering bodies, on a nonconscious level.

Bonesetters from the San Pedro la Laguna area, however, bring an additional element into diagnostics and treatment. They locate their avowed hand-based knowledge in found sacred objects as well as in their hands. These objects, called *huesos* or *baq*, "bones," are discovered by bonesetters as their roles are revealed to them (Paul 1976). The *huesos/baq* are usually small animal vertebrae or other bones, but certain stones can also be used and called "bones." Local bonesetters, such as Victorino, sometimes encounter objects such as potsherds, obsidian, and other pre-Columbian artifacts, which they also keep as sacra and use in curing.

Unlike San Pedro bonesetters, though, Comalapan ones generally report a nonsupernatural basis for their work. This aspect of Comalapan bonesetting is consistent with how, throughout Middle America, bonesetting is regarded as a pragmatic, nonreligious vocation (Cosminsky 1972; Holland 1962; Huber and Anderson 1996; Orellana 1987). Just as practical needs gave rise to bonesetting, practical methods drive it. But while the craft retains a secular character, it at times reveals supernatural aspects. Bonesetters of different Maya groups, in fact, attribute a sacred dimension to the craft (Douglas 1969; Fabrega and Silver 1973; Paul 1976; Rodríguez Rouanet 1969). As I indicate below, two Comalapan bonesetters recognize sacrality in their work, but they are the exception in their town.

Intersections with the Sacred

Different ritual specialists in Middle America such as spiritual healers and calendrical diviners carry out their work with the sense that they were divinely chosen for it (Colby and Colby 1981). Such a legitimation for working has been called divine election (Tedlock 1992), and it confers upon those elected a personal validation for exercising their specialties. This type of calling is true also for some Maya bonesetters. The vocational calling is quite common among San Pedro–area bonesetters, as shown below, but it seldom occurs among Comalapan bonesetters, and never in so dramatic a form as in the lake community.

Still, while Comalapan bonesetters seldom speak of their work in terms of divine election, they sometimes refer to their hand-based knowledge in supernatural terms. The bonesetter Lupito states simply that his abilities are a *don*, a gift ordained by God. The bonesetter Tomás echoes this about his own hands, but goes further, reporting that he received a calling to heal in a dream. Much more so than other local bonesetters, Tomás recognizes the operation of the divine in his work. He states, "My fingers, when I touch, I know that it's a gift, from God. It doesn't come from studying, it isn't a science, it's something God has given me. There's a sensitivity in my hand, when I take hold (of the body), I immediately know where the broken bone is, with my touch, [or] with my sight, I just look, and I know whether it's dislocated or broken." Tomás spells out a hand-based consciousness, attributes it to God, and asserts that it is of a different order of knowledge than what one can gain through didactic study.

This view of hand-based knowledge accords with that espoused by San Pedro bonesetters, virtually all of whom report divine election. The centrality of divine election to Pedrano bonesetting becomes apparent when speaking with local bonesetters and when reviewing the literature (McMahon 1994; Paul 1976; Paul and McMahon 2001; Rodríguez Rouanet 1969). Bonesetters' testimonies to divine election are typified by the experience of Lázaro. A dream instructed Lázaro to go to the hills where he would find a sacred object. He found the object, and months later dreamed of a man who showed him a skeleton, made it collapse, and who then instructed Lázaro to reassemble it, which he did. Having undergone this, and having performed to the satisfaction of his clients, he grew ever more certain of his divine election.

Lázaro's case highlights how Pedrano-area bonesetters value sacred objects called *huesos* or *baq* in their work. Area bonesetters use the *hueso* to carry out the initial "scan" of the injured body, placing it on the body and moving it along the skin. They then perform the primary corrective procedure, such as a fracture realignment or dislocation reduction, by pressing the object against the body. The Pedrano bonesetter then usually lubricates the body and massages the area with the hands only to make final adjustments.

When applied to a body, the *hueso* is said to move of its own accord, as long as it is held by its rightful owner. It only *appears* to be moved by the bonesetter, Pedranos stress. Some bonesetters say the *hueso* will stop abruptly when passing over a fracture. The *hueso* moves differently over dislocations or other types of injuries. Its reported magnetlike ability to hone in on injuries makes it a singular diagnostic and corrective tool. As Victorino would say, "It's a real magnet . . . because it grabs the bone."

The bonesetter usually wraps the *hueso* in a red cloth and keeps it either on his person or in a special coffer at home. Keeping the *hueso* on one's person is especially important for bonesetters who travel frequently—they want to keep it nearby. Some bonesetters never reveal the *hueso* to another person (Paul and McMahon 2001:258), while others are less strict. The latter might allow a visitor or client to see one of his *huesos* while keeping another one or more concealed.

Pedrano bonesetters remain very interested in sacred objects and stress divine instrumentality in their work. In the San Pedro area, supernatural agency is wedded to healing empiricism, unlike in other highland Maya bonesetting traditions that emphasize the secular over the sacred. Elements of both domains find their place within bonesetters' practices, although their presence has not precluded bonesetters from considering elements from still other, newer domains.

The Uneasy Encounter between Bonesetters and Technology

When the Maya bonesetter is summoned to a person's home, he does not bring along an elaborate tool kit. In fact, he carries very little, because the materials he

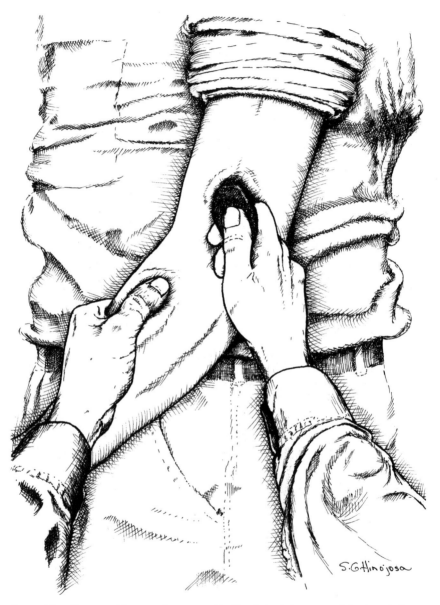

Figure 6.3.   The sacred *hueso* or *baq* as used by San Pedro la Laguna and San Juan la Laguna bonesetters. (Drawing by Servando G. Hinojosa.)

uses will probably be found at the home he is visiting. Even when injured persons arrive at the bonesetter's home, they are not brought into a special room appointed with gleaming equipment and esoteric medicine vials. They are simply helped into an area where other home activities take place, such as a reception room, the kitchen, or a patio. The bonesetters' work surroundings are quite ordinary and nonmedical. Though it might seem that Western and Maya traditions have little to offer each other, Maya bonesetting has nonetheless created a space into which select elements of biotechnology are permitted not only entry, but a role in further legitimating Maya healing. Its presence in Maya bonesetting has continued despite the tensions between practitioners of the two traditions.

Technology has affected Maya bonesetting primarily through pharmaceutical use and radiography. The challenge for bonesetters has been to weigh technological elements, which otherwise speak more to an interest in mass marketing than to concerns of natural healing, and to determine how they can be incorporated into their work. By remaining cautiously receptive toward biotechnological resources, and by keeping their ear to the ground for what the public expects them to know, bonesetters monitor the field of available resources. Pharmaceuticals are one such resource.

Pharmaceuticals

Bonesetters have been receptive toward pharmaceuticals and other commercial preparations. Those who use pharmaceuticals prefer products that are applied externally, and often keep these close at hand (see Oths 1992 on folk preferences for topical remedies). Should a client need ingestible medication, however, he will likely be sent elsewhere for it, usually to a nearby pharmacy. Among the local pharmaceutical products most recommended by Comalapan bonesetters are *Nodol* pomade (analgesic), and *Reumatan* and *Indocid* capsules (antirheumatic, anti-inflammatory). Like in Comalapa, San Pedro bonesetters seek products that can reduce their clients' pain and swelling, and speed their recovery. The ingested remedy *Reumatan* is thus also recommended by Pedrano bonesetters, as are *Dolofin* tablets (analgesic) and *Dolo Fenil* capsules (analgesic, anti-inflammatory). Bonesetters of both communities also suggest various other brands of pain relievers to their clients.

Because they must palpate the body thoroughly, bonesetters often use products that moisten, lubricate, and even warm the skin. To do this, they routinely use commercially available unguents and pomades, such as those of brand name *Balsámico GMS* and *Cofal*, and corn and olive oils. Rubbing alcohol is also used. One bonesetter in Comalapa, Armando, would sometimes apply a veterinary unguent when working. Comalapan and Pedrano bonesetters, however, do not apply these products in the same way. Whereas Comalapan healers usually apply the salves to their hands and the client's body before palpating it, their San Pedro counterparts usually work the injured area with the sacred *hueso* before applying a natural or commercial product to the area.

Some bonesetters avail themselves of pharmaceuticals more than do others. Tomás of Comalapa, for instance, counsels his clients to take very specific medications; he asserts that physicians with whom he has amicable relations have told him which drugs to use and have even encouraged him to "prescribe" the medications to his clients. As he puts it, "Even *they* [physicians] have helped me, urging me to give such-and-such medication to the patients, such-and-such capsule. So when people come for my help, I fix their broken bones and at the same time, they are to take some capsules that are sold in pharmacies. In this way, they are helped both inside and out."

Tomás reasons that the prescribed medications, among which is *Indocid*, "are like a vitamin for the bone, so that the bone will join together." He sees the visits he has received from physicians as endorsements of his work, and regards their drug recommendations as further validation of combined therapies. Like other local curers, Tomás knows that clients often feel personally reassured and empowered when they take pharmaceuticals as part of their treatments. In suggesting these products to clients, then, he validates their expectations of treatment, gaining their confidence in his method.

A similar curer–physician collaboration was reported by the bonesetter Cipriano in San Juan la Laguna, a town neighboring San Pedro and largely sharing in its bonesetting tradition. Cipriano says that a local physician, Dr. Herrera, who is Maya, and he are sometimes both summoned to treat an injured person. In the past, according to Cipriano, the physician or a nurse might give the injured person a pain injection, and then allow Cipriano to manipulate the injury. Cipriano attests that if Herrera is on duty at the department capital hospital (in Sololá), and he encounters people with fractures, Herrera sometimes recommends they go to San Juan for treatment. The referral is not mandatory for the patients, but it is usually offered to poorer ones, says Cipriano. Although Herrera and other physicians do not normally send clients to Cipriano, Cipriano says that Herrera has given him pharmaceutical advice. For instance, when Cipriano asked Herrera for a drug to reduce his clients' pain and to help them sleep, he was told to use *Neo-Melubrina* tablets (analgesic), something Cipriano still recommends. His proximity to a physician has allowed him to see how physicians use analgesics and anesthetics, and even injections. And while his contact with a physician alerted him to specialized drugs and delivery methods, other bonesetters have made use of pharmaceuticals and biomedical methods without close involvement with physicians. Cipriano's case is unusual in the extent to which he claims collaboration with a physician. As I explain below, most bonesetters would sooner avoid close contact with physicians.

The late Bartolomé of Comalapa, for example, would send his clients to a physician for analgesic injections only if they were in severe pain. Other Comalapan bonesetters also personally refrain from giving injections, but should a client of theirs want an injection and be unable or unwilling to see a physician, there are options. Persons working in pharmacies often administer injections, as do many health promoters. Given the range of people who offer injections in Guatemala, it is not surprising that some bonesetters also offer them. The bonesetter Lázaro of San Pedro stands out in this respect. Not only does he prescribe and sell *Reumatan* to his clients in several towns, he has given some clients intramuscular injections of *Dolo Fenil*. He is reluctant to talk about this, however, hoping to avoid official scrutiny. Lázaro's case recalls that of another bonesetter's in Guatemala, a Ladino (cultural non-Indian), working among Mam Maya. This bonesetter would inject a painkiller, *Lidocaine*, into dislocated joints before manipulating them (Acevedo Ligorria 1986:82–84). Although injection usage highlights the changing nature of bonesetting, it is atypical of Maya bonesetting at present.

X-Rays

Comalapan and Pedrano bonesetters have also had growing contact with radiographic technology in recent years. Injured people sometimes take x-rays of their injuries and present these to bonesetters, but bonesetters have not been quick to embrace this technology. When reminded of how important x-rays are to physicians, bonesetters point out the simple reason physicians need this technology: physicians lack hand-based diagnostic abilities. Maya bonesetters disapprove, though, of how, in their view, physicians accept x-ray technology uncritically and utilize it in flawed ways. They argue that physicians, even when viewing accurate x-ray images, fail to follow through and treat the revealed injuries. The perceived inability of physicians to treat fractures, even with the aid of this diagnostic technology, reenforces for bonesetters the sense that more is needed for effective treatment than just medical hardware. Nonetheless, Maya healers are reappraising this hardware.

Although bonesetters believe x-rays have some diagnostic usefulness (i.e., for physicians), what they really appreciate about x-rays is their confirmatory power (Hinojosa In press). This is especially evident when bonesetters must assuage clients who question what the bonesetters find through palpation of their bodies. The Comalapan Rómulo thus explains to clients that if they are unsure about his diagnosis, they should get an x-ray taken "to clear up any doubts." Another Comalapan bonesetter, Tomás, often recommends that clients bring an x-ray of their injuries to him. This enables him to visually point out to clients what injuries his hands locate in them. These and other Comalapan bonesetters, including Bartolomé, have commented that many injured persons come to them with x-rays in hand. Such persons had x-rays taken either because they were told to do so by a physician they initially consulted, or because they wanted to bring the images to a bonesetter. Some bonesetters and clients in Comalapa and San Pedro sometimes also compare "before" and "after" images of injury sites, again underscoring the persuasive, and reassuring, power of the images.

The bonesetters' cautious stance vis-à-vis x-rays indicates how bonesetters continue placing primacy on the hands to diagnose and heal. Radiography provides seemingly direct information access to physicians, but it has not persuaded bonesetters to abandon their hands. X-rays are available in the larger cities and department capitals of Guatemala, but can also be found in some provincial communities. Comalapa, for instance, has one private x-ray provider. San Pedro, on the other hand, has no x-ray facilities, even in its new Health Center inaugurated in 2001. Though radiographic facilities are widely found today and are within physical reach of those visiting Comalapa's and San Pedro's bonesetters, healers do not recommend x-rays to all their clients. Bonesetters know that x-rays are an added expense for people and, contrary to some popular Guatemalan understandings, the rays are not directly therapeutic.

Maya bonesetters have reservations about the accuracy and biomedical applicability of x-ray images, but many consider them useful in terms of patient relations. Many bonesetters are now expected to be able to view and interpret x-rays, although they are not equipped to do this. Still, x-rays buttress these healers' diagnostic and curative skills while reassuring that bonesetters are reasonably familiar with the visual currency of biomedicine. Rather than undermining the public faith in the bonesetters' abilities, x-rays, as used by bonesetters, widen the authoritative space in which they work.

Practitioners and the Professional Environment

There is no doubt that biomedical technology has entered highland Maya bonesetting, but bonesetters do not view themselves as participants in a biomedical system. In fact, they consider themselves very unlike biomedical specialists in their approaches and methods. Physicians, likewise, distance themselves from bonesetters' modus operandi. In this section, I discuss how bonesetters and physicians view each other, and show how their views shape the contact between them. Bonesetters make decisions about biomedical technology in a tense occupational environment, one in which they are marginalized. The following suggests, then, that the future of manual medicine, and the directions of its changes, will hinge on more than just the presence of bonesetters and physicians: It will hinge on the dialogue between these practitioners, a dialogue between distinct and self-validating domains, ones with unequal access to power.

Bonesetters' Views of Physicians

Maya bonesetters hold a number of opinions about physicians, revealing both respect and repudiation toward them. A thread uniting different bonesetters' views of physicians, though, is that bonesetters tend to distrust physicians and, more diffusely, biomedicine. Bonesetters convey a sense that physicians are intelligent, learned people, but that they perform certain tasks poorly and they overcharge for their services. Still worse is how, bonesetters claim, physicians show little real care to their patients. When clients tell bonesetters about how physicians unsatisfactorily treated their injuries, bonesetters remember these accounts, reinforcing their negative views of physicians. Bartolomé, for instance, heard and saw how after the 1976 earthquake, physicians treated many injured people by simply casting their fractured limbs without properly aligning them. More recently, Cipriano has treated people who were first attended by physicians. When these persons complain that their casted limbs remain very painful, Cipriano removes the casts and treats the injury himself (see also McMahon 1994).

Despite the poor iatrogenic outcomes the Maya bonesetters learn of, some bonesetters suspect that certain physicians might actually know how to treat fractures. But even of these it is said, "They know how [to treat fractures] but they don't want to do it, they don't want to fix them," according to Comalapan Tomás. His words suggest that most physicians would rather not bother with the demanding procedures fractures require. Evident, also, is the implication that Guatemalan physicians, most of whom are Ladinos, are especially unwilling to treat Indians. As it stands, the quality of medical care and options offered to largely rural Maya is below that available to urban dwellers and Guatemalan Ladinos who tend to be wealthier than Indians. This reality has not been lost on Maya who suspect that physicians, and their profession, have never had the Indians' best interests at heart. Given this, Indians are not surprised when certain physicians treat them more like personal nuisances than as legitimate customers (see Cosminsky 1987; Falla 1971; Pebley et al. 1996).

Whether or not physicians can apply their medical skills to the treatment of fractures, their abilities have not been proven to the satisfaction of Mayas or Maya bonesetters. Mayas already consider physicians ineffectual with their hands, especially because physicians cannot or will not palpate and massage the few pregnant women who consult them. This bolsters the Mayas' belief that the physician's knowledge, while authoritative in some areas, does not extend to the manual skills necessary for bonesetting. Bonesetters therefore concede a very conditional degree of authority to biomedicine, but continue operating on their own.

One way this partial concession of authority is expressed is by how bonesetters sometimes use biomedical narratives to buttress claims of their healing ability and to validate their work. Some Comalapan bonesetters describe how they have been visited by physicians who seem interested in their work. Rómulo, for one, has been visited by Guatemalan health workers and by foreigners exploring manual medicine through the lens of occupational therapy. For Tomás, visits by physicians have entailed both conversations and opportunities to treat the physicians' own injuries and get advice on pharmaceutical use. Dr. Sucuc of Comalapa affirms that, indeed, physicians from out of town come to visit local bonesetters. Even a local Maya physician, Hugo Icú Perén, made an unusual effort to learn about Maya bonesetters. Icú Perén prepared his medical thesis on Maya bonesetters of Comalapa and two other towns. In it, he suggests how medical practitioners might advance in their mission by learning about these healers (Icú Perén 1990). Bonesetters from the lake communities sometimes also mention medical workers when speaking of their own work. Recall how Cipriano from San Juan says a local physician and he have treated patients jointly, and that the physician refers patients to him from a hospital. When asked if he got along with the physician, Cipriano replied, "I have a gift from God, but I can't compete with a physician, because he's got his studies. . . . [E]veryone has his own specialty." He expresses respect for the physician, especially because this physician allegedly encourages his patients to seek traditional healers.

Although some physicians show an interest in Comalapan bonesetters, there is a caveat. In nearly all the cases wherein physicians and health workers visit Comalapan bonesetters, the visitors are from out of town, usually from Guatemala City. One virtually never hears of visits to bonesetters by Comalapan physicians. Icú Perén notwithstanding, it seems that out-of-town physicians have admitted to a healthier curiosity about bonesetting than have local physicians. Bonesetters in the San Pedro area, in contrast, while offering narratives about people unsatisfied with medical treatment, do not often speak of visits by any physicians, local or otherwise. Dr. Arana, the attending physician at the Health Center of San Pedro, admits that in his eleven years of local service, he has not been involved with any bonesetters.

The bonesetters' sometime-contact with individual physicians has helped ameliorate some of their personal antagonisms toward them, but bonesetters still distrust them as a class. At the same time, closer contact between physicians and bonesetters has made the craft more permeable to Western elements such as pharmaceuticals and x-rays. The sustained direction of influence, from physician to bonesetter, has subsequently reenforced the subordinated position of bonesetting vis-à-vis biomedicine. Today, while physicians may know and visit bonesetters, no physician looks upon a bonesetter as his equal. Personal efforts by a few physicans have not dissolved the structural tension between the two classes of practitioners, largely because of how most physicians look down on bonesetters.

Physicians' Views of Bonesetters

It is little surprise that, institutionally, physicians hold a dim view of bonesetters. Consistent with how Guatemalan physicians generally regard indigenous healers, physicians show varying levels of antipathy toward Maya bonesetters (Icú Perén 1990; Paul and McMahon 2001). When individual physicians do make positive remarks about bonesetters, they often cloak them in language that casts doubt on the bonesetters' abilities. For example, physicians who recognize how people prefer visiting bonesetters over physicians sometimes claim that "the people have more faith in them [bonesetters] than in us," as Dr. Suárez of Comalapa offers. He, in effect, reveals how some physicians attribute the high patronage of bonesetters to client beliefs ("faith") rather than to any actual skills of the bonesetters. Dr. Arana of San Pedro takes this further, claiming that injured people are misguided in going to bonesetters in the first place. As he puts it, "the people believe blindly in them, precisely because of the traditions deriving from their ancestors." In a more sanguine moment he acknowledges a certain level of technical skill among individual bonesetters, remarking, "in some cases, they might have some effect," but conveys his overall misgivings about them. Other physicians even admit that physicians have sought bonesetters' treatments, but stop short of endorsing the bonesetters.

Whereas physicians in Comalapa and San Pedro cite cases in which bonesetters did not treat a patient successfully, they admit that physicians see only a fraction of all the cases bonesetters treat. Only the most complex cases find their way to physicians who, in turn, summarily order radiographs and usually send the patient to out-of-town personnel. Still, Guatemalan physicians refuse to concede that bonesetters might be dealing well with those cases physicians do not see.

With such assessments of bonesetters, there is little ground for official recognition of them. This is significant in view of how some bonesetters have been urged by health authorities to obtain a "license" to practice (Icú Perén 1990:60). It is unclear what such a license would entitle them to, but it is unlikely that bonesetters would be thereafter encouraged to diagnose and manipulate injuries. "Licensing" would probably be intended to, as with Maya midwives, identify local bonesetters and bring them under monitoring by physicians. It would almost certainly mandate that bonesetters accept fewer cases and out-refer more, perhaps converting them into a "portal of entry" into the formal health sector. While there is evidence elsewhere in Central America for this change in the bonesetters' role (Peterson 1994), highland Maya bonesetters are not speeding their clients' entry into the formal sector, further hardening physicians' feelings toward bonesetters.

Part of the reason physicians want to monitor Maya bonesetting is, interestingly, the non-supernatural character of the craft. Physicians have often taken issue with non-Western healers, but they have been particularly disparaging of healers who work in the supernatural realm. In the case of Maya bonesetters, though, their largely empirical practices are what have prompted critiques from physicians. Because bonesetting is so empirical, physicians reason that biomedicine can provide better services than bonesetters', and this encourages them to move into the bonesetters' domain (see Cooter 1987:169). Ironically, it is because bonesetters' work is so empirical that it encounters problems with biomedicine! The very physicality of bonesetting strictures its engagement with biomedicine, an institution that otherwise promotes non-supernatural health seeking.

Each practitioner appreciates elements of the other's work only to the extent that those elements can aid the practitioner making the judgment. The prevailing view among physicians, then, is that bonesetters can best help people by referring them to biomedical personnel. Meanwhile, bonesetters value the physician's world only insofar as it can occasionally validate their work and provide useful products. The work of the "other's" world is, at best, incidental to the real curing. Unlike bonesetters, though, physicians are in a position to institutionally dissuade people from visiting bonesetters, something they have not yet done aggressively. The possibility of this, and the popularity of Maya bonesetters, ensures that the end to the troubled conversation between these domains is not yet in sight.

Conclusion

Maya bonesetting comprises multiple expressions of an old and specialized craft, rooted in the experiences of different communities. As a nonuniform body of practitioners, Maya bonesetters make use of different tools, practices, and guiding principles. They also value differently the role of the hands in diagnosis and healing, as evidenced by the arresting contrasts in technique between Comalapan and Pedrano bonesetters. In this case, wherein the latter bonesetters couple a sacred object to their hands, the former do not. Bonesetters of both places, however, consider their hands of such importance that they stress how a certain species of awareness and ability resides directly in them. Physicians, on the other hand, are said to operate without this. When this embodied agency assumes a supernatural character, the experiential gulf between Maya and medical therapeutics grows.

Although biomedicine today reaches throughout Guatemala, the bonesetting craft still exists outside of official parameters. This affords bonesetting a degree of autonomy not enjoyed by other manual therapeutics, such as midwifery. Still, biomedicine has impacted the craft in many ways, primarily through pharmaceutical and radiography use. Bonesetters engage biomedicine ideologically in different ways, and this affects how they appraise biomedical elements. For instance, some bonesetters who consider pharmaceuticals a useful adjunct to their work have made a place for these in their practices. Other bonesetters consider radiographs to be of great confirmatory power and bring them into their dialogue with clients. On the other hand, bonesetters may have little confidence in a bio-medically approved measure like casting and exclude it from their work. Likewise, depending on their views of physician efficacy and of their own personal abilities, bonesetters vary in practicing out-referral.

Maya bonesetters have been learning about different biomedical elements while limiting their contact with physicians. Physicians, for their part, have shown little sustained interest in the work bonesetters do and generally keep their distance from them. Their mutual regard, however, is not on an even keel. Bonesetters concede some health authority to physicians, but physicians are reluctant to acknowledge any real traumatological expertise in bonesetters. Still, physicians sometimes reveal an ambivalence about bonesetters, suggesting that physicians may yet rethink structural hostilities toward them. For now, though, biomedicine focuses on bonesetter limitations rather than abilities.

Bonesetters have met the institutional challenges to their legitimacy, in part, by adapting and applying certain biomedical technologies in ways that confirm the bonesetters' efficacy. This has permitted them to amplify their authoritative space in a difficult vocational environment while strengthening their claim that healing knowledge is located in the hands. It has also allowed them to demonstrate flexibility to a public mindful of new technologies. To a significant degree, then, Maya bonesetters keep their pragmatic edge by reconciling the old and the new, and by obscuring the boundaries between these when needed. Their craft draws from individuals with hand-based talents, although these individuals now struggle to remain relevant in a changing world.

Notes

Numerous persons helped make this study possible. I extend special thanks to the bonesetters and other residents of San Juan Comalapa, San Pedro la Laguna, and San Juan la Laguna, Guatemala. Also offering their assistance were Omar Rivera, Kay Brittain, and Jessica Villescaz. The content and conclusions of this paper remain, nonetheless, my own.

I. With the exception of Hugo Icú Perén, all names in this study are pseudonyms.

References

Acevedo Ligorria, Joaquín Antonio
    1986 Una aproximación a la antropología médica en Todos Santos Cuchumatán, Huehuetenango. Medical thesis, Universidad de San Carlos de Guatemala.
Anderson, Robert T.
    1981 Bonesetting: A Medical Bone of Contention. *The American Chiropractic Association Journal of Chiropractic* 15:89–100.

1983   On Doctors and Bonesetters in the Sixteenth and Seventeenth Centuries. *Chiropractic History* 3:11–15.

1987   The treatment of musculoskeletal disorders by a Mexican bonesetter (sobador). *Social Science and Medicine* 24:43–46.

Annis, Sheldon

1981   Physical Access and Utilization of Health Services in Rural Guatemala. *Social Science and Medicine* 15D:515–23.

Asturias de Barrios, Linda

1994   Woman's Hand, Man's Hand: Textile Artisan Production in Comalapa, Guatemala. PhD dissertation. State University of New York at Albany.

Bricker, Victoria Reifler

1973   *Ritual Humor in Highland Chiapas.* Austin and London: University of Texas Press.

Colby, Benjamin N., and Lore M. Colby

1981   *The Daykeeper: The Life and Discourse of an Ixil Diviner.* Cambridge, Mass.: Harvard University Press.

Cooter, Roger

1987   Bones of Contention? Orthodox Medicine and the Mystery of the Bone-Setter's Craft. Pp. 158–73 in W. F. Bynum and Roy Porter, eds. *Medical Fringe and Medical Orthodoxy 1750–1850.* London, Sydney, Wolfeboro, New Hampshire: Croom Helm.

Cosminsky, Sheila

1972   Decision Making and Medical Care in a Guatemalan Indian Community. PhD dissertation. Brandeis University.

1982   Knowledge and Body Concepts of Guatemalan Midwives. Pp. 233–52 in Margarita Artschwagger Kay, ed. *Anthropology of Human Birth.* Philadelphia, Pa.: F. A. Davis Company.

1987   Women and Health Care on a Guatemalan Plantation. *Social Science and Medicine* 25:1163–73.

Csordas, Thomas J.

1993   Somatic Modes of Attention. *Cultural Anthropology* 8:135–56.

Douglas, Bill Gray

1969   Illness and Curing in Santiago Atitlán, a Tzutujil-Maya Community in the Southwestern Highlands of Guatemala. PhD dissertation. Stanford University.

Douglass, Susan L.

1994   *Strategies and Structures for Presenting World History, with Islam and Muslim History as a Case Study.* Beltsville, Md.: Amana Publications.

Fabrega, Horacio, Jr., and Daniel B. Silver

1973   *Illness and Shamanistic Curing in Zinacantan: An Ethnomedical Analysis.* Stanford, Calif.: Stanford University Press.

Falla, Ricardo

1971   Juan el gordo: visión indígena de su explotación. *Estudios Centro Americanos* 26:98–107.

Figueroa Ibarra, Carlos

1980   *El proletariado rural en el agro guatemalteco.* Guatemala City: Editorial Universitaria.

Filer, Joyce
　　1996 *Disease.* Austin: University of Texas Press.
Foucault, Michel
　　1994 *The Birth of the Clinic: An Archaeology of Medical Perception.* Trans. A. M. Sheridan
　　　　Smith. New York: Vintage Books.
Hinojosa, Servando Z.
　　2002 "The Hands Know": Bodily Engagement and Medical Impasse in Highland
　　　　Maya Bonesetting. *Medical Anthropology Quarterly* 16:22–40.
　　In press. Bonesetting and Radiography in the Southern Maya Highlands. *Medical An-*
　　　　thropology.
Holland, William R.
　　1962 Highland Maya Folk Medicine: A Study of Culture Change. PhD dissertation.
　　　　University of Arizona.
Huber, Brad R., and Robert Anderson
　　1996 Bonesetters and Curers in a Mexican Community: Conceptual Models, Status,
　　　　and Gender. *Medical Anthropology* 17:23–38.
Icú Perén, Hugo
　　1990 Práctica de traumatología empírica en el área Cakchiquel de Guatemala. Medical
　　　　thesis. Universidad de San Carlos de Guatemala.
Instituto Indigenista Nacional
　　1978 Aspectos de la medicina popular en el area rural de Guatemala. *Guatemala Indígena* 13(3–4).
Magan, D.
　　1982 An Interview with a Somali Traditional Healer. *Somali Refugee Health Unit Newslet-*
　　　　ter 17:1–5.
Maines, Rachel P.
　　1999 *The Technology of Orgasm: "Hysteria," the Vibrator, and Women's Sexual Satisfaction.* Baltimore,
　　　　Md.: The Johns Hopkins University Press.
Majno, Guido
　　1975 *The Healing Hand: Man and Wound in the Ancient World.* Cambridge, Mass.: Harvard
　　　　University Press.
Martin, Emily
　　1992 *The Woman in the Body: A Cultural Analysis of Reproduction.* Boston, Mass.: Beacon Press.
McMahon, Clarence Edward
　　1994 The Sacred Nature of Maya Bonesetting: Ritual Validation in an Empirical Prac-
　　　　tice. MA thesis. Texas A&M University.
Nash, Manning
　　1958 *Machine Age Maya.* American Anthropological Association, Memoir no. 87.
　　　　Menasha, Wisconsin: American Anthropological Association.
Nunn, John F.
　　1996 *Ancient Egyptian Medicine.* Norman: University of Oklahoma Press.
Orellana, Sandra L.
　　1987 *Indian Medicine in Highland Guatemala.* Albuquerque: University of New Mexico
　　　　Press.

Oths, Kathryn S.
   1992   Some Symbolic Dimensions of Andean Materia Medica. *Central Issues in Anthropology* 10:76–85.
   2002   Setting It Straight in the Andes: Musculoskeletal Distress and the Role of the Componedor. Pp. 63–91 in Joan D. Koss-Chioino, Thomas Leatherman, and Christine Greenway, eds. *Medical Pluralism in the Andean Region: A Tribute to Libbet Crandon-Malamud.* New York: Routledge.
Paul, Benjamin D.
   1976   The Maya Bonesetter as Sacred Specialist. *Ethnology* 15:77–81.
Paul, Benjamin D., and Clancy E. McMahon
   2001   Mesoamerican Bonesetters. Pp. 243–69 in Brad E. Huber and Alan R. Sandstrom, eds. *Mesoamerican Healers.* Austin: University of Texas Press.
Pebley, Anne R., Noreen Goldman, and Germán Rodríguez
   1996   Prenatal and Delivery Care and Childhood Immunization in Guatemala: Do Family and Community Matter? *Demography* 33:231–47.
Peltier, Leonard F.
   1990   *Fractures: A History and Iconography of Their Treatment.* San Francisco, Calif.: Norman Publishing.
Peterson, Caroline
   1994   *Sobadores* as Integral Health Care Providers in Nicaragua. Paper presented at National Symposium on Indigenous Knowledge and Contemporary Social Issues, March 3–5, Tampa, Florida.
Redfield, Robert, and Alfonso Villa Rojas
   1962   *Chan Kom: A Maya Village.* Chicago, Ill.: University of Chicago Press.
Rodríguez Rouanet, Francisco
   1969   Prácticas médicas tradicionales de los indígenas de Guatemala. *Guatemala Indígena* 4:51–86.
Ruiz de Alarcón, Hernando
   1984   *Treatise on the Heathen Superstitions That Live among the Indians Native to This New Spain, 1629.* Trans. and eds. J. Richard Andrews and Ross Hassig. Norman: University of Oklahoma Press.
Sahagún, Bernardino de
   1961   *The Florentine Codex, Book 10—The People.* Trans. Charles E. Dibble and Arthur J. O. Anderson. Santa Fe, N. Mex.: The School of American Research and the University of Utah.
Scarry, Elaine
   1985   *The Body in Pain: The Making and Unmaking of the World.* Oxford: Oxford University Press.
Taussig, Michael
   1987   *Shamanism, Colonialism, and the Wild Man: A Study in Terror and Healing.* Chicago, Ill.: University of Chicago Press.

Tedlock, Barbara
    1987 An Interpretive Solution to the Problem of Humoral Medicine in Latin Amer-
        ica. *Social Science and Medicine* 24:1069–83.
    1992 *Time and the Highland Maya.* Albuquerque: University of New Mexico Press.
Villa Rojas, Alfonso
    1980 La imagen del cuerpo humano según los mayas de Yucatán. *Anales de Antropología*
        17:31–46, Tomo II.

Body as Teacher: The Roles of Clinical Model and Morphology in Skill Acquisition   7

JOHN O'MALLEY

THE PURPOSE OF THIS CHAPTER is to outline the process of skill acquisition in two very different healing arts, demonstrating that while each healing model provides a basis for learning, in the end skilled manipulation is a function of experience. The healing techniques of Renato Roda, a type of traditional Filipino healer (*hilot*), are compared to my chiropractic techniques; we both use manipulation and massage. Most musculoskeletal lesions treated by the *hilot* revolve around blocked blood flow (*naipit na ugat*), creating a palpable entity that to me feels like muscle spasm. The chiropractic lesion, the subluxation, is based on the idea of restricted or aberrant joint movement causing interference with the nervous system's normal function. In both cases, manipulation is a common technique used to treat the problem.

Using Heidegger's (1962) concept of *Dasein* (our personal and collective way of being in the world), it is possible to demonstrate that healing techniques are largely phenomenological, and that only in the early stages of skill acquisition are the rules of the clinical tradition important. The greatest influence on developing palpation skills is the experiencing of presentations of various palpable lesions. These are demonstrated to exist in the patient by their cross-cultural identification as palpable phenomena by both *hilot* and chiropractor. By locating the same lesion Roda and I can agree on its status as being "the thing to manipulate." Merleau-Ponty's (1962:302–303) idea that we approach the world from the perspective of gaining maximum access to our environment, and his idea that we manipulate objects through the use of maximum grip (Dreyfus 1996), are employed to demonstrate that the "know how" (learned skills) of competent manipulation will always be similar.[1]

The "just right" feeling that precedes the decision to act, the symphonic interaction between the practitioner and patient, is predicated on the morphology of the practitioner and morphology of the lesion joined existentially in the correct attitude of both participants. All skilled practitioners guide this tactile conversation, and with "know how" direct the interaction to a successful outcome by employing a similar maximal grip, the existential state that underlies competent technique.

Since in the instant of its application, the healing act is phenomenological, what then remains of the thematic knowledge of the respective sciences and to what extent does this knowledge unhelpfully influence the practitioner's perception and treatment options? Chiropractors are taught that they do what they do because their treatment rationale, or science, accurately describes the patient's problem. There is an implicit order to the relationship, suggesting that technique evolves from the science. The opposite may in fact be the case. O'Malley (1998) demonstrates that manipulative skills develop from immersion in the healing process, and that the science of each particular genre, at least in part, provides a culturally acceptable explanation through which the practitioner can communicate the purpose of treatment to the patient, fellow practitioners, and students.

This is not to say that any one paradigm is invalid, but rather that paradigms may be only obliquely relevant to the application of manipulation and massage. This begs the question: If paradigms are not essential to the application of manual therapy skills, then what purposes do they serve and from where do skills originate? The answer must explain how two differing approaches can converge at the level of application of technique. In effect, what is it that they have in common?

Setting and Methodology

I conducted three field trips to the Philippines between 1989 and 1994, spending seventeen months observing, videotaping, interviewing, and performing collaborative treatments with fifteen *hilots* in Santa Mesa, a Manila suburb. Although I am competent in basic Tagalog, I also used translators, and was helped by the fact that many of my informants had a rudimentary grasp of English. I was interested in the question: What is the relationship between the clinical model and the practitioner's touch-perception of the patient? The investigation of this question was broken into three components: the first, identifying the clinical model of the *hilot*—an ethnographic task; the second, identifying and describing the palpable lesions perceptible to both the chiropractor and the *hilot*—an ethnographic task requiring chiropractic skills; the third, establishing the relationship between the two—an analytical task involving the reappraisal of the philosophy of chiropractic (O'Malley 1998).

Renato Roda was one of two *hilots* singled out for extensive collaborative treatment investigation. What struck me was the extraordinary similarity between his method of manipulation and my own. He manipulated the low back of a middle-aged male patient, using what appeared to be a chiropractic side-posture technique. His prone manipulation of the thoracic spine of a child-patient demonstrated a high level of skill. The preparation, positioning, and delivery of the manipulative thrust in both cases would not have looked out of place in most chiropractic practices.

His massage technique was similar to chiropractic at the micro level of immediate application but showed some idiosyncrasies at the macro level of general method. These differences can be explained by dissimilarities in the clinical models of the two healing techniques.

By investigating the relationship between clinical models and experience, as the two main factors contributing to the development of technical skills, we can gain insight into the role of the body as teacher and the distorting effect clinical models may have on perception.

First, it is necessary to establish a method for cross-cultural translation of touch-mediated diagnostic and healing procedures, and then provide a detailed description of each clinical model. From these it is possible to establish how clinical models influence the learning process and trace the practitioner's journey from novice to expert. Having established the role of the clinical model, it is then necessary to look at how the morphology of the patient, combined with the intentionality of the practitioner, result in convergence of manipulative technique styles.

A Method for Cross-Cultural Evaluation of Touch Perception

The analytical tools of linguistics provide a useful analogue for interpreting the art of touch-mediated healing. In linguistics, there is a basic distinction between phones and phonemes (Hawkes 1977:23). The phone is the actual sound as it exists. The phoneme is the minimum discernible difference in sound that makes a meaningful difference in a particular language. An analogy can be drawn between the phone and the physical structure (anatomy of the patient) that exists to be felt. Conversely, the phoneme could be viewed as analogous to the minimum discernible difference that can be experienced through palpation by a competent practitioner of a particular genre of palpation. A phoneme may have meaning in one language and not be discernible in another. Similarly, that which is perceived as being felt by the practitioner of one tactile genre may be indiscernible or meaningless to the practitioner of another.

In proposing the following investigative method, I am assuming that the investigator is competent in at least one tradition of palpation (such as chiropractic). To distinguish the linguistic terms "phone" and "phoneme" from their tactile analogues, I designate tactile phones as "t-phones" and tactile phonemes as "t-phonemes." The investigation of the "language" of touch-mediated healing must logically address three issues.

First, there is the identification of familiar t-phones, a point of interest that can be felt by both the informant and the investigator from the particular cultural perspective of each—emic to etic translation. Second, there is the process of learning to feel unfamiliar t-phones that are discernible but do not have specific t-phonemic meaning in the investigator's culture—emic assimilation. Third, there is the need to describe unfamiliar t-phones and t-phonemes that the researcher cannot learn to experience—emic description.

The most in-depth and authentic way to experience the t-phonemes of a genre is as a participant. This requires that the researcher learn the specific genre similar to the way a novice would. Chiropractic clinical training is a type of apprenticeship. The clinical instructor finds an area of diagnostic interest on the patient and has the student feel, and then describe, what has been found. Often the point is tender and the patient can therefore easily identify its location. The patient is instructed to tell the student when he or she is on the correct spot. I used this approach to locate the lesion or structure that the *hilot* was attempting to describe.

Because I was experienced in another touch genre, I was capable of learning faster than a genuine novice. Nevertheless, even an experienced palpator would find that learning all aspects of a new palpatory genre has its difficulties.

Where the investigative process simply required translation, (i.e., the t-phoneme as it was described by the informant has meaning for the researcher), the process was relatively straightforward. I am not suggesting that direct t-phoneme substitution was necessarily possible, as the science and the culture of the genre under investigation gives each t-phone a t-phoneme that is specific to the genre. Nevertheless, if a *hilot* describes what a chiropractor calls "spasming muscle" as being a "pinched blood vessel" (*naipit na ugat*), chiropractors have an emic reference point from which they can assume the presence of the underlying t-phone.

The second investigative issue is the instances where the informant described a t-phoneme for which no translatable chiropractic t-phoneme meaning exists. It was necessary to learn the meaning of the new t-phoneme and how to experience it. The t-phoneme was described in terms of the t-phonemes of the genre under investigation. Where possible, contrasting descriptions in relation to similar t-phonemes in the investigating genre were used.

It is possible to learn to experience just about any t-phoneme of an underlying t-phone, except where a t-phoneme is illusory. By this I mean where a meaning is placed on an object that cannot have noumenal referent—that is, one not demonstrable to others under agreed conditions. The obvious difficulty is in proving the unreality of such an object. This cannot be done directly, as it would be arrogant to assume one person's perception is effectively superior to another's. To address this conundrum I looked at objects that could not exist as they were described because they defied anatomy as we know it. This approach can also be accused of arrogance, assuming the superiority of one anatomical model over another. While biomedicine's clinical anatomy does not exhaust bodily reality, in the area of gross anatomy it is authoritative. I stand firmly on this point against extreme cultural relativists. For this reason I can challenge the location of *ugat* (felt by me as muscles and tendons), as these are within certain definable and predictable boundaries.

This brings me to the third investigative issue. When it is not possible to experience the t-phoneme as it is described by the informant, the t-phoneme can only be described from the emic perspective of the informant. Having established a methodology for cross-cultural investigation of touch perception, it is necessary to give the t-phonemes their respective cultural descriptions, in effect providing an account of the healing genre's account of itself.

To some extent, the following descriptions are distorting in that they only concentrate on aspects of the paradigms relevant to the delivery of manual therapy techniques. Chiropractic is an extension of biomedical thinking and as such involves not only esoteric chiropractic knowledge but also other biomedical knowledge. Equally, Roda's techniques exist within a framework of background knowledge involving the common belief systems of a variety of indigenous healers and, to a lesser extent, an indigenized version of biomedicine.

The Chiropractic Clinical Model

The founder of chiropractic, Daniel David Palmer, developed his healing art at the end of the nineteenth century. He postulated that the fundamental cause of disease was the chiropractic lesion or subluxation (Palmer 1910:505). For Palmer, the subluxation consisted of a joint "whose articular surfaces have lost in part their natural connection—one in which the articulating surfaces remain in partial contact," but no longer act in perfect concert (Palmer 1910:873).[2] In addition to this biomechanical component, he emphasized the impact of the subluxation on the nervous system. Palmer posited the presence of a vitalist capacity, "innate intelligence," that dwells in each of us, acting through the nervous system to ensure our well-being. He further claimed that innate intelligence was an individuated form of "universal intelligence," an intelligence that sets the laws of nature. Palmer claimed that the subluxation interferes with the normal vitalist role of innate intelligence by blocking its flow through the nervous system, particularly at the level of the intervertebral foramen.[3] This, he claimed, leads to a state of "dis-ease," a state in which the body operates at less than possible optimum due to poor integration. The purpose of chiropractic manipulation, from a traditional perspective, is to remove the subluxation, allowing for the resolution of disease.

At present, there is debate between chiropractors who hold to Palmer's original idea or some derivative of it, and those who have a mechanistic view of the body, seeing no need for any vitalist substance or presence (Coulter 1989, 1990, 1993). The former are advocates of a uniquely chiropractic area of study called "chiropractic philosophy," which is intent on maintaining Palmer's original ideas untarnished, and through these the broad scope of practice that Palmer originally claimed for the profession (Donahue 1986, 1987, 1989). By contrast, there are those who see chiropractors as back pain specialists. These practitioners deny the need for a vitalist concept, adopting something akin to the biomedical model of disease (Brantingham 1988; Donahue 1988).[4]

Irrespective of which camp one supports, the subluxation is seen as the lesion treated by chiropractic. While the emphasis has shifted from the malposition of vertebrae to their aberrant movement, the centrality of the subluxation to chiropractic practice has not significantly changed in over one hundred years. Nevertheless, the subluxation at the level of description remains an elusive entity. Gatterman (1995:7–9) identifies over one hundred synonyms for the subluxation, indicating the breadth of opinion concerning its true nature. The actual nature of the subluxation will remain a conundrum for yet some time. However, this does not paralyze chiropractic practice—suggesting that while the definition is a problem, locating the subluxation may not be quite so difficult. Two common techniques for doing this are motion and static palpation.

Motion palpation is, as the name suggests, a process for feeling the difference in range of motion between two vertebral segments. The process consists of the chiropractor feeling for a difference in movement in one direction and comparing it to movement in the opposite direction. The direction of least-perceivable movement is designated the direction of restriction, and, once this has been established, the chiropractor can "list" the vertebra. An example of a listing would be L2-PRS. This means the chiropractor has decided that the second lumbar vertebra (L2) is fixated in a (P)osterior position with (R)ight posterior rotation and right (S)uperior wedging. Studies have shown poor interexaminer reliability for this procedure (Panzer 1992:522). O'Malley (1998) argues that this is because the listing system is a cultural construct that unhelpfully imposes itself on the patient's lesion.

Static palpation—locating a subluxation by touch—is based on the assumption that a particular motor segment is restricted, having associated muscle spasm that gives it a distinctive palpable character. In a survey of chiropractors in the state of Victoria, Australia, Walker and Buchbinder (1997:585) found the most commonly used diagnostic measure for finding the subluxation is static palpation. Similar findings were reported by Strender et al. (1997). This is not surprising considering that the most reliable finding in terms of interexaminer verification has been practitioner-elicited tenderness—a key indicator in static palpation (Boline et al. 1993). This suggests that what the practitioner is feeling has a correlate within the patient. Static palpation is the method that Roda and I used to identify the character and location of our agreed upon lesions.

To summarize, the chiropractic lesion consists of restricted movement between two adjacent vertebra resulting in neurological consequences, one of which is associated localized palpable muscle spasm, the subject of static palpation. Roda, however, while identifying the same location of a lesion, has a totally different interpretation of what he is feeling, and of what must have transpired to establish the lesion.

The *Hilot* Clinical Model

Hilot interpret what I call spasming muscle fibers as damaged *ugat* within the muscle. Such *ugat* are engorged with *dugo* (blood), making them palpable. The *hilot* model makes no distinction between arteries and veins—both are simply *ugat*. Abnormal *ugat*—in that the blood having become either stagnant or too sluggish has ceased to flow correctly—are described as being *ipit*. Although they cannot always be translated this succinctly, *ipit* or *naipit* usually mean "caught" or "pinched." *Naipit* refers not so much to a process (the pinching of a blood vessel) as to the resultant reduced or blocked blood flow. The concept *naipit na ugat* underlies several important causes of *pilay*, musculoskeletal pain, which subtend the intentionality of *hilot* touch-perception and treatment. While *pilay* usually refers to musculoskeletal pain, it can also cause abdominal pain.

Based on etiology, I have divided *pilay* into two subgroups: *pilay* caused by cold (*pilay-hangin*), and *pilay* caused by trauma (*pilay sa mga buto*—*pilay* of the bones), and *pilay sa mga litid*[5] or *ugat* (*pilay* of blood vessels).

Pilay-hangin is caused by *lamig* (cold) entering the body and blocking blood flow. *Hangin* translates as "air" or "wind," but in *hilot* concepts of illness usually refer to the characteristic of air, particularly wind, of being cold. It achieves this by moving through the *ugat* (blood vessels), accumulating at certain points where it interferes with blood flow by causing the blood to thicken or the *ugat* to swell. Where *lamig* moves in *ugat* it does not present a problem. It is where *lamig* comes to rest that the patient experiences symptoms. Tan (1987:63) notes that "blood and the circulatory system seem to form a core concept in Filipino folk physiology, perhaps because blood is known to be distributed throughout the body and its loss is correlated with weakness and death." Tan (1987:64) reports the belief that blood thickens if exposed to too much heat or cold. Roda believes blood becomes sluggish when it is too cold, while heat has the opposite effect. When the *hilot* massage, it is usually to expel *lamig*. *Lamig*, though, is more than just the absence of warmth. *Lamig* shows characteristics of both quality and substance. The quality, *lamig*, is signified by the adjectival form, *malamig*. This is the quality an object exhibits when it feels cold to touch. The noun *lamig* encompasses the quality of coldness, but it also has characteristics that would suggest that it is substancelike. *Lamig* moves by translation, not conduction, entering the body attached to a carrier substance such as *hangin* (air) or *pawis* (sweat). In the *hilot's* understanding of the "pathogenicity" of *lamig*, it requires a portal of entry such as the pores of the skin, the mouth, and the vagina.

While the effects of *lamig* may accumulate over time, several informants were adamant that *lamig* itself also accumulates, losing none of its pernicious attributes. This is more characteristic of a substance than a quality. *Lamig* often detrimentally affects a target organ that can be some distance from the point of entry.

Lamig bears some resemblance to the biomedical concept of "opportunistic pathogen." Not everybody is susceptible at all times. Rather, a confluence of circumstances allows *lamig* to enter the body. The person's state of health, the condition of the portal of entry, the nature of the carrier substance and the person's behavior all impact on the question of susceptibility. A sweating person, for instance, is susceptible because the pores of the skin are open.

The idea of susceptibility is often linked to treatment. A patient who has undergone massage is susceptible, as the treatment opens the pores of the skin and temporarily traumatizes *ugat* and *laman* (muscle), making them more susceptible to *lamig*. This post-treatment concern for the patient is commonly linked with prohibitions on potentially dangerous activities. In particular, the patient must not be exposed to cold water because *lamig* will enter through the opened pores.

Roda's patients recognize the relationship between the environment, illness, and susceptibility, but this relationship is qualitatively different from the biomedical concept. "The Filipino emphasizes not the germs plus low resistance, but rather the correct timing (*tiyempo-tiyempo*) of the two most important elements in the development of low resistance—internal predisposition and external mitigating circumstances" (Himes 1971:42). *Pasma*, an illness caused by *lamig*, demonstrates this relationship. Predictably, the person is usually tired and/or hot (predisposition) when he or she makes the mistake of coming in contact with *lamig* (external circumstance). Because of the person's "weakened" state, *lamig* enters the body, affecting the muscles and joints. The resultant pain and dysfunction are the main symptoms of *pasma*.

The treatment of *lamig* is based on the particular *hilot's* view of the cause. Treatments that involve physical therapeutics are described by the general term *hilutin*. Just as the word "chiropractic" refers to chiropractic healing techniques such as massage and manipulation, so *hilutin* refers to the physical therapeutic healing techniques of the *hilot*; the two most common being massage and manipulation, used together or individually. While manipulation and massage are used by most *hilots* who treat *pilay* or *lamig*, the rationale for treatment is totally different from that of chiropractic. Roda's massage is not simply a process of making muscles more supple and relaxed, as is the case with chiropractic massage. Rather, it is a process of moving *lamig*, associated with a carrier substance such as *hangin* or *pawis*, to a location where it can be expelled from the body. Roda describes an abdominal massage technique where the *lamig* ends up in the *sikmura* (stomach). If this is not treated, the *lamig* and the *hangin* might *mabuo* (congeal) the blood. The *lamig* attached to *hangin* is moved by massage so that it can be expelled as flatus.

When massaging limbs, the *hilot* always massages away from the center of the body. *Lamig* is pushed to the periphery where it must be expelled. The *hilot* often follows this procedure with manipulation of the toes and fingers. The explanation for the sound, that *hilots* refer to as *lagutok* and chiropractors as an "osseous release," is that *lamig* escapes with a "pop" when the joint is suddenly tractioned. The relationship between this sound and pain relief is well-accepted.

I have described *pasma* and *pilay-hangin* because they are important causes of what I would describe as pain of musculoskeletal origin. Also, they are predicated on belief in a closed circulatory system, which has a distorting effect on *hilot* palpation. By demonstrating the distorting effect of the *hilot* clinical model on palpation, it is possible to speculate that chiropractic belief in motion palpation is similarly distorting.

The second type of *pilay*, that caused by trauma, has two subcategories; *pilay sa mga buto* (*pilay* of the bones), and *pilay sa mga litid* or *ugat* (*pilay* of blood vessels). *Pilay sa mga buto* is where *litid* and *ugat* close to joints are trapped between the *buto* (bones), stopping blood flow. This lesion is not that dissimilar to Palmer's original concept of the nerve root potentially being "squeezed or crushed" as it leaves the intervertebral foramen (Palmer 1910:295).

Roda explains that when a joint is sprained, the joint "opens up" at the instant of the sprain. The *litid* and *ugat* move into the space between the bones. When the bones return to their presprain position, the *ugat* or *litid* are trapped. This causes the swelling associated with such an injury. It is not necessarily the whole *ugat* that is caught; it may be just its *gilid* (wall). When the *ugat* is full of blood, it is easily pushed against the potential space between the bones. This type of *pilay* is treated by manipulation of the involved joints. Although this process can happen as a result of trauma, it can also occur in sleep. The potential space between the joints can open due to the relaxation of sleep; part of the wall then moves in. If the sleeper shifts position, the space closes, and the wall of the *ugat* is caught causing *pilay*. Chiropractic patients will often report a case of *torticollis* (wryneck) developing overnight. The patient goes to sleep feeling fine only to wake with a painful wryneck.

Ugat can become *ipit* between the cranial plates. In one case treated by Roda, the patient suffered a depression fracture of the vomer-maxilla (nasal and cheek bones) (diagnosed by doctors at the Philippine Orthopedic Hospital). Roda's treatment consisted of realigning the damaged bone that, in his opinion, was twisted, resulting in *naipit na ugat*. Before the bones could be realigned, Roda had to "remove the *ugat* that are *ipit* at the joints of those bones, the nasal bones." This was done by a light massage technique working away from the voma-maxillary suture. Any attempt to relocate the bones without first removing the *ugat* would fail. Roda explains, "If there's still *ugat* trapped, when you manipulate that, the bone won't be able to move back because there's still *ugat* inside." Once Roda had "manipulated" the area, the patient, who had been suffering for over a year, noted considerable relief.

Manipulation of the cranial plates is widely accepted in osteopathy and chiropractic. The technique used to treat the case described above was not dissimilar to an Applied Kinesiology (AK) cranial technique for vomer-maxilla. In the AK technique, the most common lesion is where the vomer-maxilla has "moved" medially and superiorly. This is corrected by tensioning the vomer-maxilla inferolaterally on the correct part of the breathing cycle. Chiropractic explanation for the success of cranial techniques is still not widely accepted beyond those who practice AK or Sacro-Occipital Technique (SOT). While skeptical about the theoretical explanation of AK and SOT cranial technique, as a practitioner who uses AK I know empirically that cranial techniques are very effective. Like the *hilot*, the chiropractor knows empirically that the technique works and, like the *hilot*, the chiropractor develops an explanation that, even if speculative, explains outcomes from one established perspective.

Roda's treatment for *pilay sa mga buto* consists of tracking along the course of the *ugat*, freeing them from joints. His usual method is to apply traction to the *ugat* or *litid* using digital pressure, such that when the joint opens it allows the *ugat* or *litid* to spring out. He uses the elasticity of the trapped *ugat* and *litid*. Once the *litid* or *ugat* are tensioned, he moves the joint through a range of motion so that it will open, facilitating the release of the trapped tissue. It is this process of tracing *ugat* from the center of the body to the periphery that exemplifies one aspect of the *hilot* model that distorts palpatory perception. Because of the circulatory system's perceived continuity, most *hilots* who treat *pilay* believe the system of *ugat* can be traced all over the body. Roda does not consider himself to be transferring from one hypertonic muscle to another.

The process is repeated until all the trapped *litid* and *ugat* are released. The freed *ugat* must be held off to one side like untangled yarn to ensure that, as the *buto* are moved around to free more *ugat*, those already released are not caught again. The *lagutok* that sometimes accompanies this technique is the sound made when the *ugat* is released. This is associated with relief, and the area will probably still have problems if it does not occur.

For some instances of *pilay sa mga buto*, the appropriate treatment is to manipulate the joint using an adjustive (manipulative) technique that involves a short lever, high velocity thrust, in effect, a chiropracticlike adjustive technique. This type of technique was of greatest interest to me not because it is a significant part of *hilot* technique, but because it is, at a functional level, indistinguishable from chiropractic technique.

In summary, the *hilot*, like the chiropractor, uses manipulation and massage to achieve the treatment outcome, but there are differences between their techniques. It is by exploring how these similarities and differences occur that we start to understand the relative roles of thematic and experiential knowledge in the development and application of technique. By examining the learning process we see how thematic knowledge becomes incorporated within perception.

The Origin of Technique

In addressing the question of perception, the German philosopher Martin Heidegger (1962:23) starts by describing our attitude to the world. He accepts a priori our existence in the world but feels that the philosophical tradition has failed to question the true nature of this "being." He is interested in how we comport ourselves to the world of our everyday being, a comportment he describes as a characteristic of our "everyday human existence." The concept of "everyday human existence" is captured in the German Dasein, which literally translates as "being there" (Waterhouse 1980). When Heidegger uses Dasein, this human existence has a number of important defining characteristics: "The best way to understand what Heidegger means by Dasein is to think of our term 'human being,' which can refer to a way of being that is characteristic of all people [or a group of people] or to a specific person—a human being" (Dreyfus 1991:14). It therefore incorporates the way of being of our institutions. Hence it is valid to talk about the Dasein of chiropractic, or the Dasein of *hilot*.[6] We can also talk of "a Dasein." Here we refer to the individual, for instance, Roda's Dasein.

The reason Dasein can be used in these two ways is because the person, a Dasein, does not develop in a social vacuum. It is through contact with another that Dasein develops from the neonate. Common influences in the development of the individual, such as chiropractic pedagogy or immersion within *hilot* healing culture, present as identifiable aspects of the individual's Dasein. Terms such as the "Dasein of chiropractic" refer to the collective presentation of the chiropractic aspect of the individual Daseins that constitute the chiropractic profession.

Dasein's importance to Heidegger is not in its "what it is," but rather in its "way of being." For instance, when we talk of the Dasein of chiropractic, what is important is not any definition of chiropractic, but rather how chiropractic as an institution or collective lived experience has a way of "being-in-the-world." Knowing how this "way-of-being" affects touch-perception in chiropractic diagnosis is a prerequisite to understanding chiropractic's efficacy as a healing art.

When watching Roda treat, one striking aspect of his action is the fluidity and purposefulness of his whole bodily attitude to the patient. This attitude will be the starting point of our investigation of the *hilot* learning process. In looking at his actions, I noted that most of the time they demonstrated what Dreyfus (1996) describes as the "flow" experienced by athletes. This type of activity comes from orientation to the task at hand, an orientation Heidegger defined as "for-the-sake-of-which." (Heidegger 1962:118–22) In Roda's case, it is something like the "cure of the patient's problem." But this application of the idea is too broad to address the question of the origin of Roda's "flow." The "for-the-sake-of-which" in the instant of his action happens at a far more immediate level. The fluidity of his movement depends on a harmony of perception and action that shows no perceivable breaks. This harmony gives the appearance of "flow."

Heidegger does not address the impact of neurophysiology on the process of purposeful interaction with the world, concentrating instead on the immediate existential apprehension of the world. In the example of our case study, action involves another—the patient. How can Roda's attitude to the patient best be described? Here, two ideas of Heidegger's are particularly illuminating: "readiness-to-hand" and "presence-at-hand" (Heidegger 1962:100–101, 117).

The things with which we have direct intercourse Heidegger calls "equipment" (Heidegger 1962:97).[7] This orientational definition stems from the fact that we do not normally approach "an object" (equipment) from the perspective of confusion, but with an ability to manipulate it for our own purposes. This gives us a special relationship to this equipment, which is characterized as being "in-order-to" (Heidegger 1962:97).

We use a fork "in-order-to" eat, a car "in-order-to" travel. A chiropractor massages muscles "in-order-to" achieve their relaxation and a *hilot* massages *ugat* "in-order-to" expel *lamig*. Equipment, and its utilitarian nature, does not exist in and of itself, but rather in relation to an environment of equipment. We deal with this environment in a state of circumspection. We tend not to think of a hammer as an object to be held by the handle with the business end pointing toward the nail so as to hit the nail. Rather, we just pick it up and hammer with no real concern for its being a hammer, or thought of how we will use it. The hammer carries with it a relationship suggesting its "in-order-to" hit-a-nail character. "Dealings with equipment subordinate themselves to the manifold assignments of the 'in-order-to'" (Heidegger 1962:98). Before we can use equipment it must first present itself to us as being "ready-to-hand" (Heidegger 1962:100).

When we enter a room, its books, furniture, and light switch are all "present-at-hand"; it is the "in-order-to" which changes their status from "present-at-hand" to "ready-to-hand." The light switch becomes "ready-to-hand" "in-order-to" turn on the light. Once this is achieved, it drops back to being "present-at-hand." This usage of equipment is carried out with an air of circumspection. We do not really take any notice of the light switch, we just use it. When using equipment, we are not thematically aware of its characteristics. It is this "everydayness" that characterizes our use of equipment. To understand how chiropractic's everyday coping differs from the *hilot*'s, we must examine the origin of the respective Daseins of chiropractor and *hilot*.

Only by growing and learning can the neonate develop into a Dasein. The child does not learn everyday coping by internalizing societal rules, but rather by experiencing them in the context of their implementation. This experimentation elicits responses from the child's world, which in turn mold a way of "being-in-the-world," a characteristic of Dasein.

Possibly the first meaningful contact with the world, that is, the first time a perception signifies in such a way that it can be understood thematically, is contact with the mother's breast. The child learns the "language of breast contact" in the process of purposeful thematic action. While breastfeeding is initially a reflexive process, the emotional input, especially from the mother, is usually present from the start. The child's reciprocated emotions are likely to be his or her first emotional contact with "the other." Heidegger talks of Dasein's "being with" others (Heidegger 1962:153–63). The developing Dasein learns to perceive the world, aware of the perspective of others who make up his or her immediate environment.

Whatever skills the *hilot* may have learned in apprenticeship or practice were learned after he or she internalized the skills of everyday coping Filipinos normally master as part of growing up. Therefore, prior to the *hilot* is the Filipino. Before the *hilot* first palpates a body with clinical intent, he or she has acquired a way of "being-in-the-world," a particular "Filipino" Dasein.

Hilot perception relating to illness includes the possibility of personalistic and naturalistic causes of illness (Tan 1987:19). These possibilities are part of the Dasein of everyday Filipino existence. The difference between *hilot* knowledge and patient (everyday Filipino) knowledge is one of depth, not breadth. Consider a biomedical equivalent. Almost everyone is aware that smoking causes heart disease. But trained health care practitioners with specialist knowledge are aware of the pathophysiology. Similarly, the pernicious effects of *lamig* are commonly accepted beliefs in Filipino culture, but it is the *hilot* who has in-depth knowledge of its exact mechanisms.

In addition to "explanatory knowledge," the knowledge used to give meaning to the practice of a healing tradition, both the chiropractor and *hilot* use "experiential knowledge." Explanatory knowledge can be characterized as the science of a healing tradition, the "know that," and experiential knowledge as the art, the "know how." This distinction was made by Wilhelm Dilthey of the German historical-cultural school (Ermarth 1978:255) and more recently by Paul Ricoeur (1981:145–64).

From our knowledge of the development of individual Dasein, it is clear that the novice of any clinical tradition carries a prepedagogical Dasein. Like that of the *hilot*, the "being there" of the prechiropractic Dasein is not just "being anywhere," but is the "thereness" particular to the would-be chiropractic student. Consequently, chiropractic perception has, a priori, the cultural background of the prechiropractic student as an integral part of its makeup. Background, and its effect on everyday coping, has to be considered in terms of its impact on two specific levels of understanding: that of thematic involvement, a corollary of assimilating the culture of the particular Dasein, including the "know how," and that of phenomenological involvement, developed through immersion in the task of the skill being learned. This distinction explains why the *hilot* and chiropractor can locate the same lesion and interpret it thematically in two distinct ways, yet deal with it in a manner appearing appropriate to each other at the phenomenological level.

Cultural healing knowledge, such as the relationship between *lamig* and injury, is thematic knowledge. It can exist independent of a knower. Thematic knowledge is collective and recorded knowledge used in reflecting, recording treatments, writing letters of referral, and in explaining to patients the nature of their problems. A Dasein comes to this knowledge by learning the values, history, religious beliefs, science, and the like of his or her culture. An example of the type of learning that leads to "know that" is formal classroom learning.

Whereas "know that"—the knowledge of thematic investigation—comes from a discursive or intellectual understanding of the culture, "know how" comes from an embodied experience of action within the context of specific knowledge. This leads to the development of perception and action skills that are both emergent from, and a priori, to everyday involvement with the world. This knowledge can be characterized as "know how." It includes the skills of massage and manipulation as applied by the *hilot* and the chiropractor.[8]

When I observe Roda, the flow in his treatment demonstrates "know how." When I talk to him I realize also that, in terms of *hilot* culture, he has the "know that" of expert *hilot* knowledge. Knowledge and action are not totally separate. When initially learning his art, Roda would have had to massage for the first time. Presumably, at this stage, he did not have any greater understanding of the "know how" of massage than most Filipinos with similar backgrounds. In this early stage of skill acquisition, Roda would have had to apply the "know that" of his clinical art to a situation, and attempt treatment with the preclinical "know how" of his everyday coping. Roda was apprenticed to a kinsperson who taught him the skill. Through this process of apprenticeship, the "know that" of *hilot* massage was replaced by the "know how," which became the more important guiding influence.

The difference between the application of "know that" and "know how" is the difference between thematic involvement and nonthematic, or existential, involvement. Most of what I observed when watching Roda treat demonstrated the "know how" of *hilot* practice in operation. Occasionally, however, Roda stopped, looked, and wondered. Here I saw evidence of the thematic creeping back into his treatment.

When Roda finds an interruption in his flow, he takes notice at the level of thematic involvement. However, his hands continue to move with the same automatic flow, only now to a new purpose, the identification of the interruption. Perception is always existential but would appear to be under the direction of thematic involvement. Initially, Roda's thematic involvement consists of making a diagnosis and deciding to massage on this basis. His diagnosis would be something like "this patient has *lamig* which has caused *ugat* to become *ipit*. This *lamig* must be expelled from the body." Other thematic knowledge is now applied, giving Roda his starting point for action. Having made purposeful contact with the patient, this thematic knowledge moves to the background and Roda simply massages—guided by the situation.

Similarly, the chiropractor, having decided what to massage, simply massages. But there is a difference between Roda's massage and that of a chiropractor. The chiropractor, while having an existential appreciation of the spasming muscle, is also thematically aware of its anatomical origin and insertion. This thematic knowledge influences the existential appreciation of the patient by providing an approximate location at which the end of the muscle should be located. It, in effect, provides a horizon for the existential knowledge. For Roda, the *ugat* are all continuous and interconnected. His massage moves smoothly from one muscle group to another, as though they were continuous rather than contiguous. Something similar happens with speech. In a study where a cough was substituted for a sound in otherwise normal speech, the listener inserted the sound that was replaced ("phonemic restoration"), reporting it to the investigator as being present (Warren 1970:392). Similarly, I found that where the anatomy interrupts *hilot* palpation, t-phonemic restoration takes place. It is unlikely that t-phonemic restoration is unique to *hilot* practice, but rather is a natural process that reflects the use of palpatory skills.

Roda selects a direction of massage from the center to the periphery. This is evidence of the influence of the thematic on the development of *hilot* Dasein. The chiropractor, on the other hand, believes that the best way to massage is from the

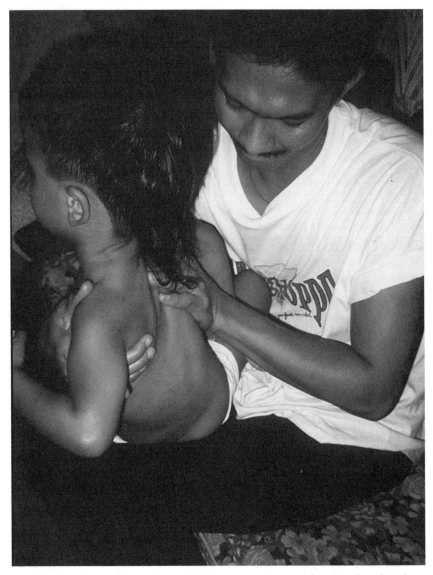

Figure 7.1.   Renato Roda adjusts a child using a sitting rotary technique. (Photo by John O'Malley.)

periphery to the center, as this aids the return of blood and lymph to the heart. The Dasein of chiropractic evolved with this thematic influence, affecting the choice of direction that, in time, "feels natural."

When attempting to massage as Roda does, I found it difficult to achieve flow massaging from the center to the periphery. Once I changed direction, flow returned. This suggests that how we learn is how we are most able to treat. When taught how to massage the back, I had already completed a course in spinal anatomy. Only after I had a firm view of the anatomy and, in particular, of the origin and insertion of the muscle concerned, did I begin to massage. I was instructed to massage from the peripheral end of the muscle to the proximal end, repeating this action while systematically moving across the muscle. When a trigger point was encountered as a slight "bumpiness" in the muscle, I was instructed to apply moderate pressure.[9] After much practice, this became the internalized "know how" of chiropractic massage. Any variation, such as massaging in the "wrong" direction or beyond the end of the muscle, does not fit in with the "know how" of chiropractic, forcing the practitioner to revert to thematic involvement, which is not the natural attitude of everydayness.

When first learning how to massage, Roda was told to trace *ugat* to the fingers or toes from whence the *lamig* could be expelled. When he massages, Roda is careful not to lose contact with the *ugat* he is following. He maintains digital contact most of the time, appearing not to notice the origin and insertion of muscles, an integral part of chiropractic massage. This results in Roda's "being-in-the-world" having a comportment that acknowledges *ugat's* continuity; it is a characteristic of his massage technique. It is clear that in developing his technique, Roda learned to emphasize some aspects of the patient's palpable anatomy and to largely ignore others.

What Roda and I located at the existential level was similar, to the extent that I could locate similar lesions and describe them using Roda's term for *ugat* caught between bones. Roda agreed with this description in each case. In Kantian terms, what we located through a tactile-based consensus could be described as indicative of a noumenal lesion of the patient, for which Roda and I had differing phenomenal interpretations. Yet we were not entirely in agreement about the lesion's existential nature. I would identify the lesion as being local, having set boundaries. Roda, on the other hand, would trace the *ugat* involved to distant locations. When asked about the possibility of restricted spinal joint motion, he simply did not understand the question. When I indicated to him that I could detect less movement in the "involved" vertebra, he said this was because of the trapped *ugat*. Even when Roda agreed with my interpretation, he applied his own etiology.

Roda's perception of the patient shows that the way *hilot* Dasein develops is influenced by the "know that" of *hilot* cultural knowledge to the extent that the "know how" reflects this knowledge.[10] Chiropractic would argue that Roda's perception of *ugat* continuity is an illusion stemming from the existential application of his clinical model. However this raises the question: Might not the chiropractor's Dasein construct and unhelpfully distort his/her perception of the body?[11]

We can see how thematic knowledge can infiltrate the process of perception, but the picture is not yet complete. We must still explore how experiential knowledge is dependent on the morphology of the patient.

Why Roda and I Can Locate the Same Lesion

The thoracic spine is one of the easiest locations on which to find evidence of subluxations by static palpation. Lesions are usually associated with a transverse process or rib head and have a prominence that makes them easily distinguishable from adjacent tissue.

I located several examples of these lesions and asked Roda to describe them. In each case the description was that of *pilay sa mga buto*—*pilay* of the bones—a subgroup of *naipit na ugat*. I also found benign transverse processes and asked him if he could locate a problem. He could not. This exercise was repeated on a second patient, only this time I was asked to describe what Roda located. It was clear by the end of this exercise that both of us could find the same type of lesion by static palpation, and that both of us saw it as important.[12]

Roda and I both found the lesion because it existed in the patient. Any practitioner who uses palpation to locate the cause of back pain, and manipulation to treat it, will have come across this type of phenomenon at some stage as being "ready-to-hand" for treatment. Prior to clinical models are patients with problems. Healing modalities evolve the "know how" to resolve these problems, finding by empirical methods what works and what does not. This "know how" is then rationalized within the "know that" of the culture of the healing modality. In the case of the *hilot*, humoral pathologies of hot and cold lead to the problem's explanation with reference to *naipit na ugat*.

Daniel David Palmer took the "know how" of bonesetting and gave it an updated "know that," which was rational and plausible in relation to the knowledge of his time. Palmer (1910:908) claimed to be the first to use short lever spinous contact in combination with dynamic thrust for the treatment of the spine. While I do not challenge the sincerity of his belief, I suspect that he primarily compared his method to osteopathy, extrapolating his findings to all forms of manipulation (Palmer 1910:139–45). In Santa Mesa I found several practitioners who, having no history of contact with chiropractic, also used short lever spinous contact in combination with dynamic thrust to resolve back pain; Renato Roda is one of these practitioners. It is likely that skills similar to the "know how" of the Dasein of chiropractic exist in many societies with a "know that" reflecting local concepts of etiology.[13]

Merleau-Ponty offers further insight into why it is that both Roda and I can locate phenomenally similar lesions. The main thesis of Merleau-Ponty's seminal work *The Phenomenology of Perception* (1962) is that aspects of perception are neither purely mental nor purely physical. Rather, perception is a product of both the mind and morphology working in concert. For Merleau-Ponty, the mind includes what Heidegger describes as background with morphology being the body. Roda and I have differing backgrounds, yet our backgrounds contain major similarities that cannot be dismissed. For example, we are, functionally speaking, physically identical. We are the same height, of similar build, and both treat with the hands. Merleau-Ponty sheds light on this morphological aspect of our capacity to perceive. The lesion I feel is a thing to be perceived by my body through my hands in the same way a painting is a thing to be perceived through the eyes, or an orchestral piece is perceived through the ears. These apparatuses determine both the limit of my ability and the bodily attitude necessary to maximize my perception. The physical limits to perception are obvious. I can see neither the infrared aspects of the painting, nor hear the ultrasonic sounds of the violin, not because they do not exist, but because they are outside the functional range of my perceptual apparatus. The bodily attitude, however, needs some exploration.

The object of examination determines the distance and orientation of the viewer. A diamond is best looked at through a magnifying lens. A mountain range only shows its full splendor when its extent can be taken into account from an appropriate distance and orientation. We see, then, that the object demands the correct attitude from the observer. Merleau-Ponty describes this demand as a tension between too much or too little of an attitude toward the object. This tension is alleviated when we achieve equilibrium between options, resulting in the maximum view. "The distance between me and the object is not a size which increases or decreases, but a tension which fluctuates round a norm. An oblique position of the object in relation to me is not measured by the angle which it forms with the plane of my face, but is felt as a lack of balance, as an unequal distribution of its influences upon me" (Merleau-Ponty 1962:302).

Similarly with the object of touch, there is tension between the options of the various attitudes we can take to the object. Only the correct attitude creates a feeling of confident interaction with the object. With the object of touch, it is pressure and area of contact, not distance and orientation, that are important. Roda and I apply similar pressure when feeling the lesion. We use the same sweeping movement with similar amplitude to feel the object's dimensions and texture. Too much pressure obliterates the nuances of the palpable lesion while too little fails to demonstrate the contrasts indicative of the lesion's character. There are some differences in our respective methods, but these appear to be superficial. The key elements of competent manipulation are found in the technique of both practitioners, and relate to such things as depth of thrust, timing, and thrust vector. The correct pressure and amplitude reflect how application of the innate and developed capacities of the perceptual apparatus are invoked by the nature of the lesion. Were it another type of lesion, such as muscle spasm (*naipit na ugat*), different pressure and movement would be needed to exhibit the lesion's qualities.

The capacity of the perceptual apparatus is ultimately set by the morphology of the perceiver. A dog's sense of smell is keener than a person's. A hawk can see further. A bat can hear higher frequencies. In each case, this is because the apparatus is morphologically highly specialized for a specific purpose. Even so, in addition to the morphology of the apparatus, perception is also dependent on the skill of the observer. An orchestral conductor would normally have a better perception of pitch and beat than a bus driver. A gymnast would normally have a more refined sense of body position than a chess player. A chiropractor or *hilot* would normally have a better sense of palpation than a bricklayer.

In each case, the owner of the apparatus of perception, having developed the Dasein of their particular skill, performs at a level of competence higher than that of the general public. This skill presents itself in the atheoretical, but not disinterested, way with which we concern ourselves with the world.

The presentation of the skill is purely existential, not intellectual; consequently, the perceptions that emerge from its application are not so much deduced, but simply known. This existential capacity is the result of repeated exposure to objects similar to the one of interest. The body then has internalized the correct attitude to gain maximum access to the object. When looking for the object, the whole sensory apparatus orients itself toward the possibility of perceiving the object. In acknowledging the possibility that the object will be perceived, we accept the actuality of the noumenal, even if it is inaccessible.[14]

The problem with the noumenal is that even if we could describe it, it is descriptively inexhaustible and infinitely divisible in itself. Only an act of mind of the perceiver can bracket off what is important and generate a phenomenal representation. Even though we can never have access to the noumenal in any absolute sense, we can infer its existence from the coincidental nature of our phenomenal descriptions. Accordingly, the object of perception in the case of Roda's *pilay sa mga buto* and my statically palpated subluxation are probably noumenally the same. We both innately know the correct orientation to the object, and, as such, can easily find it.

Why Roda and I Have Similar Technique

Although the contention might be unpalatable to most chiropractors, it is unlikely that there is much difference between the manipulative ability of the skilled chiropractor, osteopath, physical therapist, medical manipulator, or *hilot*. The key element they have in common is skill, and skill is the corollary of experience. It would appear that manipulative styles, in their application to the same parts of the body, have a lot in common, irrespective of belief.

The mastering of these attributes of competent manipulation is synthesized in what Merleau-Ponty refers to as "maximal grip" (Dreyfus 1996). Before reading on, pick up a pen so as to read the writing on the barrel. Note how you are holding it. I am right-handed, so I hold it in my right hand, between the thumb, index, and middle fingers approximately twenty-five centimeters from my eyes. All right-handed people I have asked to try this experiment hold a pen this way. We hold things in a way to attain maximum grip (Dreyfus 1996:16). Maximum grip is not the most powerful grip we might apply to an object, but one that gives the most access to it for the purposes intended. It is a result of body/mind acting with intentionality, being in this case to read the writing on the pen.

Dreyfus takes Merleau-Ponty's idea of the "I can," emphasizing that, at its most basic level, this is not a goal-directed mental state, but "simply the body's ability to reduce tension or, to put it another way, to complete gestalts" (Dreyfus 1996). This automatic orientation to the task at hand is goal-directed only at the higher thematic level. I contend that every manipulator will have at some stage experienced that preadjustive state where the situation feels "just right" for a good adjustment. This is the time to "just do it." Most will also have experienced the opposite, where there is still "tension" that should be relieved prior to proceeding. All chiropractors with whom I have discussed this agree that, in the moment just prior to the committal thrust, they know with almost total certainty whether the procedure will succeed. The feeling of it being "just right" is something I have also discussed with Roda. No description can do justice to this experience, as it is a purely existential state. However, the concept of maximum grip explains why this feeling is common to both of us.

The "just right" feeling, the symphonic interaction between the practitioner and patient, is predicated on the morphology of the practitioner and the morphology of the lesion joined existentially in the correct attitude of both participants. The practitioner guides this tactile conversation, and with "know how" directs the interaction to a successful outcome. Given that the practitioners are morphologically similar, and that they are addressing similar lesions, it follows that the "know how" that completes the equation must, irrespective of healing genre, also be similar. This is why Roda and I, and all competent manipulators, show similar maximal grip, the existential state that underlies competent technique.

Conclusion

In the moment of therapeutic intervention, chiropractic and *hilot* lesions can be characterized as being what their respective practitioners experience them to be. In this instant, the rationale—or science—is irrelevant. It is the art, the embodied Dasein of chiropractic or *hilot*, that is the determinant of success. Whether the treatment is massage of a muscle, *litid*, or *ugat*, or the manipulation of a joint to increase mobility or to free trapped *ugat*, the therapeutic act is conceived and justified thematically, but applied existentially. The actual event is decided in an instant by the practitioner based on a myriad of existential factors. The state of relaxation of the patient, the feeling of tension in the muscles, the slipperiness of the skin, and the internal perception of the practitioner of his or her own body all interact, giving rise to the circumstances leading to the habituation of action resulting in the healing event or process.[15]

While not explicitly influencing the perception of the practitioner, it impacts the practitioner's Dasein to the degree that "science" is involved. In the history of any health culture that recognizes a lesion similar to the chiropractic lesion, the phenomenal lesion must logically exist prior to its rationalization. The demand for the rationale is generated by the healing tradition's need to explain the lesion. The apprehended lesion is discursively constructed by members of the healing genre in such a way as to make it fit a plausible model—in the case of *hilot*, its relating to blood flow, in the case of chiropractic, an ability to be listed.

Interaction is a two-way process. In formal professions like chiropractic, the model influences the a priori assumptions with which the embryonic Dasein of the chiropractor first approaches the task of skill acquisition. Chiropractic perception of motion in joints may simply be a result of the impact of the clinical model. The demarcation between conceptualization and perception is never entirely clear, as perception is already either an incipient kind of conceptualization or a basis for it. Roda's perception of the continuity of *ugat* demonstrates that these a priori assumptions are ingrained in his Dasein. In the case of the *hilot*, where there is no formal pedagogy, the model is carried within the culture of practitioners through which it influences the process of skill acquisition.

Unlike the science (the "know that"), the art (the "know how") does not exist independently of the practitioner. It is particular to the individual practitioner's skill and circumstances. As such, it cannot be understood solely in terms of universalist categories. It is embedded in the practitioner's phenomenological ability to define and treat the patient's problem. It is the result of the practitioner's cumulative experience, and while there may be broad similarities in learning and the repertoire of techniques, the use of skills will be differentially ordered and applied in each treatment situation. In effect, each treatment of a patient is a work of art.

Notes

1. Dreyfus correctly credits the concept of "maximum grip" to Merleau-Ponty, but it would appear it is Dreyfus who actually coined the phrase.

2. Although Palmer did advocate the manipulation of peripheral joints (joints located in the limbs), he is usually referring to spinal joints when he speaks of subluxation.

3. Palmer's philosophy is a mix of theology, philosophy, and conjecture. He identifies four separate components that, in conjunction with the body, make up the life process—universal intelligence, innate intelligence, mind, and soul. He was clearly a dualist, yet his dualism saw the relationship between mind and body to be one of total interaction.

4. Medicine claims its practice to be superior because it is purportedly based on scientific knowledge. From this position it has acted to marginalize chiropractic (Willis 1989:164–65). This isolation is in no small part a motive for the push toward a more "scientifically" acceptable approach (Borregard 1991:151).

5. Roda often uses the term *litid*, which normally translates as ligaments or tendons to refer to a significant case of *naipit na ugat*. This is not to say that he does not also understand that there are ligaments and tendons throughout the body, but rather that the ones he is referring to are now significant because the blood vessels within them are *naipit*, or blocked, causing swelling and pain. The term is also used by Roda to describe what I would describe as large or significant areas of spasming muscle. To both of us, such muscles feel similar to the palpable ligaments and tendons.

6. The term "Dasein of chiropractic" assumes certain commonly held beliefs and skills that are found in most chiropractors, even though there are many strains of chiropractic. The term as it is used here refers to chiropractors who use static or motion palpation as diagnostic tools, and who treat the full spine but not necessarily only the spine.

7. To the extent that we objectify people for the purposes of manipulation, they become "equipment." This objectification is not necessarily wrong. For example, control of others in certain medical circumstances is important for safety reasons.

8. "A movement is learned when the body has understood it, that is, when it is incorporated into its world, and to move one's body is to aim it at things through it; it is to allow oneself to respond to their call" (Merleau Ponty 1962:139).

9. Trigger points are "small palpable nodules within soft tissues that when pressed on or otherwise stimulated cause a marked pain response by the patient" (Meeker 1992).

10. Leeper (1935) suggests that the effect of one clue influences what we find next. Thus, finding one part of the subluxation or *naipit na ugat* tends to orient the practitioner to the possibility of what would be predicted by the "know that" of the healing discipline.

11. The very point of Kant's noumena and phenomena is to demonstrate that all perception is distortion to some degree. The extent of this distortion is always a problem for us. Consequently, we can only talk of distortion as a relative concept relating to our personal idea of correctness, or in the case of a profession, our commonly held, theoretical concept of correctness.

12. The difficulty with presenting this argument is that it is impossible to determine what the other person feels existentially. Therefore, any claim to feeling the "same" lesion can only be based on the coincidence of our mutual discovery of it and the extent of our common description.

13. Schiötz and Cyriax (1975:5–27) give numerous examples of spinal manipulation across a plethora of cultures ranging from ancient Greece to China and the Pacific Islands.

In several cases, the technique involved some form of identification of a specific lesion and direct thrust to reduce it.

14. Alternatively, we are forced to collapse all reality into pure idealism, a form of perceptual solipsism.

15. In this situation, Dasein is also the continual flux between thematic knowledge and experience of the actual event at hand. That is, learning is a continual process, so that the healing act becomes teaching in the hermeneutic sense.

References

Boline, P. D., M. Hass, J. J. Meyer, K. Kassak, C. Nelson, and J. C. Keating
1993 Interexaminer Reliability of Eight Evaluation Dimensions of Lumbar Segmental Abnormality: Part II. *Journal of Manipulative and Physiological Therapeutics* 16(6):363–74.

Borregard, P.E.
1991 Belief in Science and Medicine. *Journal of Manipulative and Physiological Therapeutics* 14(2):151.

Brantingham, J. W.
1988 A Critical Look at the Subluxation Hypothesis. *Journal of Manipulative and Physiological Therapeutics* 11:130–32.

Coulter, I. D.
1989 The Chiropractic Wars or the Enemy Within. *American Journal of Chiropractic Medicine* 2(2):64–66.
1990 Of Clouds and Clocks and Chiropractors: Towards a Theory of Irrationality. *American Journal of Chiropractic Medicine* 3(2):84–92.
1993 Alternative Philosophical and Investigatory Paradigms for Chiropractic. *Journal of Manipulative and Physiological Therapeutics* 16(6):419.

Donahue, J. H.
1986 D. D. Palmer and Innate Intelligence: Development, Division, and Derision. *Chiropractic History* 6:31–36.
1987 D. D. Palmer and the Metaphysical Movement. *Chiropractic History* 7(1):23–27.
1988 Disease in Our Principles. The Case against Innate Intelligence. *American Journal of Chiropractic Medicine* 1:86–88.
1989 A Proposal for the Development of a Contemporary Philosophy of Chiropractic. *American Journal of Chiropractic Medicine* 2(2):51–53.

Dreyfus, H. L.
1991 *Being in the World: A Commentary on Heidegger's Being and Time, Division I.* Cambridge, Mass.: The MIT Press.

Dreyfus, H. L.
1996 The Current Relevance of Merleau-Ponty's Phenomenology of Embodiment. *The Electronic Journal of Analytical Philosophy.* Spring (4) 1996. http://hci.stanford.edu/cs378/reading/dreyfus-embodiment.htm (accessed May 4, 2004).

Ermarth, M.
  1978 *Wilhelm Dilthey: The Critique of Historical Reason.* Chicago, Ill.: University of Chicago Press.
Gatterman, M.
  1995 *Foundation of Chiropractic Subluxation.* St. Louis, Mo.: Mosby.
Hawkes, T.
  1977 *Structuralism and Semiotics.* London: Methuen & Co. Ltd.
Heidegger, M.
  1962 *Being and Time.* Trans. J. Macquarie and E. Robinson. London: SCM Press Ltd.
Himes, R. S.
  1971 Tagalog Concepts of Causality: Disease. In *Modernization: Its Impact in the Philippines* V. IPC papers No. 10. Eds. F. Lynch and A. de Guzman. Quezon City: Ateneo de Manila University Press.
Jocano, F. L.
  1973 *Folk Medicine in a Philippine Municipality.* Manila: National Museum.
Leeper, R. W.
  1935 A Study of a Neglected Portion of the Field of Learning—The Development of Sensory Organisation. *Journal of Genetic Psychology* 46:41–75.
Mackie, F.
  1985 *The Status of Everyday Life: A Sociological Excavation of the Prevailing Framework of Perception.* New York: Routledge.
Meeker, W. C.
  1992 Soft Tissue and Non-Force Techniques. Pp. 519–31 in S. Haldeman, ed. *Principles and Practice of Chiropractic.* 2d ed. Norwalk, Conn.: Appleton & Lange.
Merleau-Ponty, M.
  1962 *Phenomenology of Perception.* New York: Routledge.
O'Malley, J. N.
  1998 The Impact of the Subluxation Model on Perception: A Cross-Cultural Study of *Hilot* and Chiropractic. PhD thesis. Royal Melbourne Institute of Technology.
Palmer, D. D.
  1910 *The Science, Art, and Philosophy of Chiropractic.* Portland: Portland Printing House Company.
Panzer, D. M.
  1992 The Reliability of Lumbar Motion Palpation. *Journal of Manipulative and Physiological Therapeutics* 15(8):518–24.
Ricoeur, P., ed.
  1981 Explanation and Understanding. Pp. 145–64 in P. Ricoeur, ed. *Hermeneutics and the Human Sciences.* Cambridge, England: Cambridge University Press.
Schiötz, E., and Cyriax, J.
  1975 *Manipulation Past and Present.* London: William Heinemann Medical Books.
Snell, R. S.
  1980 *Clinical Neuroanatomy for Medical Students.* Boston, Mass.: Little, Brown and Company.

Strender, L. E., M. Lundin, and K. Nell
    1997 Interexaminer Reliability in Physical Examination of the Neck. *Journal of Manipulative and Physiological Therapeutics* 20(8):516–20.
Tan, M. L.
    1987 *Usug, Kulam, Pasma: Traditional Concepts of Health and Illness in the Philippines.* Quezon City: Alay Kapwa Kilusang Pangkalusugan (AKAP).
Walker, B. F., and R. Buchbinder
    1997 Most Commonly Used Methods of Detecting the Spinal Subluxation and the Preferred Term for Its Description: A Survey of Chiropractors in Victoria, Australia. *Journal of Manipulative and Physiological Therapeutics* 20(9):583–89.
Warren, R. M.
    1970 Perceptual Restoration of Missing Speech Sounds. *Science* 167: 392–93.
Waterhouse, R.
    1980 Heidegger's "Being and Time." *Radical Philosophy* 26:29–35.
Willis, E.
    1989 *Medical Dominance* 2d ed. St. Leonards: Allen & Unwin Australia Pty. Ltd.

Two Ethnographers and One Bonesetter in Bali

8

ROBERT ANDERSON AND NORMAN KLEIN

THIS CHAPTER CONCERNS AN EPISODE in the friendship and collaboration of two medical anthropologists, Norman Klein and Bob Anderson. Long after we first met as anthropologists with shared interests in alternative medicine, and more by coincidence than by design, we each temporarily detoured in midcareer from our work as professors by becoming chiropractors in order to study them. By going completely native, we were carrying participant observation to an absurd extreme, given that academicians keep busy enough without miring down in a world of scheduled patients, licenses to practice, malpractice insurance, and annual continuing education requirements. But this we did, and neither of us has any regrets. Independently of one another, we found that our added-on chiropractic training equipped us to better document bonesetters in different parts of the world—a bonesetter being defined as a body worker who does soft tissue work such as massage, but who also engages in joint manipulation, the signature modality of chiropractors (see Huber and Anderson 1996:31).

The Paradox of Discordant Cultural Constructions

The episode in question began in 1996 when Klein used a sabbatical leave to undertake fieldwork in Bali that included interviewing and observing a bonesetter (Balinese, *balian uat*). He published his findings in the form of a video documentary, *The Balian of Klungkung*. Two years later, Anderson unexpectedly discovered that he would be able to visit Bali for a couple of weeks and asked Klein if he would mind putting him in touch with the *balian* of Klungkung, which Klein was happy to do. Subsequently, in 1998 Anderson presented his findings on the same bonesetter with whom Klein had worked in a video documentary entitled *Bonesetters in Bali*.

Viewing the two videos, one might think that we had studied two entirely different men. Needless to say, we do not assume that a single informant can be taken to represent a culture *en toto*, Margaret Mead to the contrary (1953:44). Our versions are as different, the one from the other, as was Robert Redfield's (1930) vision of the Mexican community of Tepoztlán from that of Oscar Lewis (1951), the first and still most notorious example of how two anthropologists employing the same supposedly objective, dispassionate methods of field ethnography in the end wrote totally different descriptions of a single culture. It is thought that this discrepancy in part derived from the passage of two decades between the studies, and the fact that when Redfield lived in Tepoztlán, the community had just reactivated an old tradition of communal cooperation, which had again become defunct by the time Lewis arrived. Differences in temperament and personal ideology are also thought to have enhanced the contrast of their ethnographic accounts.

The confrontation between Redfield and Lewis may have been the first case of mutually incompatible ethnographic interpretations, but it was certainly not the last. In fact, disparate cultural constructions are more the rule than the exception whenever restudies are carried out. As we write, the anthropological profession is struggling with an attack on the integrity of several researchers who have worked in the Amazon rain forest among the Yanomami. The controversy stems in part from Napoleon Chagnon's characterization of these people as "fierce" and given to mayhem and murder, as contrasted with Kenneth Good's insistence that they are gentle, nurturing, and kind (Chagnon 1983; Good and Chanoff 1991). Chagnon and Good started out as friends but ended up in a hateful standoff, each accusing the other of malfeasance and ineptitude. Fortunately, Klein and Anderson remain close friends, and we see our different videos as stimulating and provocative without looking for one to be correct and good while the other is villainous and inept. We feel we can learn more about the bonesetter and about the nature of ethnographic inquiry by trying to understand how we arrived at such contrasting characterizations. To that end, in the next two sections we present the commentaries that informed our documentaries, after which we will discuss how the two divergent narratives can be reconciled. The spoken commentaries have been slightly edited for clarity and ease of reading. Our intent, however, is to preserve the verbal accounts without substantial change in order that the reader can see exactly how different our descriptions are.

The Narration from *The Balian of Klungkung,* by Norman Klein

Bali is an island enclave of approximately three million Hindus amidst the more than nine hundred inhabited islands that comprise the predominantly Moslem country of Indonesia. It is a land of contrasts where, for example, rice and tourism are primary economic forces. And despite the continuing growth of tourism (millions come each year) and all the money and business it generates, the people continue to maintain their special religion-based traditions as nowhere else.

Bali is a land of ceremony where the forces of the world must be kept in balance, where mountains are especially holy places and the sea is the place to purify the village and its gods. This is seen in the *Melasti* ceremony, which serves to restore the balance of good and evil on the day before *Nyepi*, which begins the new year.

Life in Bali consists of a constant mediation between the world of the tangible and visible, and the world of the intangible or hidden. There is the realm of darkness and mystical activity, which is difficult to understand, and the realm of light, which relates to everyday life. An illness will be viewed as having both these tangible and more opaque and mystical qualities. It is the *balian* who can move safely in both worlds and who can deal with both the spiritual and physical needs of a patient (Eiseman 1990:135).

In 1979, while the current *balian* of Klungkung's father (then the *balian*) was away from the house, a man with a broken leg came. The son asked him to come back when his father returned, but the man refused to leave and demanded treatment. After his initial reluctance, the young man, who was not yet a *balian*, relented and treated the man. For the second treatment, his father accompanied him to the man's house. At the third visit, the man and his house had disappeared without a trace and seemed never to have existed. It was decided that it had all been a test and that the man was, in fact, a spirit. So it was that this young man had become the *Balian* of Klungkung. The *balian* is a traditional healer who may address a wide variety of problems. Most often they also specialize, for example, as bonesetters (*balian tuleng*), mediums (*balian taksu*), healers whose power is based on possession of *lontar* texts (*balian usada*), and those who emphasize massage in their practice (*balian uat*) (Connor, Asch, and Asch 1986:24; Eiseman 1990:137–41).

We are observing the *balian* of Klungkung as he functions as a *balian uat*. In this scene, we see a patient who five days earlier suffered a shoulder injury lifting a heavy load, and he was unable to raise his arm above shoulder height. He is being treated with a combination of balms, massage, reflexology, and manipulation. Following this treatment, he exhibits a full range of motion in his shoulder. He also damaged his knee playing basketball ten years ago and is receiving treatment for that injury.

It is believed that all parts of the body are connected by channels called *uat*. These structures may be identified as blood vessels, nerves, tendons, or muscles. But they do not need to accord exactly with the Western concept of anatomy (Connor, Asch, and Asch 1986:188). They transmit not only tangible fluids,

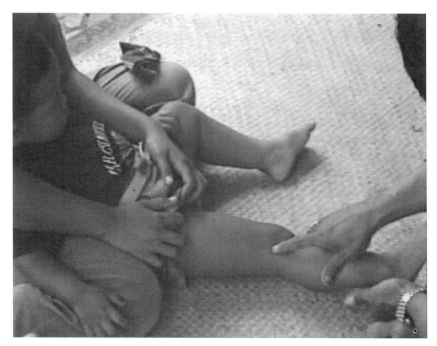

Figure 8.1.   The *balian* pointing out a child's "crossed *uat*," a traditional diagnosis. (Photo by Norman Klein.)

chemicals, and impulses, but also spiritual essences and the mystical life force. Others may perform massage, but only the *balian* can combine the two worlds of the sacred and the secular.

The *balian* of Klungkung has never stopped the learning process. Since becoming a *balian*, in addition to learning from his father, he has been influenced by several traditions as suggested by the books on reflexology and acupuncture seen here, and these and other principles are regularly applied.

Several weeks earlier, I had suffered a severe knee injury while in Singapore and was afforded the opportunity to have the *balian* treat me. Before employing massage, acupressure, and a chiropracticlike manipulation, the *balian* palpated and then performed a quite proper orthopedic test on my right knee.

The connecting channels, or *uat*, must flow freely and smoothly. *Uat* may be damaged in many ways ranging from spiritual to structural. Also, the damage may be variably characterized as, for example, stiff, frozen, knotted, or crossed. Depending on the source of the problem and its manifestation, resolution may involve manual as well as spiritual intervention.

In this next scene we see a child who had twisted his right ankle three days ago and is unable or unwilling to walk. The *balian* states that the child's problem is that

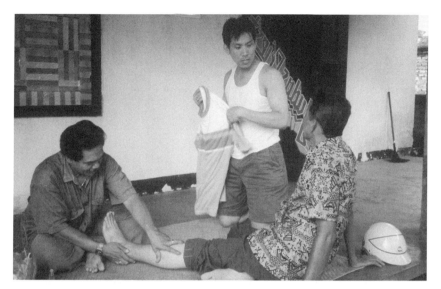

Figure 8.2.   A young man getting his injured ankle treated by the *balian*. (Photo by Elliott Oring.)

the *uat* are crossed and once that is corrected, the baby will be fine. After the treatment, the child appears to walk without hesitation.

Once every year in the 210-day calendar cycle on the day dedicated to Saraswati, the goddess of learning, science, literature, and wisdom, former patients come to the house of the *balian* of Klungkung and make offerings at the shrine to honor the spirit that allowed for their cure.

There are other health professionals and facilities available to the Balinese people. There are herbalists, acupuncturists, clinics, and medical doctors. There are also new practitioners drawn from the ranks of recently arrived expatriot foreigners. There are art therapists, expressive therapists, all manner of "new age" practitioners, and psychologists. There are now two chiropractors in Bali.

Even with the growing availability of alternative practitioners, it would appear that the place of the *balian* in Balinese society is secure. The requirement to contend with the spiritual side in effecting a cure, let alone for dealing with daily life and decisions, persists, and it is the *balian* who is best able to satisfy these wide-ranging needs of the community.

The Narration from *Bonesetters in Bali,* by Robert Anderson

Bali. Land of enchantment. Of gods, spirits, and ghosts. Of priests, shamans, witches, and sorcerers. Of supernaturalism. But also of naturalism. Of down-to-earth, get-the-job-done pragmatism. Of people solving problems of daily life in straight-forward, nonsupernatural ways.

My name is Bob Anderson. I'm an anthropologist. I'm also a medical doctor and a doctor of chiropractic. Coming out of that background of training and experience, I offer here a perspective on two characteristics of the anthropological literature relating to disease and health practices in different parts of the world.

First, anthropologists tend to describe kinds of diagnoses and treatments that are exotic and supernatural, to the virtual exclusion of naturalistic methods more akin to what we do in Western medicine. As a corrective to that tendency, I will share my experience with a kind of body worker in Bali known as a *balian uat* or *balian apun*, whose theory of treatment as applied on a daily basis is almost entirely naturalistic, comparable to that of a chiropractor, osteopath, or physical therapist.

Second, insofar as anthropologists do describe naturalistic healing, they tend not to examine whether the treatments do no harm and are beneficial in treating diseases when, in my experience, all pragmatic therapies need to be carefully evaluated because they may well be useless or even hurtful, as opposed to being valuable for psychological or social reasons, which is a very different matter.

To this end, I report here on a simple experiment in which I arranged for each of three bonesetters to treat me for the low back pain that I acquired after spending thirty hours on airplanes and in vehicles and airports while traveling from California to Indonesia.

One is the *balian* of Klungkung, whom I got to know through the ethnographic fieldwork of Norman Klein, a fellow anthropologist and chiropractic doctor who featured this *balian* in a documentary called *The Balian of Klungkung*. The second is the *balian* of Bangli, assisted by his apprentice. The third is the *balian* of Batu Bulan, the oldest and most experienced of the three.

I do not know how other bonesetters in Bali treat back pain, except to say that a fourth *balian* known as Jero Tapakan works in a different way from these three and would need to be independently evaluated. We know her work from an ethnographic film (produced by Timothy Asch, Linda Connor, and Patsy Asch in 1982).

In my experiment, I asked each bonesetter to treat me for pain in the lowest part of my spine, pointing specifically to the sacroiliac joints and explaining that it began a few days earlier as a result of a long flight to Bali.

The first discovery of note was that each of the three proceeded immediately to provide treatment, asking no questions about the nature and history of my pain and neglecting completely to examine me for limitations of movement or positions that result in pain. My self-diagnosis sufficed for them to conclude that my pain resulted from a blockage of channels or ducts in my body known as *uat*. What *uat* are is very unclear, except to say that they are not nerves, arteries, veins, or lymphatic ducts, and that no scientific anatomist has ever been able to find them.

Moving from theory to treatment, all three worked on the lower spine with their hands, directly treating the physical problem by physical means. No supernaturalism here.

In addition to massage and localized pressure, all three also attempted to adjust or manipulate joints, which they did very effectively on fingers and toes, making them crack noisily. It was essential for this experiment that I experienced treatment in my own body, and that I was able to interpret what was happening to my body based on being trained and experienced as a chiropractor.

On videotape, the adjustment of the *balian* of Klungkung looks as though it should have been effective. In actuality, it was poorly executed. I could feel no vertebral movement in my spine comparable to the way my foot and finger and toe joints moved when they were adjusted.

The *balian* of Bangli attempted what we refer to in Western manual medicine as a mobilization, a procedure that attempts to move the joint without thrusting sharply into it. He failed. Later, his apprentice similarly failed to mobilize those joints. On videotape, it looks as though each was vigorously applying pressure to

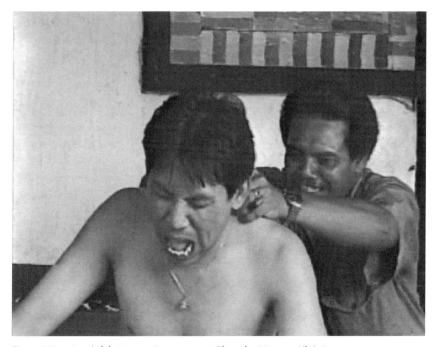

Figure 8.3.   A painful moment in treatment. (Photo by Norman Klein.)

these well-demarcated anatomical landmarks, but in fact, the knees of the one and the thumbs of the other were off to the sides of the joints, where they caused intense pain but were completely ineffective in stretching sacroiliac ligaments or breaking adhesions.

The *balian* of Batu Bulan repeatedly attempted to manipulate and mobilize the lower spine. I appreciated his gentle technique because he alone did not cause pain. Again, on videotape he seemed to be performing an effective adjustment. In fact, however, he was not accurate enough in positioning himself and me so that the small apophyseal joints in the back could release their tightness. He also failed to loosen the sacroiliac ligaments.

Also, only the octogenarian *balian* of Batu Bulan did no harm. The other two caused intense pain that can be justified by no obvious medical rationale. To help me handle what another Western patient referred to as his "torture-like physical manipulation," the *balian* of Bangli told me to exhale strongly and noisily, which I felt forced to do on several occasions (when the pain was excruciating).

The *balian* of Klungkung caused a lot of pain by snapping muscle tendons and by pressing his thumb against sensitive bony areas. He was especially harsh in mobilizing my right kneecap. I found it frightening and painful because that knee had normal function and was completely asymptomatic. It may be that he detected some slight roughness of movement, *patellar crepitus*, which is quite common in knees as old as mine. The best treatment for asymptomatic *crepitus*, however, is to leave it alone. Fortunately, the knee stopped hurting when he shifted his treatment to another part of my leg. (His diagnosis of my knee was that it was dry.)

I was not so fortunate with my neck, which, though normally pain-free, is quite stiff and looks arthritic on x-rays, the result of many years of traumatizing gymnastics. In the morning, the *balian* of Klungkung massaged and attempted to manipulate the area as part of his whole-body approach. He left me in pain. In the afternoon I was treated by the *balian* of Bangli and by his assistant. Each of them also heavily massaged the area. Neither the *balian* nor his apprentice asked or noticed that my neck was painful from the morning experience. These treatments look benign, but they caused my neck to ache for the next three days before the pain finally eased off and eventually disappeared.

So what have we learned from these bonesetters? From an anthropological point of view, it is important to realize that we were able to document a form of treatment that is naturalistic in the sense that it is based on a theory of disease that identifies physical causes thought of, in this case, as blocked ducts or channels (Connor, Asch, and Asch 1986:188; Eiseman 1990:140). Similarly, treatment was carried out by directly massaging and attempting to manipulate afflicted areas.

It is noteworthy that supernatural thinking was not entirely absent. A bit of magic was performed by the *balian* of Klungkung, who traced occult signs in massage oil over the afflicted area of the lower back before getting down to the practical business of massage and manipulation.

What we learned from a medical point of view is that all three failed to provide relief. In addition, two of them plus the apprentice caused useless pain. Why were they not effective? Perhaps because they did not treat my damaged spine. Remember, they proceeded directly to treatment without doing a physical examination, without asking questions about my movement habits, associated symptoms, the exact nature of the pain and its history as acute or chronic. What they treated was a theory of disease. It was a theory of physical causation, to be sure. But it failed to direct them accurately to the anatomic source of pain that needed to be addressed.

I do not doubt that, for the small price paid, the *balian* provides a valuable service of a psychological and social nature. My little experiment was not designed to test that possibility. It is also possible that these bonesetters are effective in treating other diseases. But, again, my experiment was not designed for that. And, finally, I strongly suspect that some bonesetters, and specifically Jero Tapakan, may in fact be more effective in treating back pain such as I had, but I was not in a position to explore that possibility.

More research clearly needs to be done, but this much can be said: The time has come for anthropologists to balance their extensive documentation of exotic, supernatural healing practices with studies of healing based on the pragmatism of ordinary human anatomy, physiology, and pathology.

The final scene shows me, without commentary, sipping a liquid medicine provided by the *balian* of Batu Bulan. I do not know what that medicine was, except that it tasted like a home-brewed aquavit. It was supposed to improve digestion because, as the *balian* explained, the physiological cause of my back pain was not merely due to the proximal pathologies of blocked channels and dry joints. Ultimately, the physiological cause was conceptualized as impaired gastric function. I know of no scientific research to validate that claim. These naturalistic concepts have their origins in the ancient Ayurvedic medical theories of India.

The Presentation of Self by a *Balian*

How could Klein and Anderson characterize the *balian* of Klungkung so differently? Part of the explanation is that we carried out observations from different analytical perspectives, as though the one used a pair of binoculars and the other a microscope. Klein used binoculars, so to speak, defining the *balian*'s approach to healing in monistic terms that merge naturalistic and supernaturalistic concepts as part of a larger overview. The *balian* is able to deal with the spiritual as well as the physical needs of the patient, Klein tells us. We are told of the *balian*'s mystical encounter when an incarnate spirit initiated him into the bonesetter's calling, and Klein highlights the annual ritual when former patients make offerings to the Goddess Saraswati.

In contrast, Anderson looked through a metaphoric microscope, defining the *balian*'s approach in dualistic terms, differentiating and compartmentalizing naturalism and supernaturalism in order to characterize bonesetting as entirely naturalistic. He insists that the *balian* worked on his joints and muscles solely by physical means. There is no supernaturalism here, he states emphatically, noting as a trivial exception that the *balian* started off by tracing an occult sign with his finger, the way a Catholic might make the sign of the cross as a transient nod to the deity.

As we talked about how we could have presented the *balian* in such contrastive ways, we came to realize that small differences in how we had each approached the *balian* provided a partial explanation. We suspect now that in each ethnographic encounter, the *balian* was motivated, subconsciously perhaps, to present himself in a way that was colored by the questions we asked and by what he thought Klein and later Anderson expected or would most admire. In each case, he activated quite reasonable choices as he selected from a complex cultural repertoire in which a *balian* sometimes fits a monistic model and at other times a dualistic one.

This explanation is consistent with the film documentaries produced by Asch, Connor, and Asch when they worked with the *balian* known as Jero Tapakan. Their best-known film is probably *A Balinese Trance Séance*, in which Jero at her altar invokes her deities with incantations and incense until she falls into a trance and is possessed by spirits of the dead who then converse with her clients in what can be characterized as a thoroughly supernatural experience (Connor and Asch 1980). In contrast, they also produced *The Medium Is the Masseuse: A Balinese Massage* in which Jero functions as a bonesetter in a normal state of consciousness, without the aid of spirits, to treat her patient in a thoroughly naturalistic way with massage and manipulation. Writing about these two films, they emphasize a contrast between how she works as a spirit medium and how she works as a "masseuse." "It is evident from the films," they inform us, "that Jero's relationship with her clients in each of the two situations is quite different" (Connor, Asch, and Asch 1986: 24).

In short, in responding to Klein, the *balian* described supernatural authentications that he did not feel compelled to offer to Anderson two years later. However, what we both actually witnessed as he worked with patients and treated each of us was thoroughly grounded in naturalistic concepts of anatomy and physiology. Bonesetting was carried out without reference to deities or spirits of the dead, without trances or possessions, and without incense or altars. But having said that, we are still left with some other sharp differences in how we constructed our documentaries, and to make sense of those differences we need to look at an additional point of divergence.

On Cultural Relativism and Critical Anthropology

In editing our videos, we constructed the culture of the *balian* in contrastive ways in part because Klein assumed the posture of a cultural relativist who describes behavior without adding judgmental commentary, while Anderson instantiated the critical anthropologist's willingness to make judgments of good and bad, right and wrong.

Viewing Klein's video, one will likely come away with the impression that the *balian* is very effective in treating musculoskeletal disorders. Two apparent successes were videotaped. The most impressive was that of a child who could not or would not walk when he arrived, but who was seen after treatment to walk without apparent difficulty. Also impressive was the man who presented with limited motion in his shoulder subsequent to an injury three days earlier. He achieved a normal range of motion in that shoulder. He was also treated for knee pain that had been treated before but still caused pain. The outcome of that treatment was not recorded. Klein himself was treated for a painful knee, also with an outcome that was not reported.

In sharp contrast, Anderson described manipulations and mobilizations that were ineffective, massage that was excruciatingly painful and unproductive, and both a knee and a neck that were subjected to therapeutic maneuvers that were contraindicated because of the harm they could do.

How could we differ so strikingly in our report of findings as a cultural relativist and a critical anthropologist? The most obvious answer is that these case studies are anecdotal, so the mere happenstance that some patients did better than others cannot be statistically evaluated. Outcomes, whether excellent or poor, must be interpreted as mere matters of chance under these circumstances. That being so, each case could only illustrate a judgment, but not compel it.

However, other more subtle factors should also be factored into this retrospective analysis because Klein and Anderson evaluated treatment outcomes or efficacy based implicitly on applying two different explanatory models or measures of success, healing of an illness versus curing of a disease (Kleinman 1980:104–118; see Anderson 1991, 1997:261–65). Klein, in effect, evaluated the *balian* in terms of whether or not he was successful in healing an illness, an approach that basically asks if patients were satisfied with their treatment. The *balian's* patients appear to have been quite pleased. Anderson, on the other hand, took as his measure the cure of disease in terms of eliminating or ameliorating anatomic or physiologic pathology. Only the shoulder injury clearly showed improvement on that level insofar as range of motion was improved. None of the other pathologies treated by the *balian* in Klein's documentary were evaluated in anatomic-physiological terms. Even an apparent success in treating the little boy is problematic because it is not clear whether or not he was able to walk before he was treated. However, we conclude that Klein's findings are not inconsistent with Anderson's negative evaluation of the treatment he received for back pain.

Emic versus Etic

To further compound differences in evaluation, Klein reports from an emic point of view while Anderson reports from an etic point of view. "Emic" refers to an approach that describes the culture of a particular society the way the indigenes themselves would do it, whereas an etic description translates or transforms local culture traits into cross-cultural categories or analytical concepts (see Anderson 1996:76–79). Thus, Klein obligated himself to present the *balian* the way the man sees himself in terms of his own local culture (the emic perspective), so he is described as spiritually gifted, as enhancing his abilities by reading books, as growing in skill, and as successful in healing illness. Explanations in terms of blocked or crossed channels were described without being questioned. Of course, Klein was aware that the loci of many of the observed manipulations were not biomechanically related to the problems being treated. He was also fully aware that a physical evaluation of each patient prior to treatment would have been necessary to effectively evaluate outcomes because he is trained and experienced in physical diagnosis and treatment. However, he chose to present an emic account consistent with a culturally relativistic approach.

Anderson, on the other hand, assumed a cross-cultural, so-called etic perspective that relied on reformulating Balinese cultural categories as medico-scientific categories of description and evaluation. He used chiropractic and biomedical concepts as a basis for commenting on culture-specific concepts such as those of channels being blocked, of joints getting dry, and of impaired digestion as the ultimate cause of musculoskeletal disorders. Further, he critiqued treatments in terms of the accuracy of manipulative thrusts, of precision in the use of mobilization, and unjustified forms of massage that caused great pain.

On Being True but Not Complete

When all is said and done, it seems that each of us presented an appropriate documentation. Each offers a correct and useful ethnographic depiction of the culture of this bonesetter, even though the findings are discordant. The problem is not that one or the other is inaccurate or wrong. The problem is that each is incomplete.

References

Anderson, Robert

1991   The Efficacy of Ethnomedicine: Research Methods in Trouble. *Medical Anthropology* 13:1–17.

1996   *Magic, Science, and Health: The Aims and Achievements of Medical Anthropology.* Fort Worth, Tex.: Harcourt Brace.

1997   Is Chiropractic Mainstream or Alternative? A View from Medical Anthropology. Pp. 555–78 in Dana J. Lawrence, J. David Cassidy, Marion McGregor, William C. Meeker, and Howard T. Vernon, eds. *Advances in Chiropractic* 4. St. Louis, Mo.: Mosby.

Chagnon, Napoleon A.

1983   *Yanomamö: The Fierce People.* N.Y.: Holt, Rinehart and Winston.

Connor, Linda, Patsy Asch, and Timothy Asch

1986   *Jero Tapakan: Balinese Healer, An Ethnographic Film Monograph.* Cambridge, England: Cambridge University Press.

Eiseman, Fred Jr.

1990   *Bali: Sekala and Niskala.* Vol. I. Hong Kong: Periplus Editions.

Good, Kenneth, and David Chanoff

1991   *Into the Heart: One Man's Pursuit of Love and Knowledge among the Yanomama.* New York: Simon & Schuster.

Huber, Brad R., and Robert Anderson

1996   Bonesetters and Curers in a Mexican Community: Conceptual Models, Status, and Gender. *Medical Anthropology* 17(1):23–38.

Kleinman, Arthur

1980   *Patients and Healers in the Context of Culture: An Exploration of the Borderland between Anthropology, Medicine, and Psychiatry.* Berkeley: University of California Press.

Lewis, Oscar

1951   *Life in a Mexican Village: Tepoztlán Restudied.* Urbana, Ill.: University of Illinois Press.

Mead, Margaret

1953   The Study of Culture at a Distance. Pp. 3–53 in Margaret Mead and Rhoda Metraux, eds. *The Study of Culture at a Distance.* Chicago: University of Chicago Press.

Redfield, Robert

1930   *Tepoztlán: A Mexican Village.* Chicago: University of Chicago Press.

Videography

Anderson, Robert

1998   *Bonesetters in Bali.* 15 minutes. For information on obtaining this video, contact Norman Klein at nklein@calstatela.edu.

Asch, Timothy, and Linda Connor

1982   *The Medium Is the Masseuse: A Balinese Massage.* 35 minutes. Distributed by Documentary Educational Resources, 5 Bridge St., Watertown, Mass., 02172.

Connor, Linda, and Timothy Asch

1980   *A Balinese Trance Séance.* 30 minutes. Distributed by Documentary Educational Resources, 5 Bridge St., Watertown, Mass., 02172. Telephone (617) 926-0491.

Klein, Norman

1996   *The Balian of Klungkung.* 11 minutes. For information on obtaining this video, contact Norman Klein at nklein@calstatela.edu.

"Getting Rolfed"
Structural Bodywork, Disciplined Deportment, and Embodiment

9

ERIC JACOBSON

CLIENTS OF A METHOD OF PHYSICAL MANIPULATION known as Rolfing® describe a variety of physical, emotional, and psychological experiences as consequences of that therapy, including sensible changes in posture and movement, autonomic responses, negative affects, emergent memories, and increased confidence in their physical and social abilities.[1] The association of these experiences with Rolf manipulation and their apparent elicitation by the biomechanical changes that it produces raise a number of issues for the anthropology of embodiment. Moreover, these phenomena are not idiosyncratic to the Rolf method, but are also elicited by other manipulative therapies, and are common as well in a wider range of nonmanipulative therapeutic and spiritual practices. Their study therefore has the potential to expand our general appreciation of the mutability of embodiment.

I chose Rolfing as a vehicle to raise these issues neither because it is unique in improving biomechanical function nor in giving rise to such experiences, but simply because it has been my occupation for the past thirty years. This affords me familiarity with its history, views, and clinical practices, and with the sorts of testimony that are typical of its clients. In what follows, I write first as a practitioner who is frankly committed to Rolf's particular view of biomechanical competence and its profound significance for the individual's experience. I then turn as an anthropologist to what this implies for the study of embodiment. In this mode, I argue that Rolfing experiences confirm the close genetic and functional links that others have noted between cultural disciplines of the body and codes of deportment, and the formation of embodied selves. Finally, I speculate that the causative links that Rolf drew between biomechanical improvement and the alleviation of what I refer to as "restrictive modes of embodiment" may be pertinent to a wider range of healing practices, and consequently deserve serious anthropological investigation.

Bodywork, Structural Bodywork, and Rolfing

Over the past thirty years, new methods of manipulative therapy have spread at an increasing rate, generally first in the United States and then in Europe and other parts of the world. Arising largely outside of established professional contexts, these have come to be known collectively as "bodywork." Although practices and brands have proliferated almost beyond counting, the vast majority falls into a few categories and traces back to a relatively limited number of sources. The most numerous general types are methods of massage, acupressure, neuromotor facilitation, cathartic therapies, and "structural bodywork," Rolfing being the progenitor of the last.[2]

Biomechanically rationalized manipulation is particularly North American in that all of its seminal variants originated here: the chiropractic of Palmer (Moore 1993), the osteopathy of Still (Gevitz 1982), and the Structural Integration of Ida Rolf (Rolf 1977). The first two were professionalized well prior to the flowering of the bodywork movement, and are therefore not usually included under that rubric. Rolfing, however, appeared more recently (*circa* 1954), and is as yet a protoprofession.[3] It has nevertheless inspired a proliferation of derivative therapies, all of which share its defining aim of improving the biomechanical functions of the body as a whole, and its defining method of increasing myofascial elasticity through direct manipulation. This species is accordingly known as "structural bodywork."

Rolf begin to develop her therapy in the 1950s, but it drew much wider attention twenty years later with the rise of the "human potential movement," a North American subculture of enthusiasm for various unconventional and innovative methods of enhancing individual well-being. By the nineties, Rolfing's reputation as an intense but efficacious mode of bodywork had expanded further into the even more diffuse "New Age movement," a polyglot of unorthodox therapies and spiritualities. Rolf's emphasis on whole-body reorganization, her interest in the consequences of "integration with the gravity field," and her proposal that "an integrated body behaves differently" resonated with both zeitgeists. As the human potential and New Age movements waned, some segments of the Rolfing community migrated away from their founder's credo of addressing the body's biomechanical totality in favor of treating specific pains and dysfunctions. This has taken them toward a distinctly more biomedical model of practice. However, a large proportion of practitioners and teachers continue to hew to Rolf's original principles.

Rolf saw individual variation in biomechanical response to the earth's gravitational force as an essential, yet largely neglected determinant of the quality of human lives (Rolf 1973, 1977, 1979). (For a detailed earlier discussion of very similar ideas, see Strauss' 1966 essay.) She developed her own vision of biomechanical excellence, one that she rationalized in terms of a central criterion of the body's competence to deal with gravity, and could therefore cast it in the purely geometric terms of "verticality," "horizontality," and "symmetry." Equally essential were the dynamic ideals of "grace" and "integration" in movement that, although subtler of perception, she also specified in biomechanical terms.

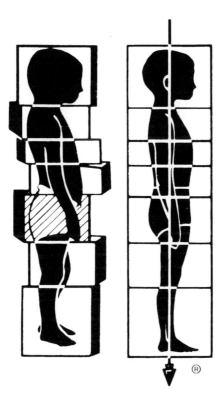

Figure 9.1. A body organized around the vertical ideal of the "Rolf line" in contrast to a "random body." (A service mark of the Rolf Institute for Structural Integration, Boulder, Colorado; used by permission.)

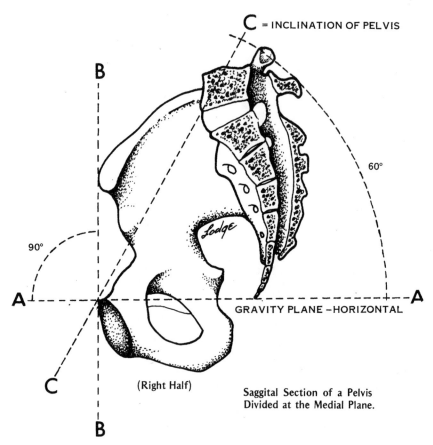

Figure 9.2.   The "horizontal pelvis" (from Rolf 1977:87).

Rolf's favored formulation of verticality was that the main segments of the
standing body—head, thorax, and pelvis—would be centered both laterally and
anterio-posteriorly on the "Rolf line," the vertical passing through the body's center of mass (figure 9.1). As she often pointed out, we intuitively define "vertical"
as the direction of the earth's gravitational force. The application of "symmetry"
to heads, shoulders, hips, and other bilateral features is equally obvious. She also
emphasized the goal of anterio-posterior "horizontality" (figure 9.2), especially of
the "horizontal pelvis" in which a line drawn from the upper edge of the pubic
symphysis to the joint between the sacrum and fifth lumbar vertebra would be
horizontal to the gravitational vertical (figure 9.3). In the dynamic realm "grace"
refers not simply to the range of joint mobility (a body with hypermobile joints
is not seen as graceful), but to the extent to which the soft tissues spanning adjacent joints participate in movement by stretching and contracting, a condition that

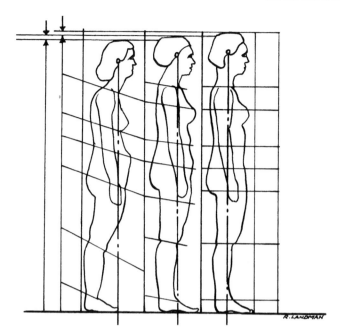

Figure 9.3. Progressive realization of the ideal of horizontality (from Rolf 1977:88).

requires an elastic and balanced tonus between functionally opposed muscle groups. This is understood in explicit contrast to the "mechanical" quality of movements that occur only at the joints themselves, with no elastic engagement of adjoining tissues. "Integration" refers to a uniformity of tonus, grace, and coordination throughout the entire body, a quality that is most easily seen in basic activities such as walking, and rising from a sitting or lying position. An especially good criterion of "integration" is the extent to which the cross-extensor reflex is activated in walking. This is a cerebellar-controlled, reflexive pattern in which the arms and shoulders swing contralaterally to the legs, hips, and pelvis. In a well-integrated body, this manifests as a graceful spiraling first one way then the other, involving every joint and muscle in an easy yet precise coordination.

Together these ideals parameterize Rolf's vision of a human body moving through the gravitational field with maximal energetic efficiency and mechanical ease. According to her doctrine, the more fully they are embodied, the less energy, stress, and strain are required to stand, walk, and perform the other bodily activities of everyday life.

The goal of Rolfing is not the impossible one of delivering each client to a full realization of these ideals, but rather to progressively approximate them. Nor is the aim a new rigidity in which the ideals must be maintained at every moment.

Although we may think of posture as static (e.g., sitting, standing, and lying down), Rolf viewed it as a continuous, dynamic behavior. Close observation of any standing body reveals a constant micromovement that continuously corrects for the subtle perturbations of balance by respiration, speech, and gesture. The goal of Rolfing is not to freeze this subtle dance into static verticals and horizontals, but to enhance the flexibility, elasticity, and balance of tonus that underlies it, thus enabling its execution with minimal effort and strain, and instinctive coordination and grace.

Rolf saw these parameters of bodily life as determined by elasticities, tensions, and rigidities in the myofascial tissues, an intricate network of sheets, bands, and cords that pervades the body. Myofascia is one of several types of connective tissue. It envelops every muscle as a whole, defining its shape as well as wrapping bundles of fibers nested two levels deep within each muscle (figure 9.4). In addition, myofascial sheets and webs spans broad anatomical areas, providing biomechanical linkage across individual muscles, joints, and even larger structures. Rolf referred to this generally neglected system as "the organ of structure." She found

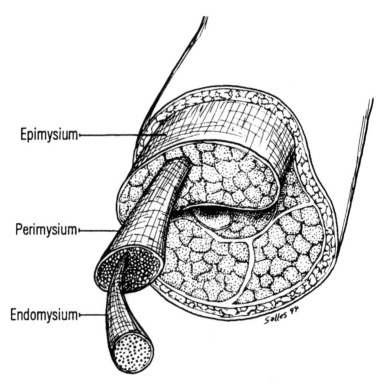

Figure 9.4.   Nested myofascial wrapping of muscle fiber bundles (from Schultz and Feitis 1996:4).

that judiciously applied manipulative force could improve biomechanical function by effecting stable increases in local myofascial elasticity, by releasing adhesions between adjacent fascial sheets, and by the consequent repositioning of myofascial structures relative to one another.[4]

An initial course of treatment consists of a sequence of ten sessions, each of which Rolf defined in terms of specific biomechanical goals, and for each of which she taught specific manipulative techniques. The usual routine is for clients, perhaps after a brief initial discussion of sequelae from the preceding treatment, to disrobe down to underwear or a two-piece bathing suit (the back must be visible) and to stand while the Rolfer inspects their posture.[5] Typically, they are asked to breathe deeply a few times and to walk back and forth across the room, allowing a visual assessment of their biomechanics relative to the Rolf ideals. Rolfers note the degree to which each client actualizes these ideals and the specific ways in which they depart through a cultivated visual inspection that their progenitor exemplified to a seemingly supernatural degree. Significant variations in treatment arise from a Rolfer's ability to discern the biomechanical significance of slight variations in surface contour and movement. Practitioners consequently regard this visual ability as most indicative of one another's level of expertise.

On that basis, the broad goals of the session are determined—which aspects of the client's biomechanics will be most effectively addressed at that time. Limiting treatment to the initial ten-session framework will broadly dictate treatment goals, but visual inspection will still inform variations in those goals and the choice of particular techniques to address individual differences.

Most of the work is performed with the client lying in various positions on a low, wide table. This allows the Rolfer to lean his or her weight into the contact to a greater or lesser degree, thus affording a wide range of pressures. Work may also be done with the client in various other postures: seated, standing, kneeling, on all fours, and so on. Palms, knuckles, fingers, and elbows are used to press into and reposition regions of soft tissue. The patient is often directed to slowly move a limb or joint in order to increase and direct the therapeutic force through the targeted fascia. While certain stock techniques are inevitably employed, the exact parameters of manipulation—whether contact is made by fingertips, knuckles, closed fist, open hand, or elbow; the amount and duration of pressure; whether and how the point of contact is moved; and whether and how the client is directed to move—are all calibrated from one intervention to the next on the basis of the visible effects of the preceding manipulation and an ongoing tactile assessment of the texture and elasticity of the fascia being worked.

The immediate effects of this are both local and wider-ranging increases in soft tissue elasticity. To the trained eye, these are visible as increases in the range, grace, and fluidity of simple movements such as the flexing of a knee or elbow. In addition, one also observes shifts in the "at rest" relationship between bones. These include changes in the contour of bodily segments (e.g., the head may widen, the rib cage may deepen front to back), changes in the positions of major segments relative to one another (e.g., the rib cage may sit more directly over the pelvis, the head over the shoulders), and increased coordination and grace in whole-body movements such as breathing, walking, or rising from a chair. Clients often experience these changes immediately as altered sensations of joint flexibility, increased ranges of motion, larger internal spaces, easier weight-bearing, and general postural relaxation.[6]

Rolf's method also included an educational component. In addition to explaining basic musculoskeletal anatomy, biomechanics, and the ideals of gravitational competence, she also provided exercises in posture and movement awareness. These are designed to enhance a client's ability to actualize the Rolf ideals once increased myofascial elasticity had given them the ability to do so. The new possibilities of bodily life are not always spontaneously occupied. Sometimes habitual patterns of inattention and contraction continue; sometimes the new freedom is used, yet in uncertain, disorganized ways. The exercises foster greater sensitivity to musculoskeletal sensations and encourage the client to permit more relaxed yet vertical posture (e.g., "imagine an angel is gently leading the top of your head skyward"), and flexibility in movement.

Yet even from its beginnings, Rolfing was not about biomechanics alone. Its inventor realized, just as all of the mentors she saw fit to acknowledge had, that the freedoms and restrictions within which each individual lives their physical life have a significant bearing on their experience of self and the social world. Rolf often voiced the hypothesis and the hope that the individual's social behavior would "mature" as they more closely approximated her indices of biomechanical excellence. This is an additional sense in which her method is holistic. Not only biomechanics, but also intero- and exteroceptive perception, one's understanding of self and others, social conduct, and even spiritual life are expected to benefit from an improved relationship to gravity. This, again, contrasts sharply with biomedical biomechanics that recognizes nothing like this intimate parallelism between gravitational and kinetic competence on the one hand, and psychology and social conduct on the other.[7]

One of Rolf's favorite maxims was "gravity is the therapist," by which she meant that the properly Rolfed client would move through the gravity field in patterns that involved less effort, stress, and strain, and more elasticity and ease, that this increased synergy would allow continuing incremental advances in biomechanical excellence, and that many local pains and dysfunctions would be alleviated in their course. In this she placed her faith not so much in the brute force of gravity's relentless downward pull as in the capacity of the human musculoskeletal and neu-

romotor apparatus, once relieved of the grossest rigidities and restrictions, to re
spond to that force in patterns that reinforce rather than degrade its structure—
that is, a neuro-biomechanical innatism. Rolf was not, of course, the only thinker
to propound an innatist doctrine of bodily liberation. There is a special ideological (and also reportedly experiential) resonance between Rolfing and other innatist
practices such as hatha yoga, Tai Chi, Qi Gong, Asian meditative disciplines, and
also with Ayurvedic, Tibetan, and Chinese medicines that emphasize the body's
ability to heal itself of local ills once overall energetic balance is restored.

The Experience of "Getting Rolfed"

The experiences clients attribute to Rolfing vary, overlap, and interlace in complex
and highly individualized ways.[8] Nevertheless, a few general types are discernible.
In order of decreasing prevalence, these are: 1) sensations of pain, 2) perceived
changes in movement and posture, 3) emergent memories, 4) autonomic responses, and 5) emergent affects. Although only a minority of clients reports all
of these, none are rare, peculiar, or even idiosyncratic to Rolfing. Virtually all
clients describe the first two, usually spontaneously, and the latter types of experience, although less common, occur often enough that they are familiar to every
practitioner and are prominent in the public lore on Rolfing. As I have already
pointed out, these experiences are also common in other kinds of structural bodywork. As anthropologists, we are, of course, interested not only in how clients describe them, but also in how Rolfers explain and interpret them.

In general, positive reports outweigh the negative and will be emphasized in
what follows. I do not mean to imply, however, that these occur uniformly. This is
an account of what Rolfing yields at its best. It is also worth pointing out that
these reports are made not only by experienced clients, but also by those who are
entirely naive to the theory and expectations of Rolfing, who perhaps anticipate
only relief from a specific pain or disability. The argument that clients phrase
these reports purely in response to the "demand characteristics" of the clinical situation—to meet their Rolfer's expectations, or because they have been inculcated
in a discourse of Rolfing that requires such reports—cannot explain their repeated emergence in the accounts of naive clients, and from individuals of widely
varying cultural backgrounds and diverse educational and socioeconomic levels.[9]

Most common, and most consistently noted in public discussions, are a variety of painful sensations ranging from "dull ache" to "sharp" feelings, which at
their extreme are "like being stabbed with a knife," to "burning" feelings, as
though a lit match were held to the tissue. Although the more extreme of these are
featured prominently in journalistic accounts, sensations of pain remain in a tol-
erable range for the great majority of clients, and virtually always dissipate as soon

as the manipulative force is removed. They seem a correlate not of any injury to the tissues, which is rare in Rolfing, but of a rapid rate of myofascial change, an explanation that Rolfers find useful when clients become anxious about the significance of painful sensations. It is interesting that the intensity and quality of Rolfing pain depends almost not at all on the degree of force or any other variables of the manipulation itself. With the exception of a few areas of the body (e.g., feet and ankles) that seem "hardwired" to interpret any unusual pressure as pain, these sensations seem to depend more on the physical quality of the connective tissue being worked on, its thickness or rigidity, its knotty, grainy, or fibrous texture. When areas with those qualities are engaged, clients frequently report acute pain, and tissues with those textures most often give rise to memories of a physical injury or emotional trauma. They seem to be textural hallmarks of past injury and strain, either physical or emotional—again, a useful item in the Rolfer's repertoire of explanations.

Greater ease and range of motion in a specific joint are often experienced when a client tests its movement immediately following a manipulation. Many practitioners have their clients stand and walk in midsession so that they have a chance to feel such changes more vividly. This often elicits spontaneous descriptions of altered sensations of both posture and movement. But sometimes biomechanical changes unambiguously visible to the Rolfer are not sensed by the client. Habitual muscular tensions may persist even when increased myofascial elasticity has made it possible for the client to relax into more flexible, more coordinated patterns of movement. Rolf's "exercises," "experiments," and "cues" are often introduced at these times to encourage the abandonment of restrictive habits and fuller occupation of new possibilities.

These are moments in which clients sometimes report experiences that are particularly pertinent to the study of embodiment. When they sense the beginning of change in their long-established ways of standing, sitting, or walking, they sometimes give voice to the "rightness" of the habitually more tense and the "wrongness" of the less effortful posture or movement. Such statements usually emerge in response to changed proprioceptive sensations alone—without the client looking at their image in a mirror. They sometimes include memories of the instructions, admonishments, or threats by which the client was taught what was "right" and "wrong" in postural life. They may recall the specific circumstances of such exhortations quite exactly, and those memories sometimes directly implicate cultural values. These memories can be elicited in multiple modalities, including proprioceptive, kinesthetic, and nocioceptive (e.g., "That feels exactly like the time I ran my thigh into the barbed wire fence"), and also visual, auditory, and affective.

Perhaps the most common of these has to do with shoulder position, which is often the first aspect of posture to become significantly freer. Many North

Americans are taught early in their lives to pull their shoulders back so that the joints are behind the anterior-posterior midpoint of the rib cage, with the scapulae approximating a "flat" upper back. There is variation in how far back the shoulders are pulled and whether they are simultaneously pulled up into the neck or down into the midback. As increased myofascial elasticity allows the client to relax the habitual effort necessary to maintain such a position, they may exclaim, "But this is slumping!" or "Now I look like a slob!" Specific instances of instruction are also recalled: "Our dad used to always shout at us at the dinner table 'Sit up straight! Pull your shoulders back! Don't slouch!'" or, "In school they always use to tell us not to sit like this!"

Similar judgments and memories emerge around other aspects of posture. One that usually comes somewhat later in the Rolfing process has to do with pelvic movement in walking. North American women who are raised WASP or Catholic are often taught to tense their lower backs and buttocks when walking so as to minimize the swaying of the hips, which would otherwise occur as weight-bearing shifts from one hip joint to the other. As one foot touches down and begins to bear weight, the hip on that side begins to move medially to more efficiently transfer the weight of the body through to that foot. As the foot reaches the back of the step and begins to lift off, the medial migration of that hip reaches its maximum, and it begins to move laterally away from the midline as the opposite hip begins to move medially. The alternation of left and right hips migrating toward the midline produces a lateral swaying of the pelvis. If movement is unrestricted enough, this is accompanied by a "figure-eight" excursion of each hip around a horizontal axis as it first lifts up and reaches forward, then drops and pushes back (Ohlgren and Clark n.d.). When increased myofascial elasticity makes it possible to permit this pelvic swaying, women sometimes ask, "But aren't I being too sexy to walk like that?" They may also describe the ways in which the importance of minimizing hip sway was impressed on them: "My mother would shout at me if she saw me walking this way!" In some cases they have learned traumatically, as when young women are sexually attacked and later permitted or encouraged to think it was their "fault" for being too provocative. North American males sometimes worry aloud that they will be thought to be homosexual if they permit their hips to sway as they walk. Sometimes they recall specific shaming or predicted stigmatization: "If you walk down the hall like that people will think you're a slob/wimp/sissy/whore/fag."

Adolescent boys as well as young men often become attached to an ideal of "bulked up" arms and shoulders, spending hours at weight machines to cultivate the requisite mass of muscle. The strain of excessive weight lifting and the general anxiety to display the resulting bulk both contribute to a habitual tension in the arms and shoulders. Typically the arms splay outward at an angle from the body rather than hanging easily under the shoulder. The shoulders are either chronically raised into the neck or pulled so tightly down and into the center of the chest as to restrict breathing. Perhaps because they expect this display to provide a significant social advantage, men sometimes maintain it even when increased fascial elasticity allows the possibility of relaxing. For some, permitting the arms to fall to their sides and the shoulders to let go of their neck and rib cage can be a moment of unexpected emotional vulnerability, as though necessary barriers around one's heart had been let down. They may also describe the new, less effortful posture as "wimpy" or "weak."

In general clients who report such memories seem to have been taught that failure to maintain the requisite posture will be read as a failure of moral character, and will lead to some degree of social stigmatization. On the positive side, the prescribed posture is often identified as a sign of their good character. "Stand up like a man!" "Sit like a proper young lady!" Both moral and social status will be determined in significant part by their achievement of these specific bodily deportments, at least in certain social settings.

However, bodily discipline occurs not only through the examples, exhortations, sanctions, and traumas imposed by others, but also through the individual's own voluntary pursuit of internalized ideals. The ambition to acquire a particular bodily shape is usually, though not always, acquired in childhood or adolescence. This is not true, however, in every case. Postural ideals can be adopted from peers and the mass media even by adults. Many men and women express a concern to maintain a certain tension in their abdominal muscles so that their "bellies don't stick out." (Rolfing in this area generally produces a more uniform tonus in the abdominal muscles that, while not providing as flat a profile as "hard abs," does significantly restrain the dreaded protruding belly.) A young woman whose unusually tight abdominal muscles challenged my manipulative abilities responded to my comment that they were unusually tight: "Of course they are! I do one hundred sit-ups every morning!" When asked why that was so important a part of her routine, she responded "I have to have killer abs. Otherwise I won't get good dates."

The distinction between postures and movements that one may be skilled in performing—but which are more or less optional depending on the effect one wishes to produce in a given situation—and those that the individual accepts as more pervasive indicators of personal value and status, is important. The latter may be the object of considerable effort even when one is alone. People look at themselves in the mirror to check the acceptability not only of their complexion, dress, and hair, but also of their bodily shape, stance, and gesture. Whether through the harshness of disciplinary sanctions or through the magnitude and chronicity of one's own efforts, some deportments become rigid and no longer amenable to variation.

Perhaps even more often than they exclaim as to the "wrongness" of abandoning postural rigidities, clients comment on the positive sensations that emerge when they do. "I can breathe more easily." "I feel so much lighter on my feet." "Now I feel like my feet are really comfortable on the floor." They may feel "lighter all through my body." "It's easier to walk now." "It takes less effort to stand up." Positive intuitions of the self's value, security, and competence are often attributed to these new pleasures: "I am much more secure on my feet now." "I don't have to defend myself all the time," or conversely, "Now I feel like I could really defend myself if I needed to." The spontaneous movement of the hips in walking and the eventual emergence of the cross-extensor reflex may elicit reports that "walking feels more natural" or "more powerful."

If we accept that less restrictive ways of standing and moving allow an increased functioning of innate neuromotor coordinations, such as those that organize breathing, balance, visual tracking, standing and walking, then these reports express a spontaneous pleasure in the fuller expression of those coordinations. Sensations of improved circulation are also reported; one's feet, hands, and face may "feel warmer." Subjective changes in temperature can also be given positive personal meanings: "I feel warm in my stomach now, like something good is happening there." Pleasurable change may also be noted in the distal senses: "The room looks clearer and brighter now."

Autonomic sensations are somewhat less common than sensations of pain or biomechanical change, and they occur in less immediate consequence to manipulation. Their onset is more gradual and they may be of longer duration, sometimes building up slowly over the course of a session. Most common are sweating, especially of the hands and feet, which is sometimes accompanied by feeling cold or anxious. Nausea, dizziness, goose bumps, or trembling are also reported, the latter often accompanied by "feeling cold," or alternatively by "feeling filled with energy." Occasionally, trembling will increase in amplitude until the client's entire body is shaking. After some minutes without manipulation, such reactions usually abate. Any of these may be explained to the client as "releases of stored up stress," or even more specifically as "releases of stored up anxiety," "disgust" (in the case of nausea), or simply "energy." Just as with sensations of postural change, autonomically driven sensations sometimes lead to the emergence of memories and dysphoric affects.

Although nothing in the theory of Rolfing requires that the client's experience have an affective dimension (beyond their comfort with and trust in the Rolfer), a significant minority of clients do report the spontaneous emergence of fear, anger, grief, or embarrassment as immediate consequences of local increases in fascial elasticity. They often have no idea at first what such affects are "about." When more or less specific memories do accompany emerging affects, they usually come more gradually, lagging behind the initial wave of emotion. Surfacing rage may eventually lead to, "Why did my father do that to me?" an eruption of sobbing to, "Nothing I did was ever good enough for her," and a welling up of intense anxiety to an anguished, "I just keep trying to think of why my brother would do that to me." When there is an accompanying memory, the recalled episode sometimes includes a physical injury to the area of the body that has just been worked on. More often, however, it is a memory of an episode in which that area had to be tensed in order to inhibit an emotional expression that was forbidden or unsafe. Rage is often reported when fascial tensions in the upper back are relieved, this being an area often held chronically tense to deaden impulses to strike out at one's persecutor, to reach out and choke off a tormenting voice. Work on the front of the rib cage can release grief at some loss or injury that could not be safely displayed when it occurred. Work on the throat may give rise to vocalized sounds that would have carried too high a price at an earlier time.

Rolf did not conceptualize the emergence of memories, affectively charged or not, as part of the therapeutic process that her methods facilitated, but many of her followers now understand such episodes in terms of a psychotherapeutic model of the catharsis of traumatic memories. According to this, Rolfing can free the client not only from chronic biomechanical tensions but also from rigid psychodynamic defenses adopted in earlier stages of life and in response to distressing, possibly traumatic situations. This can, to some degree, free them from rigid adherence to those past adaptations and allow a wider range of responses to their present adult circumstances.

In addition to their appearance during treatments, affects and memories from earlier in life may also arise hours or even days later. This is so commonly reported that one wonders whether similar cathartic processes also occur in those clients who do not report them, that perhaps they emerge in far more gradual and less conscious ways, or that some clients choose not to mention them or fail to associate them with Rolfing. It may also be that some individual difference in the organization of somatic experience distinguishes those clients who experience emergent memories and affects from those who do not. However, none of these hypotheses have been empirically assessed. Whatever the explanation, many of those who do experience significant biomechanical and even psychological improvements do not report such eruptions of memory or emotion.

Some clients also notice changes that occur over weeks and months. The most common of these are general increases in bodily sensation, increased awareness of emotional responses, and "more energy." A general sense that a more relaxed deportment is acceptable and socially defensible seems to contribute to the "maturity" that Rolf postulated as a long-term benefit of an improved relationship with gravity. As a clinical impression, clients over the long term often seem less anxious that a relaxed posture and movement might brand them as "too sexy," "a slob," "a wimp," or with some other stigma. Greater expressive range and assurance in social relations are also described—feeling "more secure," "more powerful," and even "more relaxed." The Rolfer sometimes hears that a client has become "more willing to speak up for myself," "quicker to draw my limits," and generally more willing to express irritation, desire, affection, or sexuality. Sometimes clients report becoming markedly more proactive in altering social relations that are stressful or otherwise unpleasant. Some describe increased calmness and lucidity in their spiritual practices, or more frequent peak experiences, however expressed (such as "oneness"). The potential benefits (not to imply that all are realized by each client) therefore seem to include improvements in biomechanical life, respiration and circulation, maturation of character, and enhanced spiritual experience.

Rolfers usually attribute these changes to increased somatic sensation and the generalization of improved biomechanical functioning to an experience of enhanced social competence. Feeling surer on one's feet, easier and more coordinated in everyday movements, having a more vivid sensation of muscular activity, perhaps deeper into one's bodies, clearer sensations of attraction, repulsion, and other impulses and emotions, freer to deploy a variety of stances and gestures—all of these support a reconstruction of the self as more self-reliant and secure, more accurate in intuition and taste, more trustworthy of impulse, and more capable of responding to social challenges.

In addition to biomechanical improvements and catharses of negative memories, therapeutic change is also attributed to alleviating the sequelae of musculoskeletal injury. As is well known, scarring entails a thickening and increase in the fibrousness of the myofascia for some distance around the original trauma. In addition to reducing mobility and circulation at the immediate site of scarring, injured fascia may also adhere to adjacent structures, thus compromising the mobility of larger areas. In addition, injurious impacts may cause bony malalignments. Even after wounds have closed, and bruises, swelling, and acute pain have abated, reductions in myofascial flexibility and skeletal misalignments may persist and have long-term, deleterious effects on circulation, sensation, posture, and mobility. The restoration of myofascial elasticity and mobility can contribute dramatically to the reduction of these deficits. Just as with other improvements in biomechanics, the relieving of these sequelae of physical injury often elicits feelings of greater somatosensory pleasure and expressions of enhanced self-image.

Following the initial ten sessions and whatever improvements occur in the following months, some clients are satisfied with their gains. Others become interested in the longer-term project of progressively approximating the Rolf ideals and return periodically for additional treatments. The latter are often also involved in other bodily disciplines such as sports, dance, or athletics, with spiritual practices, or with various modes of alternative health care that they see as compatible with Rolfing and enhanced by the changes it produces. These other practices often involve a similarly innatist ideology: that the body-mind can heal and better itself in extraordinary ways if it is relieved of accumulated stress and injury.

Lest I paint too exclusively rosy a picture of Rolfing's therapeutic effectiveness, I must acknowledge that some clients do not experience significant change either biomechanically or psychologically. As in any clinical endeavor, there are "hard cases" for whom the Rolfer's best efforts produce only an unacceptably glacial pace of improvement. Responses such as "I don't feel anything different" or "I feel just the same as before," although disappointing, are sometimes congruent with the absence of any but the most minor signs of biomechanical improvement. And even among those whose posture and movement do visibly improve, some are apparently unable to sense those changes, or for some reason unwilling to attend to them.

Very rarely a client will react adversely to sensations of postural change, even those that are overtly visible improvements in biomechanical function. Once, upon standing up after a session that had improved the flexibility and supportiveness of her feet, a client exclaimed, "Oh no! Now I can feel my weight in my feet! I think of myself as a dancer and I like feeling weightless!" It is interesting, however, that such definitively negative reactions occur only with extreme rarity. The predominant tendency across genders, ages, and cultural backgrounds is to experience biomechanical improvement as pleasurable and as enhancing to both physical and social confidence.

It is worth repeating that none of these epitherapeutic phenomena, neither the positive nor the negative, are unique to Rolfing, to the broader species of structural bodywork, or even to bodywork in general. Clients in "body-centered" psychotherapies also respond to skilled touch, manipulation, directed breathing, and movement with memories of distressing or traumatic interpersonal experiences, and with the reexperiencing of negative affects (Lowen 1958; Kellerman 1985; Reich 1978). The same is true of acupuncture and various Asian practices of body-centered meditation such as Tai Chi, Qi Gong (Kerr 2002, Xu 1994), and Hindu and Buddhist Tantrism. In fact, testimony of these same general kinds seems to emerge whenever an intervention that increases bodily sensation or mobility coincides with an opportunity for clients to talk about their therapeutic experience. Given the variety of body-involving practices that elicit them, and their evident relationship to changes in biomechanical flexibility, these phenomena deserve close attention by students of embodiment.

Reflections from the Anthropology of Embodiment

The preceding discussion brings some familiar theses to mind: 1) the plasticity of deportment and the lived body under the impact of cultural discipline (Foucault

1979, Mauss 1992); 2) the sedimentation of bodily discipline in preconscious or "preobjective" complexes of memory that persist over long periods of the individual's life and profoundly influence their perceptions, affective responses, and conduct (Merleau-Ponty 1962; Bourdieu 1977; Csordas 1988, 1993, 1994a); and 3) the significance of culturally disciplined deportment for the individual's position in the social order—not only for observers who interpret the meanings of their posture and movement, but also for the subject who experiences their own identity and social position in terms of their limited expressive options (Bourdieu 1977, Csordas 1994a).[10]

Although embodiment theorists have not always accorded them center stage, characteristic patterns of posture and movement have long been recognized as a key aspect of the "lived body" (Bourdieu 1977; Foucault 1979; Merleau-Ponty 1962, Strauss 1966). It is well established that in any given culture, certain visibly recognizable features of human bodies, including but not limited to deportment, are read as signifying the individual's position vis-à-vis culturally salient dichotomies and gradients such as "high class/low class," "male/female," "master/servant," "dominant/submissive," and so on. It has also been understood for some time (at least since Freud) that social attributions of the individual's position in such schemes are introjected and reflect inwardly on their experience of themselves, and that this includes their understanding of the social positions and careers available to them.[11]

One is not merely taught the cultural code according to which certain biomechanical habits are read as indications of social position and role; one is also disciplined into a repertoire of deportments, some of which are appropriate only in certain social situations, others of which are more or less permanently, rigidly impressed in the body-mind. Even the former confine one to a limited repertoire of particular positions in the ongoing play of culturally meaningful stances and gestures. One is not only aware that swaying one's hips is locally read as evidence that one is a "slut" or "queer," but one also levies that judgment on oneself or is at least anxious about or keen to deny its possible applicability. One is consequently driven to incorporate a specific, strategic attitude toward swaying the hips—it is to be rigidly suppressed, or exaggerated at all times, or performed on certain occasions in a self-consciously calculated way. The socially visible and subjectively experienced aspects of encultured embodiment thereby reflect one another. Deportment, both as a visible performance of certain possibilities in the cultural code and as a subjectively experienced identity, is both objectively and subjectively key to the reproduction of a social order.

These relationships between social training, trauma, deportment, and the lived body are usually unnoticed by subjects, and even unavailable to their introspection.

Indeed, this is part of what is meant by "sedimentation": not only that the impact of social experience is long lasting, but also that it exercises its influence from a stratum below the threshold of articulate consciousness. The experiential testimony of Rolfing clients offers an especially tantalizing glimpse into this hidden, tacit level of cultural-somatic structure. Positive or negative evaluations of specific postures and movements, the linking of these to parallel evaluations of the self, to memories of restrictive training and trauma, and to emotional responses—all seem to confirm that the formation and persistence of such complexes are key to the cultural embodiment of the self.[12]

Myofascial Elasticity, Rigid Deportment, and Therapeutic Change

The experiences discussed here arise in direct consequence to the visible increases in myofascial elasticity that Rolfing produces. This suggests retrospectively that myofascial restriction plays a major part in the sedimentation of discipline and trauma, in the maintenance of deportmental rigidity, and, consequently, in the embodiment of the self. The fact that memories of bodily discipline, sometimes accompanied by a reexperiencing the individual's original affective response, come to consciousness as bodily elasticity is restored suggests that myofascial change may be functionally involved in, if not the actual medium of, the sedimentation and release of discipline.[13] We observe that the release of the psychic and the social is catalyzed by the release of the somatic, and we consequently infer that the forces, both physical and rhetorical, that formed our clients as socialized, embodied selves inscribed their identity not only psychically, but also somatically.

Changes in myofascial elasticity, and their linkage to changes in deportment, embodiment, and the lived-body, may also have a wider anthropological significance. I have already noted that emergent memories of restrictive and traumatic episodes, and reexperienced affective responses are also reported in a wide range of other practices, both ritual and clinical. Is it possible that myofascial change plays a significant role in therapeutic outcomes, even in nonmanipulative healing practices? Oschman and Oschman (1997) and Oschman (2000) review evidence that modes of stimulation other than direct manipulation may also alter myofascia. Theories that reorganizations of bodily experience are crucial to the efficacy of healing rituals have been prominent in the anthropological literature (Levi-Strauss 1963, Desjarlais 1992, Dow 1986, Csordas 1994a). In general, they have proposed synergistic interactions between the somatosensory, affective, and semantic impacts of ritual performance. Perhaps changes in myofascia are also involved.

Summary

In this discussion I have avoided the reduction of Rolfing to an ethnotheory, a cultural discourse, or a "persuasive performance." Although each of those approaches does capture important aspects of the way in which this or any other kind of therapy works, they would tend to crowd out the very phenomena that Rolf practitioners and clients find most compelling: the immediately observable, sequential relationship between physical manipulation, changes in biomechanics, and reports of enhanced embodiment. In addition to summarizing the clinical observations and client reports that support this sequence, albeit in anecdotal form, I have also glossed the theories through which the worlds of Rolfing and body-oriented psychotherapy explain what they are alleviating—that is, the inferred causal sequence that links episodes of censure and trauma to reductions in fascial elasticity, biomechanical restrictions, and delimitation of the self's possibilities.

A second theory, which is more basic to the rationale of Rolfing, challenges the premise that cultural constructions of embodiment are entirely relativistic by asserting that a deep, metagrammar of deportmental life, incarnate in the musculoskeletal and neuromotor structure common to homo sapiens, underlies and circumscribes all cultural variation in biomechanical life and even informs the meanings ascribed to them.[14] In this, Rolf married her own notions of the psychological and existential significance of biomechanical restriction to her scientific conviction of the universality of human anatomy and neuromotor potential.

My participation in the clinical practice of Rolfing and my reflection on those experiences as an anthropologist have persuaded me that these explanatory frameworks and the phenomena they address deserve serious exploration by students of embodiment. Each suggests new approaches to central issues, and given the wide range of therapeutic practices that produce similar phenomena, may be important for the study of embodiment and healing in wider cultural contexts.

Notes

This chapter has benefited from the thoughtful suggestions of Thomas Csordas, Rosemary Feitis, Byron Good, and Alan Harwood.

1. The term "Rolfing" is a service mark of the Rolf Institute, P.O. Box 1868, Boulder, Colorado.

2. Bodywork therapies account for a significant proportion of the CAM practices currently proliferating through the cosmopolitan world. Systematic research on the therapeutic mechanisms and outcomes of CAM is funded at increasing levels. At least one major federal agency for the funding of such research, the National Center for Complementary and Alternative Medicine at the National Institutes of Health, has called for more involvement by

social scientists and anthropologists. It seems that the attention of medical anthropologists is both appropriate and timely.

3. The earliest known set of notes from a class taught by Rolf date to 1954 (Dorothy Nolte, personal communication).

4. Significant support for the variability of myofascial elasticity exists in the biological literature and is reviewed by Oschman and Oschman (1997) and Oschman (2000). More recently, an alternative theory of a neuromotor mechanism for the changes produced by Rolfing has gained adherents in the Rolfing community (Schleip 1994).

5. Rolfers often record changes in standing posture by taking "before" and "after" photographs. Jeff Linn of the Guild for Structural Integration has adapted imaging software provided by the NIH to the analysis of postural changes in "before" and "after" digital images of Rolfing clients.

6. Although epidemiological links between biomechanical disabilities, depression, anxiety, and certain patterns of cognition have been documented, these are not comparable to the anatomically and functionally more specific linkages that Rolf proposed.

7. The general descriptions and anecdotal examples of these experiences that follow come from my personal clinical experience and memory. They are not the result of any systematic research activity. IRB approval was not, therefore, involved. Many of these same types of experiences are described in the narratives of Rolfing collected by Anson (1998).

8. This is not to suggest that there is no cultural variation in such experiences, but that it seems to involve the way in which these various experiences are expressed, not the wholesale absence of any of the basic types.

9. The first of these theses finds a philosophical precedent in Merleau-Ponty's (1962) dictum that experiences of bodily motility are the prereflective ground of human meaning. As a corollary, one would expect chronic restrictions of biomechanical motility to effectively reduce the range of felt meanings available to the individual. The latter is a variant of one of the major theses of Reich's Orgonomic Therapy (1978), that chronic muscular rigidities are keyed, again on a specific, local level, to memories of social interactions that were traumatic or otherwise restrictive of the expression of the self, and that releasing those restrictions will allow a catharsis of those memories and their accompanying affects.

10. This is implied in Merleau-Ponty's (1962) understanding that embodiment is already cultural even at the "preobjective" level. It is explicit in Bourdieu's (1977, 1984) accounts of *habitus,* and in Csordas' (1988, 1993, 1994a, 1994b) integration of the semiotics and phenomenology of therapeutic embodiment.

11. Here, as in Csordas' study of Charismatic healing (1994a), the evidence suggests a close integration between culturally specified meanings of bodily life and the phenomenology of the self. It may be that a close study of any therapy or discipline that alters the body must address this integration.

12. The identification of myofascial adhesion and rigidity as the physical correlate of postural restriction closely parallels Reich's (1978) identification of "character armor," chronic patterns of muscular contraction, as the somatic basis of chronic emotional inhibition. In fact, the role accorded myofascial variability in this discussion parallels almost

exactly the role that Reich attributed to character armor vis-à-vis the formation, mainte-nance, and therapy of rigidities in the individual personality. He wrote extensively on the systematic cultural imposition of particular patterns of character structure, an aspect of what we now call "embodiment." Other influential formulations of links between chronic patterns of bodily tension and personality occur in the writings of Kellerman (1985), Lowen (1958), Perls et al. (1977), and Schilder (1993). In general, these theorists con-tinue, like Reich, to be ignored by the anthropological community (excepting Csordas' [1994a] reference to Schilder).

13. In his discussion of Catholic charismatic "leg-lengthening," Csordas (1994a) sug-gests a biomechanical component, but subordinates it to change in a cognitive schemata, the "postural model" (a construct proposed by Schilder 1993).

14. This thesis neither precludes nor denies the importance of research on cultural variations in posture and its meaning (exemplified by Hewes 1955, 1957). It only asserts that the underlying structure of the human body sets some limits on the range of varia-tion in biomechanical life, and also determines that certain kinds of variations will entail significantly more stress, strain, and eventual breakdown than others. While cultures may interpret the meanings of the more mechanically stressful deportments in different ways, one might expect that levels of stress and disability that interfere with the tasks of daily life would be recognized, at least on a practical level, as deficits of the self.

References
Anson, Briah
  1998 [1991]. *Rolfing: Stories of Personal Empowerment.* Berkeley, Calif.: North Atlantic Books.
Bourdieu, Pierre
  1977 *Outline of a Theory of Practice.* Cambridge, England: Cambridge University Press.
  1984 *Distinction: A Social Critique of the Judgment of Taste.* Cambridge, Mass.: Harvard Uni-versity Press.
Csordas, Thomas J.
  1988 Embodiment as a Paradigm for Anthropology. *Ethos* 18:5–47.
  1993 Somatic Modes of Attention. *Cultural Anthropology* 8(2):135–56.
  1994a *The Sacred Self: A Cultural Phenomenology of Charismatic Healing.* Berkeley: University of California Press.
  1994b Introduction: The Body as Representation and Being-in-the-World. Pp. 1–24 in Thomas Csordas, ed. *Embodiment and Experience: The Existential Ground of Culture and Self.* Cambridge, England: Cambridge University Press.
Desjarlais, Robert
  1992 *Body and Emotion: Aesthetics and Healing in the Nepal Himalayas.* Philadelphia: Univer-sity of Pennsylvania Press.
Dow, James
  1986 Universal Aspects of Symbolic Healing: A Theoretical Synthesis. *American An-thropologist* 88:56–69.

Foucault, Michel
  1979   *Discipline and Punish: The Birth of the Prison*. New York: Vintage.
Gevitz, Norman
  1982   *The D.O.s: Osteopathic Medicine in America*. Baltimore, Md.: John Hopkins University Press.
Hewes, G.
  1955   World Distribution of Certain Postural Habits. *American Anthropologist* 65:1003–26.
  1957   The Anthropology of Posture. *Scientific American* 196(2):122–32.
Kellerman, Stanley
  1985   *Emotional Anatomy: The Structure of Experience*. Berkeley, Calif.: Center Press.
Kerr, Catherine
  2002   Translating "Mind-in-Body": Two Models of Patient Experience Underlying a Randomized Controlled Trial of Qigong. *Culture, Medicine, and Psychiatry* 26(4):419–47.
Levi-Strauss, Claude
  1963   "The Sorcerer and His Magic" and "The Effectiveness of Symbols." Pp. 167–205. *Structural Anthropology*. New York: Basic Books.
Lowen, Alexander
  1958   *The Physical Dynamics of Character Structure: Bodily Form and Movement in Analytic Therapy*. New York: Grune and Stratton.
Mauss, Marcel
  1992[1934]   Techniques of the Body. Pp. 455–77 in Jonathan Crary and Sanford Kwinter, eds. *Incorporations*. New York: Zone.
Merleau-Ponty, Maurice
  1962   *Phenomenology of Perception*. Evanston, Ill.: Northwestern University Press.
Moore, J. Stuart
  1993   *Chiropractic in America: The History of a Medical Alternative*. Baltimore, Md.: John Hopkins University Press.
Ohlgren, Gail, and David Clark
  n.d.   *Natural Walking* (mimeograph). Boulder, Colo.: Rolf Institute.
Oschman, James
  2000   Structural Integration (Rolfing), Osteopathic, Chiropractic, Feldenkrais, Alexander, Myofascial Release, and Related Methods. Pp. 165–74 in James L. Oschman, ed. *Energy Medicine: The Scientific Basis*. Edinburgh: Churchill Livingstone.
Oschman, James, and Nora H. Oschman
  1997   *The Scientific Basis of Bodywork, Energetic, and Movement Therapies*. Dover, N.H.: Nature's Own Research Association.
Perls, Frederick, Paul Goodman, and Ralph Hefferline
  1977   *Gestalt Therapy: Excitement and Growth in the Human Personality*. New York: Dell.
Reich, Wilhelm
  1978[1933]   *Character-analysis*. New York: Simon and Schuster.

Rolf, Ida P.

1973   Structural Integration: A Contribution to the Understanding of Stress. *Confinia Psychiatrica* 16(2):69–79.

1977   *Rolfing: The Integration of Human Structures.* Santa Monica, Calif.: Dennis-Landman.

1979   Structure: A New Factor in Understanding the Human Condition. *Somatics* (Spring): 6–8.

Schilder, Paul

1993   *The Image and Appearance of the Human Body.* London: Kegan Paul, Trench, Trubner & Co.

Schleip, Robert

1994   *Talking to Fascia: Changing the Brain.* Boulder, Colo.: Rolf Institute.

Schultz, R. Louis, and Rosemary Feitis

1996   *The Endless Web: Fascial Anatomy and Physical Reality.* Berkeley, Calif.: North Atlantic Books.

Strauss, Erwin

1966   The Upright Posture. Pp. 137–65 in *Phenomenological Psychology: The Selected Papers of Erwin W. Strauss.* New York: Basic Books.

Xu, S. H.

1994   Psychophysiological Reactions Associated with Qigong Therapy. *Chinese Medical Journal* (England) 107(3):230–33.

A WIDER LENS   III
THE BONESETTER'S CONTRIBUTION
TO COMMUNITY HEALTH

MOVING FROM CLINICAL ENCOUNTERS to a broader perspective, the final section presents four case studies that underscore the embeddedness of bonesetting practices in local contexts and the health benefits of these practices for the wider communities they serve. In this section, chapters are not concerned solely with the efficacy of treatment for individual patients, but also with the productivity of the tradition in general—that is, the volume of effective services provided overall relative to other health care providers.

The four sites of inquiry in this section envelop the globe—from the Rolfer in San Francisco, to the *componedor* in the Peruvian Andes, to the *chiressa* in the Kenyan bush, and the bonesetter in a Welsh port town. In no case is the manual medical specialist working in isolation of a larger medical system. Each country has a pluralistic medical system—a complicated array of health care services from which a patient can theoretically pick and choose. Granted, bonesetters are never central to the system, but rather are found at the margins of a powerful, authoritative biomedical industrial complex, no matter what continent or corner of the world. All four of the healers in this section, as with most in the book, practice in the private, not public, sector.

In all four accounts, we see indigenous healers interacting with biomedical specialists, at times antagonistically, at times to their mutual benefit. Despite the competition from other often unsympathetic modalities, in each case presented, the bonesetter provides an efficacious service otherwise not readily available—or in most instances affordable—to peasant, pastoralist, and working class, as well as urban elite, populations.

Aspects of community life engender the specific types of musculoskeletal distress experienced (backaches from harvesting potatoes, broken bones from defending the community cattle herds, leg injuries from rugby, facial paralysis from work stress) and specialists emerge in each community to handle the problems with which they have intimate knowledge based on their own immersion in the culturally patterned activities of daily life. At the same time, the authors here have spent lengthy intervals living and working in the communities they study, and thus also have a firsthand appreciation of the bodily ailments in question.

In chapter 10, Kathryn Oths depicts the hardscrabble existence in an Andean peasant hamlet, where musculoskeletal injuries from work, play, and accidents are a routine occurrence. Life is lived so close to the margin that without the services of the various bonesetters (*componedores*) in the community, the people would not be able to carry out the tasks necessary for survival. In the highlands, as in other contexts where people labor manually, efficacy of a treatment is measured by its ability to manage pain and disability, which allows one to continue working to make a living under precarious socioeconomic conditions.

Andean *componedores* are in high demand. Visits to them account for one in five healer visits, and as often as not, *componedores* are resorted to concurrently with other healer types as part of a comprehensive health care strategy. For example, in the treatment of one major illness episode, a person may visit a *componedor* on one day for manipulation, a health post another day for pain pills, and an herbalist later for a topical remedy. While satisfaction with other healer types in the community was mixed, in no case in the study did the client of a *componedor* rate them anything but effective and indispensable. Andean bonesetters are shown to use a wider variety of methods than typically depicted in the literature. They are recognized as a limited but essential specialty alongside other healing modalities.

Various healers play an integral role in restoring a peasant to health after a musculoskeletal or other disease incident; the *componedor* should be respected as one whose contribution to maintaining community health and social relations in the rural Andes is unparalleled. The low investment in technology keeps the cost of bonesetter services affordable; deferred payment is common; the bonesetter, unlike health post personnel, is highly mobile and can make house calls when physical injury impedes a person from walking long distances over mountain trails to get to a clinic. The constant assault on the body by highland agricultural life under precarious socioeconomic conditions insures that *componedores* will have a prominent place in Andean medical systems well into the foreseeable future.

In chapter 11, Isaac Nyamongo describes conditions for the pastoralist Borana in rural Northern Kenya, where the mobility of the people would make it difficult for the state to offer biomedical services even if it *were* a priority. He contends, "In parts of Northern Kenya where pastoral communities are constantly moving in search of pasture and water for their domestic animals, it is particularly problematic for health authorities to put in place a meaningful health care infrastructure."

As a result, bonesetters fill a vital gap in the delivery of health care. While their *materia medica* supplementing their manual techniques consists primarily of locally available natural products, they, in a fashion not unlike that of the Maya bonesetters (chapter 6), have managed to take advantage of the dominant system's facilities to secure x-rays. The matter of seeking out a bonesetter is clearly not entirely an issue of lack of access to biomedical facilities because clients often go to the hospital first to get free x-rays, which they then spirit away for their bonesetter's use.

Borana communities cohere strongly along kinship lines. Nyamongo makes clear how an injury to a Borana is never an individual matter, but necessarily involves the wider family and community in decision-making. For instance, full recovery from an injury is marked by ritual celebration for which clan members, acting corporately, must provide animals for slaughter. In a small-scale society, the welfare of each and every member is of vital interest to the community, but all the more so in the case of its young men, who are entrusted with care of their most valuable asset, the herds, and who fulfill a military role in protecting the community against outside aggression.

Though doctors will set broken bones presented to them, bonesetters in Kenya and throughout sub-Saharan Africa are viewed as the most competent musculoskeletal therapists available, even by those in the modern health sector themselves, despite the attendant risks of improper setting or gangrene. The payment of the bonesetter (*chiressa*), more than monetary, is in terms of the higher social status and political capital he gains by sustaining community members.

In the next chapter, Simon Leyson portrays the life of a dockworker and bonesetter, Jack Leyshon, against the backdrop of the gritty Welsh industrial port town in which he lived and died. Endowed with tremendous skill and charisma, Jack left such a profound impression on his community that Leyson, a chiropractor himself (and no relation), came to hear of Jack many years after his passing through testimonials of his surviving clients. He shows that not only Jack, but bonesetters in general across British history, "have enjoyed the confidence of the people," although they often had to contend with the calumny of biomedical professionals. If a person had an injury, they simply "went down Jack's" without a second thought.

Leyson borrows Williamson's (1982) notion of community to portray a sense of Jack's hometown and his place in it: "The notion of community embraces not just the idea of locality or social networks of particular kinds; it refers to the rich mosaic of subjective meanings which people attach . . . to the place itself and to the social relationships of which they are a part." Religion, sport, and manual labor interwove to create a seamless fabric of social life in Port Talbot. Jack was molded in his sensibilities by his religious mother, got his therapeutic start as a masseur for the local rugby club, and gained clients from the docks and—as his reputation grew—even the surrounding towns. Rumor had it that he even received referrals from and personally attended to physicians.

"His skill as a bonesetter was vital for the men who relied on [manual] work for their living," notes Leyson. "Security of tenure for such a job depended only on one's ability to turn up fit for work." With the delay in time it took to get treatment from the National Health Service (NHS), manual laborers preferred the fast and effective treatment of Jack, where one could simply show up without an appointment, especially because "catching the problem warm" insured a speedier recovery. Furthermore, he attracted many clients whom the NHS had failed. Thus, Jack performed a public service to his community, one that did not go unrecognized. He was indeed a community treasure. As one former client put it, "He was a man of the people. He cared about people and he cared for people." One finishes this chapter with a sense of having known and been treated by Jack personally.

In the final chapter, when Rolfer Marc Weill claims "it takes a village," he is suggesting that the modern-day bonesetter is embedded in a larger system of communication and information flow than might be apparent. Due to modern technology, which allows a high level of interaction between physically distant persons, the larger community in which he practices, San Francisco, becomes a "functional village" with characteristics not unlike that of a peasant village. That is, one's credibility is quickly established (or destroyed) by the word of mouth of those who have witnessed one's work. Internet referrals earn clients from around the Bay Area, even around the world. The alternative community finds itself under the microscope, scrutinized by biomedical professionals who might be eager to denounce its practices or at best fail to acknowledge its victories. The Rolfer must sell his or her methods to a dubious public culturally conditioned and financially encouraged by insurance coverage to seek out biomedicine without questioning the options. The success of his practice relies heavily on the social support afforded his clients by community members who have experienced and have faith in his healing approach.

A few of the chapters conclude with reflections on how, though meritorious in the ideal, there are major difficulties inherent in attempting to integrate traditional and biomedical body workers under one hospital roof (Oths, Nyamongo). These four contributions demonstrate the bonesetter's ability to treat not only the individual, but to support the functioning of an entire social system as well.

Reference

Williamson, W.
   1982 *Class Community and Culture: A Biographical Study of Social Change in Mining*. London: Routledge & Keegan Paul.

The *Componedor's* Place in the Pluralistic Andean Health Care System

10

KATHRYN S. OTHS

THE ARDUOUS NATURE OF MANUAL LABOR in the Andean highlands, aggravated by harsh climatic conditions and an exploitive, or "macroparasitic" (Brown 1987), political-economic system (Oths 1999), results in a high incidence of musculoskeletal disorders. Published studies show the frequency of bodily ailments in the Andes to be between 14 and 26 percent of all illness episodes (see Oths 1998 for review). In this study, one-fifth of all visits to healers were to a *componedor*, as those doing bodywork in the Andes are called. *Componedores*, loosely translated as "those who fix or repair," are in high demand because their treatments are seen as the most effective for managing musculoskeletal pain. These healers mobilize joints and reposition the minor movements or major dislocations of the vertebrae, joints, muscles, and even organs whose improper position may cause pain, discomfort, and disability (Oths 2002).

This chapter describes the variety of healing methods that *componedores* employ and the way in which *componedores* are utilized alongside other healers as part of a comprehensive health care strategy. The available social science research on bonesetters gives little if any description of other methods beyond physical manipulation and immobilization that they employ in their practices. Furthermore, the complementarity that might exist between the roles of the bonesetter and other healers has not been a subject of inquiry. To explore these issues, this chapter attempts to situate the Andean *componedor* practice within the larger context of the health care system.

Musculoskeletal problems are an illness of antiquity for sierrans. In the 1500s, Inca Garcilaso de la Vega, the New World chronicler of mixed descent, describing what northern Peruvian highlanders nowadays call *flotación*—that is, a rinsing or rubdown with a liquid or unguent (Oths 1992:79; also see Classen

[1993] on the symbolic power of fluidity in bodily representations)—mentions the Inca practice of passing a substance over their body "as if to cleanse with it, to rid their bodies of all of its illnesses" (1973:20–21, my translation). This practice is identical to one that accompanies joint manipulation by modern day Andeans to reduce swelling and infection. Valdizan and Maldonado (1922) mention *componedores* in their classic compendium of Peruvian traditional medicine. While a tone of condescension inflects their portrayal of all manner of Andean healing, they grudgingly attest to the efficacy of "famous bonesetters" (1922:123, my translation) and quote the highlander's belief that "doctors do not understand bones" (126, my translation). Valdizan and Maldonado devote an entire chapter to the home remedies, both plant and animal, bonesetters use in conjunction with manual therapy.

Setting and Methods

Chugurpampa, the site of this research, is a highland peasant hamlet (*comunidad campesina*) in northern Peru dispersed over an altitude range of approximately 9,000 to 13,500 feet above sea level and covering about 1,000 hectares. The principal crop is the potato and market participation is extensive. While the peasants speak only Spanish and display minimal "Indian" style in their clothing and ritual, they are clearly indigenous and socially separate from the mestizo class, which occupies the town of Julcan and other urbanized areas. Julcan, the district capital, takes one to two hours to reach by foot, and is where the Ministry of Health health post and Sunday market are found. The treacherous mountain terrain is difficult enough to walk along without falling (most nonhighland born decline to attempt it), much less to navigate when the surface is wet and/or one is carrying a heavy load. This ecological factor is salient in the genesis of musculoskeletal distress, as will be shown.

The case illnesses examined here were collected over six months among a random sample of thirty-two households (166 persons) representing about 20 percent of the population. Whereas most treatment choice research consists of a one-time rapid assessment based on an epidemiologic model of acute infectious disease, this data collection entailed repeat visits to the same household to take into account the chronic and recurring nature of highland illnesses, a pattern typical of musculoskeletal problems. On average, ten visits were made at two-week intervals to all houses in the sample, at which time I collected the details of all recent illness episodes, including the etiology, type, severity and duration of symptoms, number of workdays missed, the remedies and/or healers employed, the hot/cold nature of the illness and remedies, the success of treatment, and its cost.

In addition to over one year's residence and ongoing participation in the life of the community, my repeat visits to households helped establish investigator–

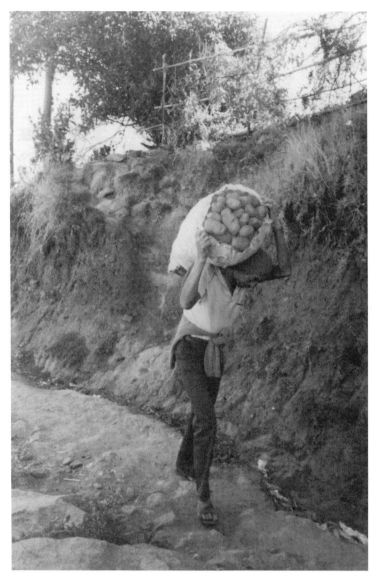

Figure 10.1.   Highland peasant carrying a load twice his weight over rough
terrain. (Photo by Kathryn S. Oths.)

informant rapport. Over time, additional details of the cause and course of the
various illnesses were revealed, creating a robust understanding of the families'
health conditions and their interpretations of them. I also established a close
relationship with Don Artemio (pseudonyms are used throughout), the region's

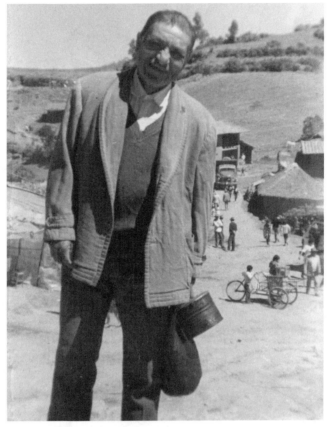

Figure 10.2.   Don Artemio, the most renowned of the region's bone-setters. (Photo by Kathryn S. Oths.)

most renowned bonesetter, and accompanied him on many of his patient visits. I also visited frequently with other *componedores* to discuss musculoskeletal manipulation and, on occasion, to observe their practices or receive adjustments myself. Furthermore, community members learned of my interest in musculoskeletal health and would avidly and informally discuss their aches and pains with me.

The Pluralistic Medical System
Leslie (1976) first defined a pluralistic medical system as a treatment context in which a population had access to both modern and traditional types of healers. Young (1983) later refined the concept to include the notion of a nested *system* of health care delivery that encompassed various medical *sectors* (basic philosophical

orientations to health, such as professional biomedicine, traditional, home care), within each of which were embedded one or more medical *traditions* (e.g., biomedical might include physicians and lay practitioners, among others, while traditional might include herbalists and bonesetters, among others). Baer (1989) later emphasized the difference between pluralistic systems in which the various sectors have relatively equal status and power and those, like in the United States and Peru, in which the biomedical sector is dominant.

In the Peruvian highlands, besides using home remedies, people may resort to a variety of traditional and modern healers when they fall ill. On the traditional side, these include the bonesetter (*componedor* or *huesero*),[1] herbalist (*yerbatero*), curer (*curioso*, who specializes in internal medicine), midwife (*partera*), traveling medicine vendor (*remediero*, usually found at Sunday market; Amazonians are considered the most powerful), soul caller (*llamador*, who cures *susto*, or soul loss), and shaman (*curandero*)— while on the biomedical side one encounters the health promoter (*promotor de salud*), health sanitarian (*técnico sanitario*), lay pharmacist (*topiquero*; both formal and informal pharmacies sell drugs over the counter that would require a prescription in the United States), lay practitioner (*practicante* or *doctor particular*), nurse, dentist, and physician. If relief is not obtained with one option, another will invariably be sought. This at times can result in a long series of different treatments, especially in the case of chronic and recurrent problems, with diagnoses frequently changing along the way. Also, at times more than one healer may be sought concurrently for the complementary aspects of relief they can provide.

The Peruvian state subsidizes health care through health posts, clinics, and hospitals operated by the Ministry of Health. Though not cheap, the price of their consultation and medicine is generally more reasonable than that of the private lay or professional biomedical practitioners, the latter being available only on the coast and extremely expensive. The health sanitarian, a local Ministry of Health employee assigned to each health post, while only having received two years of training in public health and basic medicine, is viewed as superior in competence and trustworthiness to the "greenhorn" clinic doctors to whom he is officially subordinate. His skill comes from long-term residence and experience in the community in which he lives.

Apart from the public sector, the private sector of professional biomedicine in Peru is a key factor in the delivery of health care, providing a substantial proportion (22.6 percent) of services received (Murillo Alfaro 1998). *Practicantes* are judged by highlanders to be more skilled than professional doctors in treating common sierran illnesses such as respiratory or kidney infections, and their stocks of medicine are much better maintained than those of Ministry of Health entities, which suffer from budgetary restraints and graft. The *practicante* simply visits Trujillo to buy supplies from a preferred pharmacist while the health posts must wait for state distribution. The *técnico sanitario* is unique in that he serves in both a public and private capacity, fulfilling his official capacity then moonlighting by making house calls on his own time. *Componedores*, like other traditional healers, can rightfully be considered part of the private sector (Harrison 2001:279).

Traditional and modern medicines the world over have parallel specialties that respond to the typical health needs of humans (see the introduction to this volume, and Coreil 1983). Curiously, however, within biomedicine physicians have all but ignored the treatment of everyday muscular and skeletal disorders to focus on highly specialized orthopedic surgery. The care of the body is primarily relegated to lower-status, allied health disciplines such as physical and occupational therapy and in the United States largely opposed (or at best treated as suspect) when delivered by nonbiomedical specialists such as chiropractors (see Anderson 1983). In the Andes, the *componedor's* practice is analogous to that of a physical therapist or chiropractor. Highland *componedores*, however, do not practice full-time, instead dividing their attention between their crops and their clients. As they, too, toil as peasant farmers, the embodied experience *componedores* have with the same types of stresses and strains afflicting their clients—in essence their shared habitus (Bourdieu 1977) or existential experience of "being in the world" (Csordas 1994)—helps them understand and accumulate knowledge about the nature of the physical problems on which they work.

The Andean *componedor* is the sole provider of musculoskeletal therapy in the Andean health care delivery system. As they do not duplicate biomedical services, bonesetters are left ample room to practice and have, in the Northern Peruvian Andes, created a truce rather than competition between physicians and themselves. Health post physicians are prone to refer patients to a local bonesetter rather than deal with the problem. This acceptance of bonesetters is widespread among the general populace as well. In a 1997 Peruvian national household survey, bonesetters were considered the most efficacious of all traditional healers, with over 50 percent of respondents stating a preference for these healers in the case of injury or other trauma of the bones and over 63 percent acknowledging their curative efficacy (Murillo Alfaro 1998).

The position of biomedicine vis-à-vis bonesetters in Peru stands in stark contrast to that reported elsewhere in Latin America. Hinojosa has documented active resistance by physicians to the perceived encroachment of bonesetters on their turf in Guatemala, and the bonesetters' clever utilization of medical technological resources in spite of this (Hinojosa 2002; Hinojosa, this volume). One of the primary themes of the edited collection on Mesoamerican healers by Huber and Sandstrom (2001) is the very conflict between biomedicine and most indigenous "alternative" healers, including bonesetters, and the extant barriers to the two traditions working in concert.

Treatment Modalities and Patterns of Resort

The manner in which people navigate the various medical options available to them is referred to as a pattern of resort (Nichter 1978; Kleinman 1980). Resort can be simultaneous, that is, seeing two specialists concurrently, or it can be sequential, wherein a person consecutively uses more than one practitioner for the same illness (e.g., first visiting a *curandero* then later a doctor) (Young 1983). In my entire sample of illness episodes (not just musculoskeletal), more than one healer was sought in one-fifth of all cases in which a healer was employed, with more than one healer being sought in nearly half of cases involving a *componedor*. In only a handful of cases were healers sought simultaneously, that is, on the same day, though again this situation was more prevalent when a *componedor* was sought. The use of more than one healer for an illness episode might be viewed by the patient's family as essential to cure the emotional concomitants of the problem as well as its physical dimensions. The patient is satisfied because both the illness and disease dimensions are addressed (Kleinman 1980). But physical ailments can also be addressed jointly, as in the case of a sick person going to a *componedor* for an adjustment and to a *practicante* for kidney pills, both treating the same lower back problem (*dolor de la cintura*).

Componedores in the Andes employ various styles of treatment and often mix bonesetting and manipulation with other therapeutic modalities in their quest to heal patients. The variation in treatment styles is a product of self-teaching, born of the inconsistent manner of recruitment into the profession. Most claim to have received their healing skills as a gift from God, while some at the same time have descended from healers from whom they likely absorbed techniques unreflexively. This variability in recruitment to the bonesetter role, with an emphasis on divine inspiration, has been well-documented by others (Hinojosa 2002; Paul and McMahon 2001; Klein, and Leyson, both this volume). A manual therapy treatment is called a *compuesta*; manipulative techniques in the Andean highlands include having the patient lie face down, kneel, sit in a chair, or be rolled in a blanket while the healer "closes" or puts the body back in order by gently palpating, kneading, stretching, and pulling the muscles, bones, and connective tissue. Sharp, quick jerks and pops are uncommon. After a treatment, the affected area is covered with a salve and bandaged (see Oths 2002 for a full description of types of injuries treated and styles of treatment).

It is important to recognize that, beyond simply moving bones and massaging muscles, the *componedor's* specialized knowledge, like that of other healers, is broad and grows by accretion. Any method, technique, or even technological equipment (see Anderson and Klein, Hinojosa, and Nyamongo, this volume) that bonesetters learn or acquire access to that improves their success in healing will be incorporated into their armamentarium without concern as to whether it violates some precept of "traditionalism" or disciplinary purity. Bonesetting skills have been found combined with midwifery, shamanism, and internal medicine-type curing roles in other parts of Latin America (Lipp 2001:99, 106). This catholicity of methods among traditional body workers previously has not been noted.

The frequent blending of approaches on the part of many bonesetters parallels that of U.S.-based chiropractors, who have historically been divided into "straights" and "mixers" depending on whether or not they employ additional methods. Nowadays, the majority of chiropractors incorporate into their practices modalities such as hair analysis, nutritional supplements, herbal remedies, electrical muscle stimulation, biofeedback, acupuncture, homeopathy, and other techniques in an attempt to deliver more generalized primary care. Many have come to recognize the limited value of solely moving bones, that is, eliminating subluxations, without the support of other fundamental physiological shifts (also see Weill, this volume). Likewise with the Andean *componedor*. As will become evident in the following case studies, *componedores* use a variety of techniques, with some even integrating two or more healer roles into one practice.

All of the *componedores* included in the study employed other remedies in addition to massage and skeletal adjustment, ranging from the suggestion of herbal teas to prepare to the use, preparation, resale, or prescribing of topical treatments, primarily over-the-counter salves of the Bengay variety or traditional remedies such as snake alcohol (*alcohol de culebra*) or *chuncho*, a humorally "hot" ointment, both available from Amazonian *remedieros*. It is worth noting that I never encountered a healer advocating stretching or exercise, as one might anticipate in the United States, possibly because peasant life affords more than ample opportunity for this. Frequently, in fact, the advice was to stay in bed under warm blankets for at least the rest of the day after a *compuesta*, so as not to chill the body or risk reinjury while the body was still tender and loose from the adjustment.

While all of the *componedores* in this study utilized remedies in conjunction with manual therapy, two of them actually held dual healing roles. Don Artemio, in addition to his bonesetting renown, was also a noted herbalist and the designated community health promoter. He received Ministry of Health certification for the latter, though not before he had earned a reputation for giving injections of antibiotics and other medicines. Sra. Laura, a prominent midwife, was frequently sought by women for her spinal manipulation skill for reproductive-related conditions. Varying levels of healing knowledge notwithstanding, bedside manner was consistent across all healers. A client would usually show up at a healer's house unannounced, or in serious cases, a relative would arrive and request a house call. The *componedor* would set about attending with the calmness and amiability characteristic of everyday Andean social interaction, in a collaborative rather than authoritarian style. Treatment was conducted in a polite, perfunctory manner, with the client usually on his or her way within twenty to thirty minutes.

Besides the mixing of modalities, another facet of Andean bonesetting that deserves attention is the complex pattern of resort into which they fit. That is, a *componedor* is often consulted alongside other healers, such as an herbalist, midwife, curer, shaman, pharmacist, nurse and/or doctor, to achieve the best possible result for the patient. In most cases, home remedies are also administered before, during, and after visits to specialists.

The bonesetters' modalities, their place in the patient's larger quest for relief, plus the relative costs and final outcomes of treatments are illustrated within the context of case studies of individual sickness episodes.

Nine Family Case Studies

Nine cases were chosen to represent the full spectrum of complaints and complexity that appeared during the illness collection period. Though all peasant families in Chugurpampa are poor vis-à-vis those of the larger society, and socioeconomic class distinctions within the hamlet are nonexistent, some wealth and status difference between families is inevitable, as the case studies make apparent. The vignettes should be read with the awareness that the case illness collection covered the months of July 1 through mid-December of 1988, a period that saw the best and the worst of times. For the first three months, a bountiful harvest was in progress and money was flowing. In October, the worst economic collapse in the country's history decimated the value of the highlanders' annual savings. Therefore, while living standards varied to begin with, midway through the study all households alike began to suffer economic stresses, and this limited their ability to spend on medical services (Oths 1994).[2]

Case 1

Juana and her husband were both 46, with her two surviving daughters aged 20 and 9 still living at home. Atypically, she had lost three children at the ages of 2, 10, and 13, the only woman under 50 in the sample to have lost a child older than 5. A 15-year-old nephew rounded out the household, providing the balance necessary to the gendered Andean division of labor (Oths 1999). They led a quiet life farming their twelve hectares. Their one-room thatched cottage was modest, and her husband had occupied no religious, political, or communal office. The family's one source of wealth, however, became the source of Juana's health setback.

One day in late July, while Juana was handling one of their bulls, it gored and then chased her. Her emotion when retelling the story was evident and remained high across my many visits to the household. She received bad bruises on her right arm and left ribs. Her lower back was knocked out of place (*cintura movida*, see Oths 2002), her left side felt "asleep," and her abdomen hurt. For two days she neither got up nor walked. Her difficulty moving subsided substantially after she received her first *compuesta* from Sra. Maria, her *comadre* (honorific designating ritual kinship between a mother and godmother), a 72-year-old neighbor and *componedora* of average skill. Sra. Maria would not treat her on the day of the accident because she was in too much pain, and she advised Juana to wait until the swelling had receded a bit more before the second *compuesta*. She was charged 50 intis for the service (approximately US$0.30; see note 2).

At the same time, Juana had been self-treating since the day after the incident with humorally cool remedies suggested at no charge by a *curioso*, José Eduardo. These included the application of ground wheat with alcohol to the area of the blows, herbal teas locally known as *mongo* (translation unknown), *pie de perro* (culantro), *pulipunche* (cinchona bark), and a *flotación* of Milk of Magnesia with *pisco* (anisette) for both the blows and her back.

The bull had attacked her between my first and second visit. When I spoke with her six days after the injury, she was sitting quietly in the shade knitting, as she could not yet resume work in the fields. Two weeks later, after another *compuesta* at no charge (though Sra. Maria could not get the upper back to adjust) and a continuation of the herbs (adding a new one, *raiz de ortiga negra*, or black nettle root), she felt much better and was back to work, although the lower back and left side were still a problem. In the interim she had also gone to the health post in Julcan, where she was attended by Nurse Linda. She was diagnosed with "infection" and grief (*pena*), and given eight capsules that the nurse went out and purchased for her at the pharmacy, but which did not sit well with her. The total cost for the consultation and pills was 140 intis. She was advised to travel to Trujillo to get a cast for her back, and return to the health post, but she did neither. She couldn't return to Julcan, she explained, because she was too weak to be exposed to the sun.[3] Two months later, her wounds and bruises were gone and her lower back hurt only very mildly. She continued with the home remedies, using grated potato and herbal *flotaciónes*. She also went to another *curioso*, Agustino, for a *flotación* for her lower back, which cost 200 intis. She said it was too strong for her to use, but by my next visit she was using it and claimed it worked well. In early October, in little pain but still not able to exert much force, she purchased 440 intis worth of capsules from a *topiquera* in Julcan for "infection from the blow," which she rated as very good. Until my last visit in December, she continued to have mild lower back pain, which she attributed to not taking it easy after receiving her *compuestas* (see Oths 2002). She received no more *compuestas* and for muscle aches was using *chuncho* from a *remediero*, which settled her.

Meanwhile, in late August, Juana's husband, Elmer, hurt his arm and shoulder splitting wood and subsequently getting chilled. He could not work for four days, though he was not in bed. When I first saw him, shortly after the injury, he could hardly move his arm. He used *flotaciónes* and received a *compuesta* from a friend, both of which helped. The problem oscillated between mild and moderate through December, getting better for a few days when he was "composed," and worse when he worked. Not taking care of himself when he worked caused him, in his words, to *descomponer* (get out of alignment). In November he had expected the *componedor* to visit his house, but he didn't. Elmer moves and stretches his body until he self-composes the best he can. He has been sharing *chuncho* and other *flotaciónes* with his wife.

Analysis: Both of the partners had to work, as there was insufficient labor in the household to otherwise allow them to rest and heal. The mother's injury, the more severe of the two, resulted in a pattern of resort that was quite varied, with simultaneous as well as sequential help seeking. She included home remedies, several traditional healers, a lay pharmacist, and biomedicine. Emotional fragility seemed to complicate her experience of the injury, possibly having originated in the earlier losses of her children (see Oths 1999). Both rated their *componedores'* interventions, among other remedies, as helpful in easing their pain and keeping them working. For both, the *componedor* was the first healer resorted to after the injury occurred.

Case 2

Graciela is the forty-year-old mother of four boys living at home, ranging in age from 4 to 15, plus three older children. She and her 57-year-old husband, Alberto, are stable economically, with twelve hectares of property and ample livestock— four bulls, two burros, and assorted pigs, sheep, and smaller animals. She is plagued off and on by chronic pain in the lower and upper back (*dolor de cintura* and *dolor de espalda*, respectively) caused by a fall several years ago. She considers the gravity of the illness to be light, but it impedes her walking up steep hills or doing heavy work without rest.

Graciela's problem persisted across the entire case illness collection period, with symptoms at bay on some visits, and light to moderate at other times. Lower back pain was the most consistently elicited of her complaints. She received a *compuesta* in April from Sra. García, a neighboring *componedora*, three months before I first talked to her, but the healer was not there when she returned later for another treatment. The Señora diagnosed her with having a "fallen" or "dropped" abdomen (*barriga bajada*), a culture-specific illness in which the organs, including the uterus, shift out of place. Graciela was charged a nominal fee of one inti. In the interim she had also been applying over-the-counter pharmaceutical preparations such as Mentholatum as *flotaciónes*. Mainly, her strategy was to rest when she could, which calmed her.

By my next visit she had had a setback due to harvesting potatoes, which requires a full day of filling, hoisting, and carrying large sacks of produce, weighing about a hundred pounds each (see Oths 1999). The intense sun and later the cold had aggravated her condition. She had still not returned to Sra. García and was continuing to use a variety of manufactured salves. At the end of August, she visited Mercedes, a *componedora* far down the mountain, who adjusted her spinal column. She was told she had a kidney infection, and prescribed baths, herbal teas, and a vaginal enema. She felt somewhat better. She needed to return for another *compuesta* and to have her pulse diagnosed, but it was too far for her to walk. At her worst point, in early October, she complained that her lower back "hurt as if I were going to give birth." By the middle of October, she had done the baths and herbs, plus various other *flotaciónes* that included mother's milk, limes, and cow butter. She did not take the enema, however. The problem always seemed to return when she walked or worked strenuously. From that point on, she was feeling considerably better and did not report more treatments of any type.

Graciela's husband provided a study in contrasts. Alberto was one of a handful of men in Chugurpampa with a history in the Quiruvilca mines, entailing brutal work at high altitude in freezing, wet conditions (see Nash 1979). These same men were substantially more ill with serious chronic conditions than others in the sample, and all, not coincidentally, were the only ones with evident alcohol abuse.[4] They also showed a marked preference for biomedicine, shunning traditional remedies as useless, which, given the severity of their conditions, they may often have been. Their medical treatment preference was engendered by their reliance on biomedicine during the years at the mines, where a hospital was located and all biomedical attention was free of charge.

In an odd coincidence that can only occur when one is enmeshed in daily participant observation of the life of a community, I witnessed a horrible scene. One Sunday afternoon in late August on the way back from the Julcan market on a rarely used road, I came upon a man on his back being trampled by a mounted horse. The fallen man writhed like a snake, bellowed, and somehow rose and stumbled off wildly. Only then did I realize it was Alberto and that he was drunk. I never did learn what precipitated the event, but the scene began to make sense when I interviewed him a short time later. On that visit, his myriad prior ailments were complicated by sharp pains (*punzadas*) on the left side of his chest and his eyesight going dim when he exerted himself. He at first uncertainly attributed it to a fall, then at a later visit explained he was going to take an herb for bruising, *pulipunche*, "because maybe I was beaten." He may not have remembered what happened, or preferred not to admit it to me or his family. The point is that in October, he stated "it wasn't getting any better," that his "ribs were sunken" (i.e., displaced), and that "it felt like a tumor," yet apart from home remedies, the only healers he resorted to were doctors and pharmacists, not *componedores*, though his wife recently had employed two.

Analysis: Graciela had no female help in a household of males, so she had to work even when it aggravated her ailments. She was able to carry on with periodic attention from a *componedor* and over-the-counter and herbal remedies. Her husband, on the other hand, accustomed to biomedicine from his years as a miner, did not seek what on the face of it would be the most logical and accessible treatment. He may have been trying to communicate a higher status or more mestizo identity through his use of biomedicine (see Crandon-Malamud 1991), though such behavior would have been unusual in Chugurpampa (Oths 2002).

Case 3

Shy ten-year-old Amable was the third of seven children in an economically strapped household. Her father was another former coal miner with many serious health problems. On July 2, she slipped while carrying a sack of potatoes and wrenched her upper and lower back (*espalda* and *cintura movida*) badly enough that she couldn't walk or sit. Four days later, the Julcan Health Sanitarian, in Chugurpampa for a vaccine drive, could not examine her because "he didn't have his equipment with him." He advised that she visit the health post in Julcan; her condition, however, precluded her walking there. The next day, her mother's *comadre*, Mercedes, composed her at no charge and sold her an unguent (*pomada*) from a Julcan herbalist for 100 intis. Shortly after, her teacher at school told her it was her kidneys and gave her some pills. She felt both the *compuesta* and the pills were effective. Three weeks later, she felt fine, but a week after that she slipped again while carrying water.

Amable could walk this time, but it hurt to sit or get up. In addition to a return of the previous symptoms, her thighs were involved this time and she vomited on two occasions. A week later, she received a *compuesta* from her "aunt" (fictive kin), Tia Petra, who was visiting from the city of Trujillo, and she felt a little better by the next day. She had not gone back to Mercedes as she was supposed to "because too many people watch and it embarrasses me." (That the *componedora* had a very attractive and popular teenage son likely had more than a little to do with it.) She had not been ingesting any home remedies because they made her nauseous. She had no interest in going to Julcan. "The doctors in Julcan don't do me any good" she concluded, after having gone to them for arm pain several months before. Her father promised to take her to Trujillo if the problem continued.

Three weeks later, she was fine except for some residual kidney pain. Another consult with the *técnico sanitario* (no charge) prompted the purchase of some kidney pills by her father when he was in the city (10 for 30 intis), which helped. Unfortunately, two weeks after that, Amable was thrown from a burro, adding her shins and feet to the previous ailments. Her lungs then became involved, as her back was "open." Her grandmother diagnosed *aire* and she received a puppy rubdown (*soba de perro*)[5] for her back and lungs, which helped. She would like to have taken more kidney pills but the bus fare was too expensive to travel to Trujillo for more. She was still unable to carry loads or gather firewood. Three months after the initial accident, she was feeling well except for her feet, which would get hot at night and cold in the morning. She treated this symptom off and on for the next two months with home remedies such as the unguent, a guinea pig rubdown (*soba de cuy*), an occasional *flotación* of lime with alcohol, or a drink of her mother's vitamin tonic, until it eventually alleviated.

Analysis: A total of five months of treatment, seeking the most economical and available resources in a cash-poor situation, cost Amable only 130 intis and appeared to resolve her ailments. The *compuestas* from two bonesetters were an integral part of a series of measures that also included home, herbal, and pharmaceutical remedies—the latter on advice from a teacher and a biomedical specialist. She had little faith in a physician's ability to help her.

Case 4

Rosita was twenty and lived with her mother, stepfather (himself a healer of a culture-specific illness), and older half-brother. During the first week of November, she suffered a grave episode of stomach illness of unknown origin, with colic, vomiting, and high fever. The health promoter/herbalist/bonesetter, Don Artemio, paid a midnight emergency visit to the house and gave her Antalgina (an over-the-counter pain and fever reducer), penicillin, and aspirin, and "floated" her with vinegar for fever reduction. This improved her condition, but didn't cure it. A week later she was gravely ill again with the same symptoms plus constipation. She took the rest of the health promoter's remedies. Three days later, when the symptoms had subsided some, and again a few days after that, she was given a *compuesta* by seventy-year-old Sra. Teófila, who now diagnosed the problem as a dropped stomach. Rosita improved as a result. She also applied masticated wheat with alcohol externally for fever, which helped some. Also on the day of the second *compuesta*, Rosita visited the health promoter's home, and in his absence was given *pulipunche* tea for fallen stomach by his wife. A month after the initial episode, she was fine. While her family paid 100 intis for the emergency attention, the *compuesta* and second visit to Don Artemio were "gifts."

Analysis: Rosita's case shows that bonesetting may also be a useful adjunct to the healing of (apparent) infectious illness, something that Valdizan and Maldonado alluded to (1922:123). In this case, in contrast to the first three, the services of the *componedor* were not the first sought because the illness was not perceived as primarily musculoskeletal. Nonetheless, the benefits of a *compuesta* were recognized. Distressed organs move out of situ, as do bones, and returning them to their proper place is necessary for a rapid and full recovery. Though she was being seen by an herbalist who was at the same time the best *huesero* in the region, her treatment for fallen stomach, a "female problem," came from a female *componedor*.

The next five cases are more brief and thus will receive a joint analysis at the end.

Case 5
Amelí was a twenty-one-year-old single woman, the third of six children all living with their parents. On the last day of September, she fell down some stairs and for a week and a half had mild pain in her hip and lower back and a dropped abdomen (*barriga bajada*). On the eleventh day, she received a *compuesta* from Sra. Teófila, who lived nearby, at a cost of 100 intis. The Señora diagnosed her as being "open" (*abierta*) in the hips, advising her to eat and drink humorally cool foods to quell the irritation and to use a *flotación* of alcohol and *pisco*. She followed the former advice with *pie de perro* and *unquia* (sedge) but not the latter, and was healed within two days.

Case 6
Hernesto, at thirty-five, was married with one young son and a child on the way. In addition to the sale of his potato bounty, he had a large herd of animals and was a meat dealer on the side. He was currently the community treasurer. He sustained a swollen, dislocated (*tronchado*) right elbow and shoulder from a fall. The next day at the Sunday market he received a *compuesta* from Mercedes at no cost and immediately felt better. He intended to buy some *chuncho* to apply to the area. I did not follow up the case, as it was recorded on my last home visit in December, but the pain had receded from moderate to mild the day after his treatment.

Case 7
Imelda was a sixty-eight-year-old widow whose daughter and youngest son and his family lived with her. In mid-October, she moved her shoulder slightly out of situ (*embagado*) while putting on her sweater. When after five days it continued to bother her, she decided to seek a *componedor*. She was going to visit Sra. Teófila but

when her uncle from the distant hamlet of Yamobamba visited, he gave her two *compuestas* and recommended a *flotación*, which she used. That worked well and she had no further problems.

Case 8

Paco, a young man of modest means, twisted his foot (*pie torcido*) while playing soccer in early November and it swelled. The next day, his mother's uncle from the next hamlet gave him an adjustment for 100 intis. Along with that he took a tea of *trigo blanco* (white wheat) with *ortiga negra* (black nettle), and rubbed Mentholatum on the foot. The treatment worked, and for another few weeks he continued to treat the bruise and knot it had caused with snake alcohol and an unguent.

Case 9

Pancha, thirty-six, lived in a hard-working, prosperous extended household with her parents, several siblings, her husband, and their three young boys. Lifting and carrying sacks of harvested potatoes in July caused her abdomen to drop. Her illness was of moderate severity as she could not lift or work for four days and had to urinate frequently. Her first action was to apply cocoa butter and guinea pig fat. She then went to Sra. Laura, a midwife, who adjusted her and bound her abdomen with a sash. The Señora repeated the ministration the following day. There was no charge, as the two were *comadres*. A week after the incident, the problem returned when Pancha received excessive exposure to the sun. Sra. Laura gave her another *compuesta* and a *flotación* with *pisco* and she made a full recovery.

Analysis: The last five uncomplicated musculoskeletal cases are evidence that everyday injuries, quickly and efficiently treated by a *componedor*, do not linger. After a brief period of ignoring the pain, and/or applying home remedies, the *campesinos* resorted to a musculoskeletal specialist to alleviate their problem. None of the injured even contemplated seeking biomedical care. All clients rated the treatment of the *componedor* as effective. Whether injured in work or at play, people—young and old, male or female, of all socioeconomic levels—needed to return to work. They were quickly able to function again after the low-cost treatment of their local *componedor*.

The *Componedor*'s Contribution to Community Health

As with peasants everywhere, the musculoskeletal problems that confront the highland peasant on a daily basis range from something as simple as a dislocated finger, to sprains from a fall, to being trampled by livestock. No fractures occurred during the study period, but the hamlet's *huesero*, Don Artemio, would have treated any that occurred. He held regional fame for his healing of a compound leg fracture that an astounded physician, after having declined to treat the case, later x-rayed and found to be successfully mended (Oths 2002:84).

As the case studies illustrate, *componedores* are in high demand in Chugurpampa because their treatments are seen as a quick, available, and efficacious means to manage aches and pains—that is, to alleviate them for a time, if not permanently. Some cases that call for a *componedor* are uncomplicated, usually acute episodes that are resolved quickly, while the more complicated cases are often either that of a serious injury or a chronic condition that is not amenable to permanent cure. Thus, traditional remedies in many cases must be repeated continually, even on a daily basis. In this event, efficacy is measured by a management of pain and disability that allows one to continue working to make a living under precarious socioeconomic conditions. The chronicity of mild and moderate bodily complaints is occasioned not by the ineffectiveness of local palliatives, but by the constant assault on the body by highland agricultural life.

These case studies demonstrate that the duration of illness was shortened, symptoms were alleviated, and fewer days of work were missed due to the *componedor*'s attention. The cost of treatment was typically quite reasonable, if not free. Since the *componedor* works primarily with the hands and with locally available herbs and medicaments, little investment in equipment or technology is needed to deliver and maintain services. Of particular relevance to public health, the *componedor* is usually available to visit the injured in their homes; biomedicine is often not even considered because the degree of bodily ailment and immobility does not permit a person to walk the long distance to the health post. Andean body workers provide gendered services that are culturally appropriate, as well. Highland women are notoriously modest about submitting to a physical examination—especially of their reproductive organs, especially by a man, and even during birth with a midwife. Thus, all of the women with *barriga bajada* were able to receive treatment from women practitioners with whom they felt comfortable.

Both the acquisition of funds to purchase care and the choice of healer were often guided by kinship relations (also see Carey 1988). In over 60 percent of the households I visited, people called upon a close relative or *compadre* to assist them with gifts or loans for medical treatment. If a healer and patient are kin by marriage or ritual, the sick person pays little to nothing for services. Healer kin are additionally attractive as choices because they are familiar, confidential figures who can be trusted not to harm or humiliate—significant concerns where sorcery is possible and modesty the rule. Also, as healers of all sorts are generally busy people, one is likely to get prompt and more careful attention from relatives. Even if healers are not kin, they are known to defer charges until the patient is satisfied that the treatment has worked. The payment of fees to non-kin local healers through delayed exchange is the equivalent of "easy credit terms," a long-term, low-interest loan. The Julcan *técnico sanitario* was also considered by many as "a good friend," a term rarely used in the highlands and one that describes a relationship bordering on ritual godparent status (*compadrazgo*) in its reciprocity. Though he did not provide manual medicine, he was the only one of the Julcan health personnel who made house calls when a patient was confined to bed. Early in my research when accompanying the *técnico sanitario* on a childhood immunization campaign, I was puzzled to witness him seeming to arbitrarily suggest he would like a duck he saw at the home of a family. He later explained that he had treated their young child for serious bronchitis some time back, implying that they owed him.

With an argument now constructed for the contribution of the *componedor* to community health, some policy recommendations may be put forth. Given the chronically underfunded Peruvian public health sector, persons like *componedores* who provide an unparalleled service must be relied on and promoted by the state, or at minimum left unobstructed, for the benefit of the less advantaged segments of the population. The case studies demonstrate the integral role of many types of healers in restoring a peasant to health after a musculoskeletal or other disease incident. The services of the *componedor* should be respected as one important, if partial, contribution to maintaining health in the Andean pluralistic medical system.

The integration of traditional and biomedical services has been widely discussed as a solution to health care delivery problems in developing as well as developed countries (Stone 2001; Young 1983). In the case of the Andes, however, integration would not improve the current system of musculoskeletal care for numerous reasons. The centralization of the Peruvian public health system makes it inaccessible to peasants and low in productivity (Young 1983), so moving traditional healers to the health posts would only distance them from their client base. A healing office in the Andes requires one to be somewhat itinerant. A healer with a specialty or good reputation may be called to attend the sick in other communities on a daily basis. In Chugurpampa, the traditional healers (and the health sanitarian in his private capacity) are mobile, but the health post personnel are not.

An integrated arrangement would be disadvantageous to bonesetters, who would be politically and professionally dominated by physicians (Baer 1989). They would risk losing their autonomy and having their theories of disease etiology and treatment denigrated. State funding for the healers would dictate formal training and systematized practice (Stone 2001:51); the current method of self-teaching and apprenticeship allows many the opportunity to learn who would otherwise be shut out of professional schools. The flexible payment schemes for *componedores* at present (barter, gifting, delayed, etc.) would come under regulation.

Nonetheless, there does exist the potential for *componedores* and physicians to develop a closer, more collaborative relationship, short of integrating their services.

By the same token, the answer to Andeans' bodily health care needs will not lie in the privatization and decentralization of biomedical services, as some suggest (Zwi 2001). Physicians, whether private or public, have little interest or competence in treating everyday aches, sprains, and breaks, so one would not anticipate an increase in the quality of care available. Furthermore, peasants could hardly afford the fees for services—and indeed might end up further impoverished—if they were offered (Crowley 2002). The long-term musculoskeletal health of Andeans will depend on communities continuing to supply and nurture bonesetters generation across generation.

Conclusion

In the Andes, weakness and vulnerability are characteristically feared and hidden from others. Add to this the intensity of the work ethic of Andean peasants and the prestige attached to their productivity, and one finds that visible bodily disability is avoided at all costs. The *componedor* helps restore persons to full functioning so that they can fulfill responsibilities to family and community and enhance their personal status. The therapy they provide is accessible, affordable, culturally consonant, efficacious, technologically appropriate, articulate with the larger health care system, and unavailable from other sources. Thus, the services of the *componedor* are a significant resource for maintaining community health and social relations.

Patients count on the *componedor* to treat their illness problems caused by overwork, physical stress, and falls, whether they use componedores alone or in combination with other healers and treatments. That traditional *componedores* have endured in the face of modernization pressures attests to an inherent efficacy of their practice of bodily attention, an efficacy that may be psychosocial, economic, and cultural as well as physical. *Componedores* provide an unparalleled contribution to health care in the rural Andes.

Notes

I wish to acknowledge William Dressler, Bob Anderson, Servando Hinojosa, and several anonymous reviewers for their helpful comments and suggestions. This research was funded by grants from the National Science Foundation (#8813774) and the Inter-American Foundation (#FI-135-AI).

1. The *huesero* is the more skilled of the two practitioners, setting broken bones in addition to performing skeletal manipulation and massage. There was one *huesero* in this study, but for simplicity, I consider him along with the others as a *componedor*.

2. At the start of the study, 100 intis equaled US$0.60. Due to the devaluation of the Peruvian currency, a male laborer's daily wage of 200 intis was worth roughly US$1.20 at the beginning and US$0.20 by the end of the case collection period. Prices did not rise so much as there was a general paucity of available household cash (i.e., the latter worse than the former). Given a lag time, costs of traditional healers' services in Chugurpampa rose relatively little compared to professional health services and consumer goods. During this period, as before, healers who were acquaintances of the client often agreed to a delay of payment.

3. The environment is a common etiological factor in highland sickness, with babies, the elderly, and the sick particularly susceptible to its effects (Oths 1996). The powerful radiation of the sun at high altitude causes or complicates many illnesses. For example, not wearing a hat can cause severe headache and nausea, for which it is said *le ha dado el sol* (the sun has affected one). Extremes of cold and wind (*aire*) are also illness-generating.

4. As assessed by the Cornell Medical Index, witnessed by me, and attested to by family and others.

5. In a *soba*, an animal, usually a guinea pig, is passed over the body to absorb the sickness. It is then cut open and its entrails examined to diagnose the patient's illness in the manner of an x-ray (Morales 1995).

References

Anderson, Robert A.
    1983 On Doctors and Bonesetters in the Sixteenth and Seventeenth Centuries. *Chiropractic History* 3(1):11–15.
Baer, Hans
    1989 The American Dominative Medical System as a Reflection of Social Relations in the Larger Society. *Social Science and Medicine* 28(11):1103–12.
Bourdieu, Pierre
    1977 *Outline of a Theory of Practice*. Cambridge, England: Cambridge University Press.
Brown, Peter J.
    1987 Microparasites and Macroparasites. *Cultural Anthropology* 2(1):155–71.
Carey, James
    1988 The Significance of Informal Social Support Networks for Rural Household Health in the Andes. *Michigan Discussions in Anthropology* 8:119–35.
Classen, Constance
    1993 *Inca Cosmology and the Human Body*. Salt Lake City: University of Utah Press.
Coreil, Jeannine
    1983 Parallel Structures in Professional and Folk Health Care: A Model Applied to Rural Haiti. *Culture, Medicine, and Psychiatry* 7:131–51.
Crandon-Malamud, Libbet
    1991 *From the Fat of Our Souls: Social Change, Political Process, and Medical Pluralism in Bolivia*. Berkeley: University of California Press.

Crowley, Philip
  2002 Strong Public Provision Is Only Hope for Health Care in Developing Countries. *British Medical Journal* 324:47.
Csordas, Thomas, ed.
  1994 *Embodiment and Experience: The Existential Ground of Culture and Self.* Cambridge, England: Cambridge University Press.
Garcilaso de la Vega, Inca
  1973 [1617] *Comentarios Reales de los Incas.* Lima, Peru: Ediciones Peisa.
Harrison, Margaret E.
  2001 Mexican Physician, Nurses, and Social Workers. Pp. 270–306 in Brad R. Huber and Alan R. Sandstrom, eds. *Mesoamerican Healers.* Austin: University of Texas Press.
Hinojosa, Servando
  2002 "The Hands Know": Bodily Engagement and Medical Impasse in Highland Maya Bonesetting. *Medical Anthropology Quarterly* 16(1):22–40.
Huber, Brad R., and Alan R. Sandstrom, eds.
  2001 *Mesoamerican Healers.* Austin: University of Texas Press.
Kaptchuk, Ted. J., and David M. Eisenberg
  1991 Chiropractic: Origins, Controversies, and Contributions. *Archives of Internal Medicine* 158(20):2215–24.
Kleinman, Arthur
  1980 *Patients and Healers in the Context of Culture.* Berkeley: University of California Press.
Leslie, Charles, ed.
  1976 *Asian Medical Systems.* Berkeley: University of California Press.
Lipp, Frank J.
  2001 A Comparative Analysis of Southern Mexican and Guatemalan Shamans. Pp. 95–116 in Brad R. Huber and Alan R. Sandstrom, eds. *Mesoamerican Healers.* Austin: University of Texas Press.
Morales, Edmundo
  1995 *The Guinea Pig: Healing, Food, and Ritual in the Andes.* Tucson: University of Arizona Press.
Murillo Alfaro, Felix
  1998 Demanda de Atención en Servicios de Salud, 1997. Peruvian National Institute of Statistics and Information (INEI).
Nash, June
  1979 *We Eat the Mines and the Mines Eat Us.* New York: Columbia University Press.
Nichter, Mark
  1978 Patterns of Resort in the Use of Therapy Systems and Their Significance for Health Planning in South Asia. *Medical Anthropology* 2:29–58.
Oths, Kathryn S.
  1992 Some Symbolic Dimensions of Andean Materia Medica. *Central Issues in Anthropology* 10:76–85.

1994 Health Care Decisions of Households in Economic Crisis: An Example from the Peruvian Highlands. *Human Organization* 53(3): 245–54.

1996 Ecologic and Macrolevel Influences on Illness in Northern Peru: Beyond the International Health Paradigm. Pp. 107–29 in Janardan Subedi and Eugene B. Gallagher, eds. *Society, Health, and Disease: Transcultural Perspectives.* Upper Saddle River, N.J.: Prentice Hall.

1998 Assessing Variation in Health Status in the Andes: A Biocultural Model. *Social Science and Medicine* 47(8):1017–30.

1999 Debilidad: A Biocultural Assessment of an Embodied Andean Illness. *Medical Anthropology Quarterly* 13(3):286–315.

2002 Setting It Straight in the Andes: Musculoskeletal Distress and the Role of the Componedor. Pp. 63–91 in Joan D. Koss-Chioino, Thomas Leatherman, and Christine Greenway, eds. *Medical Pluralism in the Andes.* New York: Routledge.

Paul, Benjamin D., and Clancy McMahon
2001 Mesoamerican Bonesetters. Pp. 243–69 in Brad R. Huber and Alan R. Sandstrom, eds. *Mesoamerican Healers.* Austin: University of Texas Press.

Stone, Julie
2001 How Might Traditional Remedies Be Incorporated into Discussions of Integrated Medicine? *Complementary Therapies in Nursing and Midwifery* 7:55–58.

Valdizan, Hermilio, and Angel Maldonado
1922 *La Medicina Popular Peruana.* vol. I. Lima, Peru: Imprenta Torres Aguilar.

Young, Allan
1983 The Relevance of Traditional Medical Cultures to Modern Primary Health Care. *Social Science and Medicine* 17(16):1205–11.

Zwi, Anthony B., Ruairi Brugha, and Elizabeth Smith
2001 Private Health Care in Developing Countries. *British Medical Journal* 323:463–64.

Borana Bonesetters

Integrating Modernity and Tradition in a Northern Kenyan Pastoral Community

11

ISAAC K. NYAMONGO

THIS CHAPTER FOCUSES on two aspects of treatment regarding musculoskeletal injury in a rural northern Kenyan pastoral community. First, I deal with the special role played by Borana bonesetters (locally known as *chiressa*) in the provision of health care in northern Kenya. They use locally derived materials such as herbs, roots, leaves, gum/resin, and other natural products to provide care to patients. However, the bonesetters have also, in line with the changing times, adopted some modern practices that serve to enhance their ability to provide improved service to clients. Using x-ray pictures is not uncommon. Of their own initiative or as a result of urging from the *chiressa*, patients personally visit health care facilities to obtain x-rays, which they then take to the bonesetters to use. Of course, these x-rays are taken without the knowledge of formal care providers within those health care facilities.

The second topic this chapter explores is the decision-making role played by the extended family and the community in the event of a bone injury. Health care decision-making among the Borana goes beyond the immediate family. The extended family and the community at large are important components of the decision-making process. They constitute a therapy management group (Janzen 1978) that makes decisions regarding the type of care to be made available to individuals.

The distribution of the health care system in Kenya is widely varied, with rural areas generally being underserved. In parts of Northern Kenya, where pastoral communities are constantly moving in search of pasture and water for their domestic animals, it is particularly problematic for health authorities to put in place a meaningful health care infrastructure. As rainfall patterns change, the composition of the communities also shifts to reflect the demands exerted on the environment by the people. For example, young men, who constitute the militia that protects the community and livestock from raids, go further afield with the dry

221

animals. They leave behind small stock and some milking cows. The livestock left behind is taken care of by boys and women. In severe droughts that cause the death of stock, some of the community members emigrate to faraway towns (see Odegi-Awoundo (1990) for a discussion of the effects of drought on family and community composition in Turkana). The Borana are no exception to the demands exerted by the environment.

During bad times when pasture and water are scarce, the pastoralists' transhumant movements take them into neighboring areas that are normally considered socially dangerous. They become risk takers. Also, as sources of water diminish due to drought, different groups converge at the remaining few watering points, which increases competition among users. Such movements frequently invite hostilities from the Borana's neighbors who ordinarily protect the areas under their jurisdiction. War between these communities often results. In addition to provoking these movements, the loss of livestock caused by drought must be remedied. Replenishment of livestock takes the form of raids into neighboring communities that, in turn, furthers hostilities between the groups. The resulting confrontations have occasioned serious health risks, including injuries. For example, the rough terrain occupied by the Borana community often contributes to dislocations and fractures, particularly during raids to or by neighboring communities.

Frequent migration also entails other problems in establishing a meaningful health care system. Infrastructure is usually built in areas where its would-be users will have access to it. In the face of many competing demands such as education and agriculture, the Kenyan government has given relatively low infrastructural priority to areas occupied by pastoral communities. The compelling argument usually advanced is that having infrastructure in areas characterized by the constant movement of people would constitute a waste of resources given the enormous cost of setting it up and the likelihood of its underutilization by the migratory target community. Pastoral communities thus find themselves in a state where they have to devise ways to enhance their personal and communal comfort.

As a result, modern health care facilities in areas occupied by pastoralists are few and widely dispersed. For example, in Marsabit there are thirty-one health care facilities serving an area of about 78,078 square kilometers (see table 11.1). Of these, six are small and privately managed by individuals, while the majority of the remaining twenty-five facilities are managed by the Catholic Church. The medical facilities in the district lack senior medical staff, especially in remote areas. For example, there was one qualified government medical doctor located at the district hospital in 1997. The more remote areas lack trained personnel as well as basic facilities such as furniture and equipment. The bed ratios range from 1 for every 286 and 1 for every 300 in Leisamis and Central divisions, to 1 for every 3,086 in North Horr (Kenya 1997). Communication infrastructure such as telephone ser-

Table 11.1. Distribution of Health Care Facilities in Marsabit District (excludes six managed by individuals)

Division	Hospitals	Health Centers	Dispensaries	Bed Ratio
Central	1	0	11	1:300
Leisamis	1	0	7	1:286
North Horr	0	2	3	1:3,086
Loiyangalani	0	1	1	1:784
Maikona	0	0	3	Data not available
Total	2	3	25	

vices is similarly underdeveloped, and access roads are nonexistent or are inadequate and poorly maintained. In turn, the poor infrastructure makes the unit cost of service delivery very high (Kenya 1997). When it is absolutely necessary, patients may walk days on end to reach a modern health care facility.

Due to this poor health care infrastructure, the indigenous health system of Borana pastoral communities—which developed over many generations to deal with community health problems—has persisted (Haraldson 1975). This system consists of individuals, both male and female (Swift et al. 1989:11), who provide specialized care for different health conditions, including musculoskeletal care, obstetric care, male and female circumcision, and those who care for other health problems such as snakebites, insect bites, and burns. These are not full-time occupations. The provision of care is undertaken by the different specialists on a need-by-need basis. The specialists stick to their areas of specialization.

The practice of bonesetting runs in families among the Borana community, and it is also a gendered practice. A male child learns from his father through apprenticeship over a period of time. There are no conventions regarding which of the sons in the family will become a *chiressa*. Often, it is a result of interest developed by the children. There are no women bonesetters among the Borana. Women may only be involved in massaging dislocations after the *chiressa* has treated the patient. However, the only women allowed to massage are those who have given birth to twins or who have had a breech birth. It is believed that such women are blessed, hence they can perform this duty (Nyamongo 1992). Cultural and emotional reasons are cited by informants for not allowing women to perform bonesetting. Chief among these is the Borana belief that "women are a weaker sex" and "cannot withstand" the psychological and emotional strain of seeing a badly injured patient. This view comes from largely male-centered ethnography.

The Setting

This chapter is based on data collected on the Borana pastoralists in Marsabit district (figure 11.1). The Borana are a part of the Oromo-speaking group whose origin

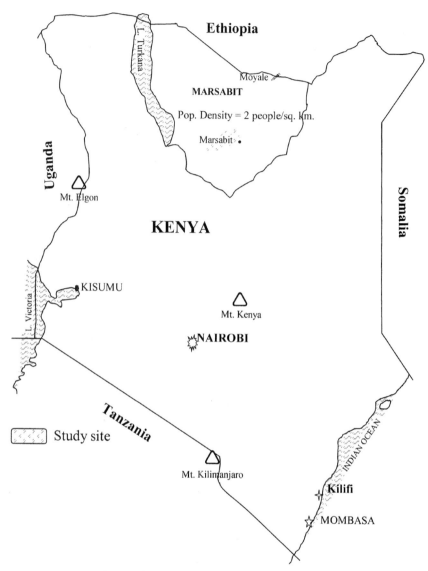

Figure 11.1.   Map of Kenya showing Marsabit district and study site.

is traced to Ethiopia. The people speak the Borana language from which they derive their name. The Borana today are most concentrated in two Kenyan districts—Marsabit and Isiolo. In 1999, the population of Marsabit district was more than 121,478. With a population density of 2 persons per square kilometer, Marsabit district is one of the most sparsely populated districts in Kenya (CBS 2001). The latest information on the major ethnic communities of Marsabit (CBS 1991) indicates that in 1989, the Borana comprised a third of the district's inhabitants. Large population movements from different areas within Kenya have remained static. Consequently, the proportion of the Borana in relation to other inhabitants has likely remained unchanged.

Natural conditions differ widely. Vast lowlands ranging from 400 to 700 meters above sea level are interspersed with several mountain ranges that reach altitudes of more than 2,700 meters above sea level. Rainfall varies from less than 200 to over 1,000 millimeters in the Mt. Marsabit region. Therefore, distribution of rainfall is not uniform throughout the district.

The Borana economy is based on pastoralism, although those who occupy areas such as Moyale and Mt. Marsabit and the higher altitudes (approximately 1,865 meters above sea level) grow some food crops. Livestock is, therefore, an important subsistence resource for the Borana. It also plays an essential role in law, ritual, and religious ceremonies, being used, for instance, to pay fines in the traditional courts of law and to pay bride price. In marriage ceremonies, the bride's parents may receive in excess of fifty cattle and camels as compensation for the loss of their daughter's productive and reproductive rights.

Cattle are the basic form of subsistence; like in many other pastoral communities, livestock are an important indicator of wealth among the Borana. The significance attached to livestock in the Borana ethnography is expressed in the relationship between a child and his first heifer. A male child is presented with a heifer at his naming ceremony, which takes place when he is approximately a year old. The heifer is known as *handura* (navel). When the boy grows into a young adult, the heifer will form the nucleus of his own independent herd (Baxter 1966:125). Livestock, most importantly, is a major food source for the Borana. They consider it vital that a man should establish his own herd as soon as possible. Women are not allowed to own cattle. They may have access to the milk, but may not have control over the animals or even where to take them for grazing purposes.

Through careful husbandry, the herds are managed to ensure their growth in number. Replenishing stock, particularly if depleted following prolonged drought, is done through raids on other communities. Herding units, usually consisting of extended family members, care for and protect the animals with the efforts of the young and energetic men in the warrior age group. They protect the herds from wildlife attacks and against raids from neighboring communities. Theirs is a job with considerable personal risks.

Marsabit is marked by low precipitation, erratic both in timing and distribution, making the district the most arid in Kenya. Vegetation is scanty, with occasional tall trees (except in the region around Mt. Marsabit); when present these trees form less than 10 percent of the overall crown cover (Schultka 1991). The most common shrubs and bushes found in these settings include *Acacia* species, *Rhamnus prinoides*, *Ry-tigynia neglecta*, *Euclea schimperi* and to a lesser extent *Commiphora* species (Schultka 1991). The latter species is relevant to the discussion in this paper. Myrrh, the plant whose resin is used by bonesetters, belongs to this group of plants.

Data Collection

The data presented here result from qualitative interviews with ten traditional male bonesetters. The data were collected in December 1991 from the Central division of Marsabit district, which occupies the area around Mt. Marsabit. The *chiressa* were selected using snowball sampling (Bernard 1995)—that is, I asked twenty-five male and female potential health care seekers to identify the traditional bonesetters they knew. The health care seekers were selected with the help of a local Borana research assistant who knew the local people and conditions. Informants were then asked to name those people they considered the most competent bonesetters. The definition of competence was deliberately left open so that the community members would use their own criteria rather than a researcher-derived measure of competency. Next, I asked the named *chiressa* to identify those they considered to be the most competent among them. Through this procedure, it was possible to identify ten traditional bonesetters considered very competent by both potential clients and by other bonesetters. The identified bonesetters ranged in age from 31 to over 75, and had experience ranging from 6 to 50 years.

Using an interview schedule, I then performed in-depth interviews with each of the ten *chiressa*. The topics of interest generally focused on actions taken by bonesetters to manage fractures. Some of the questions and issues covered are shown in table 11.2. Each of these questions was followed by probes to elicit more information from the bonesetters.

Treatment

This section presents data pertaining to the treatment of patients, first focusing on the actual treatment of patients with bone related injuries, then on the role of

Table 11.2.   Some of the Questions Asked in the Interviews with Bonesetters

1. What are the common bone-related problems you routinely manage in your practice?
2. Could you describe the general procedure for managing patients with bone injuries?
3. What is your relationship with the other health care providers? Specifically, what is your relationship with the modern health care providers and facilities?
4. In what ways, if any, have you integrated use of modern technology into your practice?
5. Are there other health problems, other than bone-related ones, that you manage?
6. What role do women play in the management of bone-related injuries?

the community. This sets the stage to better focus on the interaction between the patient and the *chiressa*. Lastly, environmental issues in relation to bonesetting activities are discussed.

Treatment of Patients with Bone Injuries

Traditional Kenyan bonesetters typically deal with long bones such as the femur, tibia, fibula, humerus, radius, and ulna, the more common sites of injuries and dislocations, which are easier to handle. In their provision of services to patients, the *chiressa* interact indirectly with the modern health care facilities. They specifically provide care to patients with bone-related injuries, but they may also be called on to treat fractures in domesticated animals (see Mesfin and Obsa 1994).

The interaction between hospital medical personnel, traditional bonesetters, and the patient is summarized in the form of a flow chart in figure 11.2. When injured, a person has three options, either to go to a modern health care facility (a hospital), to a traditional bonesetter, or to forego treatment altogether if the injury is not serious. Interviews with the medical staff at the hospital reveal that many of the patients who initially opt for hospital treatment abscond after obtaining an x-ray image(s). At the district hospital, the examining doctor and the x-ray room are not in the same building. After examining the patient, the doctor issues him or her a written note to take to the x-ray room for images to be taken. Once the x-ray image is processed, it is given to the patient to take back to the referring doctor. After obtaining the x-rays, however, instead of taking them to the referring doctor, the patients often leave the hospital and take them to a *chiressa* out in the village. Bonesetters confirmed that patients sometimes come with x-ray images—something that bonesetters consider a blessing. As I highlight in this chapter, access to this modern technology helps improve the bonesetters' precision.

If the patient does not abscond with the x-ray image, though, the referring doctor will diagnose the type of bone injury. The bone is then set and plaster of Paris is applied to keep the injured bone in place. Another x-ray image is taken a few days later to assess whether the setting was done properly and has remained stable. Actually, it may have been properly done, but the question is whether the bone ends have moved. If the setting was proper and has held, the patient is then either discharged or kept longer at the hospital, depending on the seriousness of the injury. At this point, if the x-ray shows a defective setting, the patient is likely to blame the health personnel and may resort to a traditional bonesetter.

Community perception of the competency of the health care personnel and the bonesetters is a product of two different factors. On the one hand, if outcome of treatment in the health care facilities is not what the community expects, the patient and therapy management group's opinion of the personnel in the health

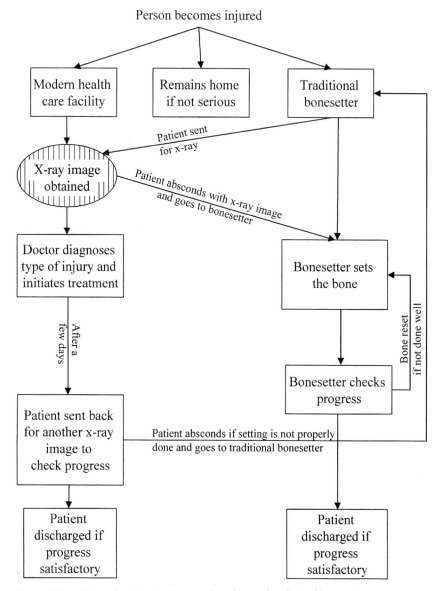

Figure 11.2. Patient decisions in the use of modern and traditional bonesetters.

care facilities will change. On the other hand, performing treatment in a culturally expected manner helps foster the confidence of the community in a particular bonesetter. These two factors act synergistically to reinforce community perceptions of services rendered by health care facilities and bonesetters. Eventually, the two factors influence decisions made in the process of seeking health care services.

When a patient chooses to go directly to a traditional bonesetter (figure 11.2), the *chiressa* will determine the nature of the bone injury by feeling with his hands and assessing the x-ray image, if available. Some of the traditional bonesetters actually encourage their patients to go to a hospital first so that they get an x-ray image. For complex injuries, a *chiressa* may send the patient either to a hospital or a more experienced bonesetter. The latter is usually the case. Complex injuries include multiple fractures, for example where a bone has broken in two different places, often requiring greater skill to set. Experience is a judgmental term, and usually there is no clear-cut way of determining experience. Often it is linked to perceived good results.

The use of the imported x-ray images helps the bonesetters determine the location of the injury instead of feeling with their hands. However, the more subtle problems are less likely to be diagnosed because the bonesetters lack adequate knowledge to correctly interpret the x-ray images. In terms of reliance, younger, more enterprising bonesetters are more likely to use x-ray images, while older bonesetters, less familiar with them, are more likely to abstain.

In order to decide whether he can handle the injury, the traditional bonesetter must first assess the injury's complexity, his physical strength, and his competency to handle the patient. Some cases may require the use of force, such as when a bone has been dislocated from its joint. If he decides he is capable, he sets the bone. Otherwise, the patient is referred to another, usually younger, bonesetter. Thus, there is always the challenge of making the decision of whether to send a patient to a more experienced or younger bonesetter.

A few days after setting the bone, the *chiressa* checks the patient's progress. Like with hospital personnel, the traditional bonesetter must determine whether the bone has been properly set. Unlike with hospital personnel, though, he does not always have the aid of an x-ray machine to do this. Accordingly, the patient may be discharged or have the bone reset by the same bonesetter.

Two examples here illustrate the actions of bonesetters in the management of injuries. In the case of fractures involving long bones, splints are used together with a string to stabilize the affected part. Animal skin may also be used together with the splits for additional support. The materials used in this process are described below. Dislocations are handled by manipulating the affected part so as to reduce the discomfort. As another example, in the case of the upper arm, the bonesetter will slowly rotate the arm or pull it in a series of controlled, quick jerks.

In the actions, several people may be involved—the bonesetter himself, the patient's relatives, and people who may be called in to provide a helping hand. Those who are asked to help need not necessarily be known by the patient. Indeed, the bonesetter's neighbors may be called in to lend a hand.

Community Involvement in the Treatment

As is the case of many communities associated with nomadism, the social networks among the Borana are strong. In nomadic communities people and resources are widely dispersed and the dangers of being raided by neighboring groups are many. The members, especially the men, must ensure a strong standing militia that can be mobilized to repulse any livestock rustlers. Since individuals are expected to defend the group's interest against outsiders, the survival of an individual also concerns the entire clan.[1] The clan must therefore collectively ensure that its sick or injured members regain health in the shortest time possible.

Due to the wide dispersal and scarcity of resources, however, the members of a recovering patient's family may not be in a position to provide the required animals to be slaughtered for the patient (see below). The patient must make a quick, steady, and complete recovery, though, so as to boost the overall manpower of the community. Therefore, the clan, acting corporately, must help in providing the required animals. Recovered individuals contribute their productive and reproductive capabilities to the community, thus helping sustain the group. These considerations of injury, resources, and recovery are necessary for the survival of the community.

The Borana bonesetters do not demand payments for services rendered. Other than *darara*, prepared from dried and crushed tobacco leaves and usually chewed for pleasure, and given to the bonesetter as a social obligation, nothing else need be given by the patient for the received services. Patients may, on their own volition, compensate the *chiressa* for his services. In return for his aid to the community, the Borana accord the bonesetter high social status. In addition, bonesetters acquire influence and occupy important decision-making positions in the community. This affords the bonesetters important political capital, which they use to influence the direction of events in the community. For example, they are often consulted and involved in solving disputes among community members. Due to the position bonesetters occupy in the community, their opinions are rarely challenged by disputing parties.

Interaction between Patient and Bonesetter

The interaction between the patient and bonesetter is shown in figure 11.3. On the first visit, a patient gives the *chiressa darara* as a token of goodwill. *Darara* is not limited

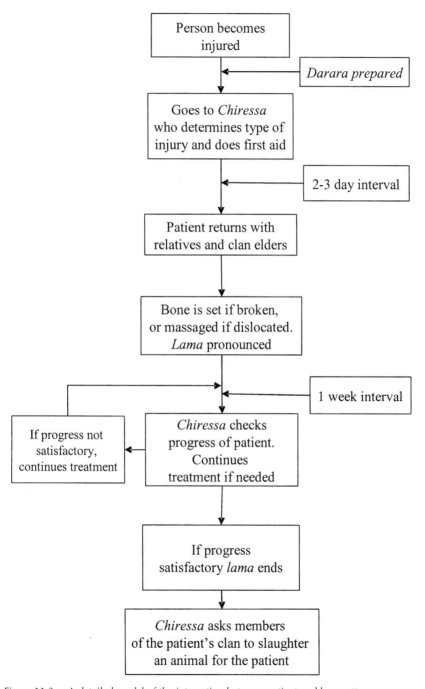

Figure 11.3. A detailed model of the interaction between patient and bonesetter.

to activities associated with health care provision, however. It is also given in other ceremonies, such as during betrothment. The *chiressa* shares *darara* with any elders present during this first encounter. He then administers first aid, if needed, to the patient. This allows for the patient to return home for consultations with family members. It ensures that consensus is reached regarding who will provide the services to the injured. The patient is asked to return after two or three days with parents and/or relatives and clan elders. Ordinarily, the bonesetters do not keep at the ready all they need to perform bonesetting because this activity is not a full-time occupation. Thus, letting the patient return to family also allows the bonesetter to make necessary arrangements to ready the materials required for bonesetting. However, the bonesetters have to draw the line between patients who cannot realistically wait for a longer period and those whose injuries may not require immediate attention.

At the second meeting, the bone is set and a period is pronounced during which food consumption is restricted. This period is known as *lama*. During *lama* the patient should not drink tea, milk, or cold beverages such as water, or eat oily foods, as these are said to interfere with proper healing of the bone. Joint massage, if the injury is a dislocation, may begin at this time.

The *chiressa* monitors the progress of the patient at weekly intervals. Satisfactory progress toward full recovery ends the period of *lama*, which is marked with ceremonies. The *chiressa* directs what animal(s) is to be slaughtered for consumption by the patient, which ensures that the individual gets the best of the available nutritious foods for a fast and satisfactory recovery.

Environmental Considerations

The Borana recognize plants that are important for the treatment of various health problems. For example, myrrh (*Commiphora myrrha*) is used extensively by bonesetters because it produces a resin they use as gum. Together with other materials also obtained from the immediate environment such as animal skin, splints, and a string prepared from the bark of local plants to tie the materials together, myrrh gum is used to make a plaster that hardens to form a protective support for the set bone, much like the plaster of Paris used in hospitals. The resin is extracted directly from the myrrh tree. Alternatively, it may be obtained commercially in dried form from local markets. In its dry form, the resin is reconstituted (sometimes using milk) to produce gum.

This resin-producing plant is an important component of Borana health care practices, something made ever more evident because commercial exploitation of the resin now threatens the plant. Competition among traders has caused the wanton destruction of myrrh plants. In fragile ecosystems such as the one occupied by the Borana, destroyed plants take several years to be replaced. The plants do not usually recover. This destruction, coupled with other environmental factors, may lead to an acceleration of desertification, which will eventually deprive the bone-setters of this important natural resource. Its loss also robs the land of much-needed cover and vegetative matter, which would otherwise counter erosion and assure aeration of the soil.

Discussion

The role played by traditional health practitioners cannot be overemphasized. In rural Africa, medical doctors are outnumbered by traditional health practitioners. In 1994 in Zimbabwe, there were more than 45,000 traditional health practition-ers but roughly 1,400 medical doctors. Thus, the traditional health practitioners reach far more people. Furthermore, the traditional healers are located in places where the community has easy access. This makes them popular and reliable among communities (Abdool Karim et al. 1994). In areas where communication facilities are poorly developed and access to modern medical facilities is difficult, indigenous medical practitioners such as bonesetters play an even bigger role in health care delivery (Haraldson 1975). These specialists are regarded with high es-teem for the services they provide.

In cases involving human bone fractures, traditional bonesetters are regarded as more competent than modern health care personnel. This belief is also held by some workers in the modern health care sector. In one case, there was a health worker at the district health hospital whose child had a fracture of the upper arm. Although he had gone through medical training college, he did not bring his child for treatment at the hospital. Being a hospital employee, it was easy to obtain an x-ray for use by the traditional bonesetter. Asked why he did not bring his child to the hospital, he said, "I have lived all my life with bonesetters. I know their competence."

Belief in traditional bonesetters is not confined to the Borana alone. In Nige-ria, traditional bonesetters are popular (Thanni 2000). In one study, out of 180 adults and adolescents surveyed, over 50 percent of them judged traditional bonesetters favorably. Thirty-seven percent of the respondents believed that the bonesetters were indispensable, while 32.8 percent believed that the bonesetters were desirable (Thanni 2000). Sixty-seven percent of the bonesetters were con-sidered as either competent or very competent (43 percent) or as performing their work satisfactorily (24 percent). The popularity of the bonesetters is not confined only to the Borana and Nigeria. Their popularity is also documented in other parts of Africa such as Morocco. Choffat (1979) argues that the services provided by bonesetters in Morocco are decentralized, socially integrated, and economical. In addition, the poor medical infrastructure is unable to replace the benefits of bonesetters. These factors have helped propagate the services of bone-setters in Morocco, as elsewhere.

Despite the popularity traditional bonesetters enjoy, their work sometimes poses risks to patients. In certain regions, like in Zaria, Nigeria, the major pathology leading to amputation is trauma and gangrene often linked to inappropriate splintage of fractures by traditional bonesetters (see Garba and Deshi 1998). The Borana, too, perform splintage with sticks and nontight resin extracts, and likewise their use of splints may not always be a successful operation. Sometimes, it is realized too late that the bone was not properly aligned and the fractured part has joined. When this happens, the bonesetter occasionally may insist on repeating the procedure—and resetting the bone is done at considerable pain to the patient because bonesetters have no access to anaesthesia. Under these circumstances, one cannot rule out the likelihood of wounds becoming gangrenous.

Conclusion

There is great potential for indigenous health care to work with and complement modern health care, as I and others (Bishaw 1990 and Odebiyi 1990) have argued. One aspect of this complementarity could develop with respect to x-rays. The Borana study reveals that x-ray images are much welcome among traditional bonesetters. Interviews with *chiressa*, in fact, revealed that they would like to have access to x-rays before and after bonesetting. This kind of venture would require considerable cooperation between personnel trained in biomedicine and indigenous health care providers. Rather than allowing patients to abscond x-rays, hospitals could provide facilities that encouraged patients to stay by assuring them access to both x-rays and traditional bonesetters. If such cooperation were emphasized, hospital attendance would likely improve, and the quality of medical care provided to bone injury patients by the traditional bonesetters would be greatly enhanced.

However, for proper integration of the two systems, the manner in which each operates should be well understood by both planners and health seekers. This will enable planners to determine the effect that the two systems would have on the quality of health care. Any perceived or real misgiving concerning the modern medical care system could alienate potential health care seekers such that they increasingly begin to consult only one (non-Western) group of providers. However, leaving traditional bonesetters on their own without providing them with basic sanitary facilities could compromise (Western) health standards. Careful planning is therefore required to formulate relevant health policies that would likely bring about an amicable integration of indigenous and modern health care services.

It is apparent that sociocultural and environmental dimensions are important in sustaining an indigenous medical system among the Borana. Borana communities, remote from urban areas, are cohesive and exhibit very strong kinship bonds. These bonds contribute to the kinds of social relations observed among these pastoralists, and ultimately condition the traditional care of bone injury patients. Environmental factors remain central to Borana bonesetting because the traditional bonesetter, the patient, and other group members all are intimately connected with the natural environment. It is the source of many of the risks faced by the Borana and provides the solutions to counter those risks.

Notes

I wish to acknowledge reviewers who have made invaluable comments on earlier drafts of this chapter. I am most grateful to the bonesetters who provided the data on which this chapter is based. Funds for this work were provided by the Japan Ministry of Education, Science, and Culture through the Supplementary Scientific Research Fund. The Institute of African Studies, University of Nairobi, provided logistical support.

1. The Borana community is divided into two moieties, the *Sabbo* and the *Gona*. Marriage between these two groups is based on the rule of exogamy. Thus a *Sabbo* is expected to marry a *Gona*. The *Sabbo* are subdivided into three submoieties (*Digalu, Karrayu,* and *Matarri*) while the *Gona* have two submoieties (*Fullelle,* and *Haroressa*). Each of these submoieties is divided into clans. A more detailed treatise of the Borana moieties may be found in Legesse (1973).

References

Abdool Karim, S. S., T. T. Zigubu-Page, and R. Arendse
    1994 Bridging the Gap: Potential for a Health Care Partnership between African Traditional Healers and Biomedical Personnel in South Africa. *South African Medical Journal* (Suppl.) 84:1–16.
Baxter, P. T. W.
    1966 Stock Management and Diffusion of Property Rights among the Boran. Proceedings of the 3rd Conference of Ethiopian Studies. Addis Ababa, Ethiopia.
Bernard, H. R.
    1995 *Research Methods in Anthropology: Quantitative and Qualitative Approaches.* 2d edition. Newbury Park, Calif.: Sage Publications.
Bishaw, M.
    1990 Attitudes of Modern and Traditional Medical Practitioners toward Cooperation. *Ethiopian Medical Journal* 28(2):63–72.
Central Bureau of Statistics (CBS)
    2001 1999 Population and Housing Census. Volume 1. Ministry of Planning and National Development, Nairobi, Kenya.

Central Bureau of Statistics (CBS)
    1991 Economic Survey—1991. Ministry of Planning and National Development,
        Nairobi, Kenya.
Choffat, F.
    1979 Treatment of Fractures by Traditional Healers in Morocco. *Sozial und Praven-*
        tivmedizin 24(2–3):172–78.
Garba, E. S., and P. J. Deshi
    1998 Traditional Bone Setting: A Risk Factor in Limb Amputation. *East African Med-*
        ical Journal 75(9):553–55.
Haraldson, S. R. S.
    1975 Socio-medical Problems of Nomad Peoples. Pp. 531–42 in W. Hobson, ed. *The*
        Theory and Practice of Public Health. 4th edition. London: Oxford University Press.
Janzen, J. M.
    1978 *The Quest for Therapy in Lower Zaire.* Berkeley: University of California Press.
Kenya, Republic of
    1997 Marsabit: District Development Plan 1997–2001. Office of the Vice President
        and Ministry of Planning and National Development, Nairobi.
Legesse, A.
    1973 *Gada: Three Approaches to the Study of African Society.* New York: Free Press.
Mesfin, T. and T. Obsa
    1994 Ethiopian Traditional Practices and Their Possible Contribution to Animal Pro-
        duction and Management. *Reviews in Science and Technology* 13(2):417–24.
Nyamongo, I. K.
    1992 Traditional Bone-Setting in a Pastoral Community: Does It Complement Mod-
        ern Health Care? Paper presented at conference on Ethnomedicine and Health
        in the SADCC Region. Maseru, Lesotho.
Odebiyi, A. I.
    1990 Western Trained Nurses' Assessment of the Different Categories of Traditional
        Healers in Southwestern Nigeria. *International Journal of Nursing Studies* 27(4):
        333–42.
Odegi-Awoundo, C.
    1990 *Life in the Balance: Ecological Sociology of Turkana Nomads.* Nairobi: African Center for
        Technology Studies Press.
Schultka, W.
    1991 Vegetation Types. Pp. 25–50 in *Marsabit District Range Management Handbook of Kenya.*
        Vol. II–I. Nairobi, Kenya: Republic of Kenya, Ministry of Livestock Development.
Swift, J., C. Toulmin, and S. Chatting
    1989 *Providing Services for Nomadic People.* Nairobi, Kenya: UNICEF.
Thanni, L. O.
    2000 Factors Influencing Patronage of Traditional Bonesetters. *West African Journal of*
        Medicine 19(3):220–24.

A Man of His People
A Concise Ethnography of
a Welsh Bonesetter

I2

SIMON LEYSON

THIS CHAPTER LOOKS AT THE LIFE of Jack Leyshon, a man who lived and worked in a coastal industrial town in South Wales from 1895 to 1980. Using an ethnographic approach, biographical details of his life are set against the industrial and social fabric of his community. His main occupation began in the early 1920s as a coal trimmer in the local docks and ended with their closure as a coal exporting facility in the early 1960s. The nature of this work was arduous and dirty, but developed strength in his arms and hands through work with a *cybe* (coal shovel). In contrast to this type of work, he had another occupation as a bonesetter. At first, he was a masseur to the players of a local rugby club and then later practiced bonesetting from rented rooms in the town. Later in life, he saw the occasional patient at his own home until just before his death at the age of eighty-five, after sixty years of practice.

He first came to my attention after I had started work in the nearby town of Neath in 1978 as a chiropractor. Many of my patients assumed we were related because of our similar surnames. Evidently, many patients had visited this man at some time or other, and all were keen to tell me of their experience of him. Their profound respect for him made me curious not only about the nature of his method, but also the man behind the public face. Why had he devoted sixty years to such an activity and under what conditions had he worked? It was clear from his former patients that this man had many qualities that inspired respect, even awe.

To clarify whether the fine memories of him depended on his bonesetting skills, his own personality, or both, I sought the accounts of his patients. I interviewed a small sample (n = 20) of his former patients to recall their encounter with this bonesetter. The patients remember his quiet, unassuming manner, his friendliness, and his reassuring nature. In marked contrast to his coal trimming

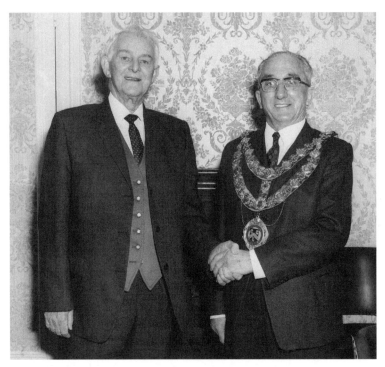

Figure 12.1.   Jack Leyshon with the Mayor of Port Talbot, Tom Rees, 1970. (By kind permission of the Mayor's Department, Port Talbot Civic Centre)

work, they recall his clean, well-kept, but immensely strong hands and well-groomed appearance (figure 12.1). His manipulations were carried out with great finesse and he treated a wide range of musculoskeletal conditions. Some patients also mentioned his charismatic quality outside of his bonesetting skills. Emerging themes were the quality of care and devotion to his patients. I suggest that he represents the type of bonesetter who, though lacking any family tradition of the craft or any training, was secure and settled within the community. This is at odds with some of his more flamboyant predecessors noted in the literature who gained notoriety by clashing with orthodoxy.

A Brief Review of the Literature

Analyzing the literature will help define the role and place of European bonesetters in a historical context, examining why bonesetters have remained largely on the fringe of mainstream medical practice. It can then be determined if Jack Leyshon was a typical or unorthodox bonesetter. The literature has focused on descriptions of bonesetting methods and its flamboyant, sometimes eccentric, practitioners. Some of it, produced at the end of the nineteenth and early twentieth centuries, was plainly confrontational and more to do with defining medical spheres of influence. For instance, in 1906, Herbert Barker, a famous London bonesetter, challenged the medical establishment by asserting that his methods of treating displaced bone, muscle, and cartilage were superior to theirs (Anderson 1981). A lengthy correspondence followed in the *British Medical Journal* with accusations, counteraccusations, and challenges for Mr. Barker to display his skills before a jury of qualified surgeons, or at least describe his methods (Anderson 1981). In March 1911, Mr. Barker was accused of professional negligence. The plaintiff sought damages of £400 because Barker undertook "to treat him for some affection of the knee, treated him without the amount of skill which he was entitled to expect from Mr. Barker." The evidence during the trial focused around whether an examination of the joint under anaesthesia as claimed by Mr. Barker could be reconciled with the injuries caused (the limb was eventually amputated). Medical evidence suggested that the knee joint must have been manipulated, not merely examined. The court found in favor of the plaintiff (Darling 1911:604). The prejudice shown toward Herbert Barker and his anesthetist, Frederick Axham, who was struck off the medical register in 1911 for associating with Barker (Smith 1979:287), reflects the published position on bonesetters. Other work was descriptive of the actual methods used by bonesetters (Hood 1871). Much of the latter was written by medical practitioners anxious to appropriate the art of bonesetting into their own therapeutic regimes. Only a few have attempted extensive cross-cultural histories of the subject from a medical or anthropological perspective (see Lomax 1975; Anderson 1992)

Bonesetting in Britain

The precise origins of British bonesetting are obscure, but Keith (1918:362) suggests that in the mid-eighteenth century, there may have been a class of practitioners scattered throughout England, particularly Wales, who were the "legitimate heirs and sturdy representatives of the British craft of Orthopaedic Surgery, known to the public as bonesetters."

Some bonesetters were descendants of long family traditions of bonesetters. The Huttons of Westmorland, the Matthewses of the Midlands, the Taylors of Whitworth, and the Thomases of Anglesey are notable. Others, such as Joseph Crowther of Wakefield (aged seventy-seven in 1884) and "Burbidge" (d. May 1875), whose father and grandfather were celebrated bonesetters, are recorded by Bennett (1884). Three female bonesetters are noted in the literature. Sally Mapp, the Doctress of Epsom, was the daughter of a well-known Wiltshire bonesetter. Mrs. Maltby of Nottingham was a descendant of a bonesetting family practicing in 1877 (Smith 1979). Ann Thomas, the daughter of Richard Evan Thomas, himself the son of Evan Thomas Y Maes, carried the art to Wisconsin (Cooter 1987:170). In the United States in general, the Reeses of Eastern Ohio, the Tieszens of Dakota (Janse 1976:75) and the Sweets of Rhode Island (Joy 1954) carried on this family theme. These "natural" bonesetting families often had other occupations. The Sweets and Taylors were blacksmiths, while Hutton was an upholsterer. For some families, there came a gradual metamorphosis from irregular to regular practitioner, the Sweets of Rhode Island and the Thomases of Anglesey being good examples. But this change does not account for all bonesetters.

Perhaps the first British bonesetter to gain notoriety was Sally Mapp, who was making her name in Epsom in 1736. Bennett (1884:7) recounts her history as being "very contradictory." She was the daughter of a Wiltshire bonesetter called Wallin and, despite success in 1736, died in 1737 in "miserable circumstances." Her success was featured in a comedy played at the Lincoln's Inn Fields theater aptly named, "The Husband's Relief; or The Female Bonesetter, and the Worm Doctor." A song dedicated to her goes:

> You surgeons of London who puzzle your pates,
> To ride in your coaches and purchase estates;
> Give over, for shame, for your pride has a fall,
> And the doctress of Epsom has outdone you all.
>
> Dame nature has given her a doctor's degree,
> She gets all the patients and pockets the fee;
> So if you don't instantly prove it a cheat,
> She'll loll in a chariot whilst you walk in the street. (Bennett 1884:9)

It would appear that the Doctress of Epsom was famous enough to warrant attention by playwrights who noted her financial success and her triumph over the established medical hegemony by her natural talent. Obliquely, it challenges them to discredit her for cheating and poaching patients. All of these themes were to be repeated over the next 150 years.

The medical literature on bonesetting is confined to an era in which the emerging orthopedic specialty in medicine began to take an interest in the work of bonesetters. Paget (1867) published a paper in the *British Medical Journal* under the title "Clinical lectures on cases that bonesetters cure," first given at St. Bartholomew's hospital. His most famous remark came when he warned that "few of you are likely to practice without having a bonesetter as your enemy; and if he can cure a case which you have failed to cure, his fortune may be made and yours marred." This lecture was reprinted twice more in 1875 and 1877 in the first and second editions of his *Clinical Lectures and Essays* (Marsh 1911:1232). Whatever friendly relationship had been enjoyed by orthodox and lay practitioner, the scene was set for confrontation and conflict.

Bonesetters of the day though, had a more whole-hearted champion. George Matthews Bennett published "The Art of the Bonesetter: A Testimony and Vindication" in 1884 (Bennett 1884). He was the descendant of a long family of bonesetters, the Matthews, who had lived and worked in the Midlands for over two hundred years. Succeeded by his son, Bennett set out a spirited defense of his work. He was stung enough by the insults that bonesetting had endured to reply,

> Before the publication of this work [Hood's in 1871], the poor Bonesetter had to endure contumely and insult at the hands of the faculty. Through their organs in the press they were denounced either as charlatans or quacks—as ignorant or presumptuous individuals who traded upon a "lucky" case to the detriment of the general practitioner. There were some indeed who by intercourse and observation knew that Bonesetters pursued their calling with success; that the principles which they followed were sound, gained by experience and improved by constant practice; that they possessed, in the different parts of the country where they lived, the confidence of the people, though they were not educated in medical or surgical schools. (Bennett 1884:3)

This passage sums up the problems of this period—disparagement and denunciation of bonesetters by the establishment, with their vilification as quacks in the press, but at the same time an affirmation that the art of the bonesetter is gained by experience, is improved by constant practice, and, most importantly, enjoys the confidence of the people. These are themes I return to when discussing Jack Leyshon. If the medical literature of this period could be described as confrontational, there is one contribution that stands out for its realism and directness. Marlin (1932) approached the thorny problem of what manipulations really consist of rather than what is claimed. With almost prescient accuracy, he described the physiology of the joint crack, which is characteristic of a successful manipulation. He moves on to the question of whether a bone really is out of place and can thus be replaced by the act. Using x-rays, he demonstrates that no bone is shown to be dislocated; therefore there is none to replace. Instead of leaving the reader to leap to the conclusion that manipulators' claims are manifestly false, he explains with remarkable clarity that manipulations work by restoring movement to stiff joints. He contended that bones were not "out of place" but "out of order"—that is, they suffered a loss of function.

Welsh Bonesetting

Bonesetters native to Wales have also received attention in the literature. Hywel provides an account of a family of bonesetters descended from Evan Thomas Y

Maes (1734–1817). Dr. William Hywel, a descendant of Evan Thomas, gives an account of his ancestor's origins, acknowledging that it might be unreliable. As a ten-year-old boy, he was shipwrecked off the coast of Anglesey in North Wales and was found by a local smuggler. He was raised as the adopted son of a local medical practitioner, Dr. Lloyd, who recognized his precocious talent for setting bones (Hywel 1984b). Perhaps the most famous of his bonesetting descendants was Hugh Owen Thomas (1834–1891), who held a medical degree and pioneered orthopedic surgery in Liverpool in the latter part of the nineteenth century. Neither Hugh Owen Thomas nor his father, Evan Thomas, were strangers to controversy. The father, a bonesetter, had nine brushes with the law (Hywel 1984a:17), which enhanced his reputation but surely infuriated the medical elite who saw him as a direct threat to their sphere of influence, not to mention their livelihoods (Cooter 1987:160–61).

The nephew of Hugh Owen Thomas, Sir Robert Jones (1857–1935), followed his uncle and became famous as an orthopedic surgeon (Watson 1934). An account of this family of bonesetters of Anglesey, "Meddygon Esgyrn Môn" (Bonesetters [or Bone Surgeons] of Anglesey) (Hughes-Roberts 1935), won a prize at the 1934 Eisteddfod (a cultural festival with competitions in music, drama, and poetry). The theme of a bonesetter's family history is continued by Joy (1954), who describes a family of bonesetters descended from James Sweet, who in 1630 emigrated from Wales and settled in North Kingstown, Rhode Island. As with the Thomases of Anglesey, this line of bonesetters was eventually absorbed into the medical fraternity as practicing orthopedic surgeons until the twentieth century.

More recently, Stephens (1993) described an ancestor of his called Silver John (John Lloyd) who lived and practiced bonesetting in Radnorshire in the early eighteenth century. He gained his nickname because he preferred to accept small pieces of silver as payment for his services, which were then sewn onto his clothing. His waistcoat, hat, trousers, and greatcoat were soon covered with silver. This walking advertisement of his success was soon to be his undoing because he was murdered for the silver. In 1814, his body was discovered in a lake (Llyn Heilyn) without the silver-adorned clothing. Stephens maintains there are still Lloyds who practice in the area today.

Evolution of British Bonesetting

The literature does not provide enough evidence for the demise of bonesetting, its complete takeover by its proponents in orthopedic surgery, or a gradual merger of the two. It does provide us with a glimpse of media activity at the end of nineteenth-century Britain, which is without reply from the bonesetters except Bennett's contribution in 1884. It also showed that the recently organized occupational groups now considered to be orthodox or regularized medicine could and did use their learned journals to negatively influence others, hence Bennett's anger that the faculty used their organs of the press to insult bonesetters. The bonesetting fraternity could not use such an approach because it was neither an organized occupational group, nor may it have perceived that such a threat existed from another occupational group far removed from its own societal domain.

In contrast to the professionalization of the occupation of medicine, British bonesetters never became organized and were probably unaware of the benefits of doing so. The thrust for professionalization was entirely absent. Perhaps medical practitioners denied bonesetters their status on the grounds of "caste" (Anderson 1981). With few exceptions, bonesetters were regarded as uneducated, rough, and unscrupulous. They were denounced as quacks and, as with Herbert Barker and Evan Thomas of Liverpool, prosecuted for their practice.

While the bonesetter's method was described (Hood 1871) and copied by those interested in its effects, the traditional bonesetter remained stigmatized and outside the ranks of the learned medical profession. Even if the methods of bonesetting could be copied and legitimized, its practitioners—despite the eloquent, respectable, and well-versed such as Bennett—could not cross the cultural and occupational Rubicon. Nonetheless, even without professionalization, bonesetters have survived, rooted in local communities, reliant on local patronage, and free from intraprofessional tension.

With the professionalization of the chiropractic and osteopathic communities, it would be natural to assume that the old style of bonesetter might die out in Europe. But in Finland and Denmark, there is still an active body of bonesetters whose methods and outcomes have been studied (Hemmila 1997, 2002; Anderson, chapter 1). The results suggest that traditional bonesetters compare favorably with physiotherapy and light exercise in terms of quality of life they can provide patients with chronic back pain.

As opposed to the more well-known bonesetters already described, there may be a group of bonesetters whose methods were not copied or appropriated, remaining "authentic" perhaps from before the days of Richard Hutton in the 1860s to the present. Staying out of the limelight and being unorganized might make them less occupationally noticeable, but it does not invalidate their work or weaken their contribution to their own communities' health care. The bonesetter I describe belongs, I believe, to this latter group: authentic, settled, and community-based.

South Wales Docks and Coal Trimmers

Employment in Port Talbot, and therefore the communities that depended on it, revolved around four interlinked industries—power (coal and coke extraction/

production); transport (coal, coke, finished products, extracted minerals); metallurgy (smelting of iron and copper ores; steel and copper rolling/milling); and labor (skilled and unskilled, direct and indirect). The town's economy, based on smelting and tinplate works, gradually declined at the end of the 1800s with the development of a steel industry. The docks had been extended in 1894 to cope with larger vessels both to bring in iron ore and to export coal from the Llynfi valley. In October of 1962, coal exports were switched to nearby Swansea so that the Port Talbot docks could concentrate on the iron and steel trades and in particular the import of iron ore. This meant the end of most jobs associated with coal transport and export.

The types of workers needed to service ships that called at these ports included: timber workers (porters and deal runners); general goods workers; coal workers (tippers and trimmers); iron ore workers; patent fuel workers; riggers; lightermen; and hobblers/strappers. Further up the Llynfi valley, coal mining employed substantial numbers of men, women, and children.

Coal trimmers had a specialized task of evenly bunkering coal in steamships so the boat was balanced. Unlike other gangs who worked at the docks, these groups considered themselves more skilled and so enjoyed better bargaining power than others. Over the period of Jack Leyshon's life, port workers became organized into unions, were exploited by some but not all employers, and exercised their right to strike on many occasions (Leng 1981). This history of an occupational group's development is marked not only by militancy, but also by a progression of improvements in the wages and living conditions of this group. Day rates for Port Talbot dockworkers in 1914 were 8 shillings. This rose to 15 shillings and a penny in 1919. Many coal trimmers in Newport were earning over £30 per week after piecework and overtime, with some earning up to £60 (Leng 1981:79).

Jack Leyshon's roots were firmly planted in this community of working people. Williamson (1982:6) suggests that:

> the notion of community embraces not just the idea of locality or social networks of particular kinds; it refers to the rich mosaic of subjective meanings which people attach . . . to the place itself and to the social relationships of which they are a part. . . . It is in terms of such meanings that the community can be recognised and the people who live there can recognise themselves. The pattern of these meanings is what constitutes the culture of the community.

Port Talbot has evolved from four small villages into a fully industrialized town. It still maintains this status, albeit with a lower profile, and by its very survival deserves its sense of community.

Methods

The problems of undertaking a life history of any individual are reviewed by Burgess (1982:133). He raises questions concerning the reliability, typicality, and representativeness of the sources of life histories such as autobiographies, letters, diaries, court records, and so on. Mandelbaum (1982:146) defines a life history as being merely an "account of a life, completed or ongoing," but adds that this is selective since it would be impossible to recount all aspects of that person's life experience. This impression is reflected by Honigman (1982:79) when he suggests that, "An ethnographer cannot avoid selecting some people, objects or events for study, thereby renouncing, for a time at least, the possibility of studying others."

One of the major difficulties in this study has been obtaining accurate information on Jack's life. Documentary sources are few and only two local newspaper clippings have been found that specifically mention his bonesetting activities. This lack of documentary evidence is not surprising given that there may not have been a professional need to maintain clinical records or other practice information. It hampers our appreciation of exactly how large his bonesetting practice was, in terms of numbers of patients and the range of conditions he treated. As far as his life as a bonesetter is concerned, the principal source of information about his working methods was former patients.

A total of twenty interviews were conducted between November 1988 and July 1989. Former patients accounted for eighteen interviews, 12 men and 6 women. A single interview was done with his two daughters and one with his nephews. Only four men interviewed were not former patients of mine but had been patients of Jack's. Their names were supplied by some of the other patients who thought they might be useful to me. I already knew most of the interviewees, so there was no need for any formal introductions beyond explaining the need for such a study and its relevance.

Two studies in the field of health and illness have used an informal interview method to produce accounts that extend beyond a mere description of the selected cases. Cornwell (1984:1) has studied twenty-four people living in East London with a focus on their "commonsense ideas and theories about health, illness, and health services." Her case study approach tries to avoid reducing subjects to "ciphers" and concentrates on elucidating what is of concern to local people in a specific community. Concepts of the private and public accounts of illness and health emerge, which support the idea of medicalization being a particular form of rationalization and legitimization. Crawford (1984) interviewed sixty people in the Chicago metropolitan area with an expressed interest in health. He wanted to find out how people there describe certain categories of concern. Health as self-control, as release, and as opposition emerged as themes for discussion. His open-ended interview technique, while allowing for the free flow of the interviewees' thoughts, had to indirectly elicit information on how people think about responsibility for health.

Both of these studies, using a qualitative approach, produced information that illustrates how people think about health and illness. They show that the experience of both health and illness is mediated, not in biological or even medical terms, but in commonsense terms. The extension of this common sense into the fabric of our social bodies is as profound as the experiences that produce them. The ethnography of Jack is better informed by this qualitative "common sense," as it was the medium of exchange between the bonesetter and his patients.

Ethnography of Jack Leyshon

Apart from local industry that provided work for so many, there were also strong community traditions in religion and sport. These three interests of work, religion, and sport occupied Jack for much of his life. The foundation for all of these interests came from his near family.

Undoubtedly, the person who influenced him most in his formative years was his mother. She was reputed to be religiously strict and was a devout member of the Ebenezer Welsh Baptist Chapel. Until his marriage in 1920, his life, apart from work, would have involved many social activities organized through the Chapel. With his brother, this would have meant sport. In the summer, cricket would have been played while in the winter and spring months, rugby union dominated. The Chapel had numerous teams depending on the number of eligible youngsters it had in each age group. These teams played each week against other Chapel sides in the area.

Apart from sporting activities, there were regular periods of worship on Sundays, including Sunday school, and it is probable that the Chapel ran many other social events to involve the congregation. Running parallel to Jack's involvement with the church was his connection with Aberavon Rugby Football Club. He joined the club in 1924, not as a playing member but as the trainer. All teams had different names for this special character: spongeman, bagman, rub-a-dub, trainer. His principal duties were to see that players received first aid if injured on the field. Many injuries were the result of collisions, collapsed scrums, and the like, with injuries such as concussions, cuts and bruises, broken or dislocated bones, and sprains and strains of muscles and tendons. Occasionally, there would have been more serious injuries such as severe spinal injuries requiring medical attention.

His association with the club covered many decades and his availability on "Monday mornings" and "between tides" (ships could not berth when the tide was out), coupled with his growing skill as a bonesetter, won him many friends both on and off the field. His reputation extended because he was always willing to treat players of visiting teams. He was visited by players of international rugby status as well as "exiles," those Welshmen who had gone "North" to play the professional game of Rugby League.[1]

Jack Leyshon's father was employed as a tinplate man at the Mansell Tinplate Works, although he occasionally worked in the docks. It is natural, therefore, that he should follow in his father's footsteps to gain a trade. Jack initially worked as a rollerman in the light plate mill of the old Port Talbot Steel Works. Later however, he moved into dock work and became a coal trimmer.

This involved the manual redistribution (bunkering) of coal loaded into coal export and coal-powered ships. Coal was loaded initially into a ship's hold by conveyor belt. Coal trimmers, working as a team, then shoveled the coal into the outer reaches of the hold. The trimmers tossed shovelfuls of coal from one person to the next until the last man was reached. His job was to build a wall of coal away from the hold wall, and then gradually fill in the gap behind the wall until the ceiling was reached. This process of redistribution balanced the vessel by equalizing the weight of the coal. This work was necessarily dirty, dusty, and very strenuous. Since team work was involved, there could be no letup in the pace once work was started. The use of a coal shovel for so many years and the volume of coal handled gave Jack the massive, strong hands he was famous for. His skill as a bonesetter was vital for the men who relied on this work for their living. Security of tenure for such a job depended only on one's ability to turn up fit for work. The process of turning up for work and signing on even if there were no ships to be handled was termed "being on the blob," so-called because the dockers would receive a blob (an official stamp) on their cards to record their willingness to work. This was done twice a day.

His employment in the docks remained until they started to close in the early sixties. Shipping, just before the Second World War, had started to use oil instead of coal to drive the steam turbines. The war itself saw the conversion of many ships to this new fuel because it was cleaner, more space efficient, and easier to load, as well as less time-consuming and labor-intensive.

In complete contrast to his work as a coal trimmer, Jack had another occupation as a bonesetter. Although it is likely that the majority of his earlier work as the Aberavon Rugby Club trainer was carried out at the ground or near the dressing rooms used by the players, he later expanded his activities into rented rooms, which allowed the nonplaying public better access to his skills.

He worked entirely on his own—without the support personnel necessary to the practice of orthodox medicine. He did not employ a nurse or receptionist to organize his appointments, and apart from a simple infrared lamp and couch, his practice lacked the usual paraphernalia of orthodox medicine. These premises were unsuitable for some patients because access involved climbing some stairs to get to his room. It was sparsely furnished and divided into three cubicles, each partitioned by a curtain. Jack would proceed from one to the other to treat his patients. In one, there may have been a patient having heat treatment delivered by an ancient heat lamp. In another, he might have dealt with the patient directly. Patients waited on chairs provided in the room itself. There was no receptionist and no telephone to make appointments. If he was too busy to see someone, the patient would either come back later or another day. His later premises at Station Road, Port Talbot, were initially located upstairs, but he then moved to a room on the ground floor at the rear of the property, which was fronted by a travel agency. The setup was similar, except that there was only one room, so patients were seen one by one. Again, there was no receptionist or telephone to make appointments. It was a question of turning up at the premises and seeing if he was busy or whether his job as a coal trimmer (and therefore the tide) had detained him. It was at the entrance to this practice that a brass plaque bore his name and the inscription "Bonesetter." It is also not known whether he called himself a bonesetter before his move to the location on Station Road. With his death, we shall probably never know the reason why he adopted this title rather than one of physiotherapist, which would have been widely understood by more of the community.

Of immediate note is the contrast between his work as a coal trimmer and as a bonesetter. It is not clear why he embarked on another part-time occupation in such a way. The wages he received at the dock may not have been enough to support his family adequately, but this cannot account for the fees he charged his patients, which were nominal. Another contrast is in the actual physical nature of the two jobs. Coal trimming is dirty, dusty, and physically demanding, especially on the shoulders, arms, and hands, whereas bonesetting demands strength but finesse (in manipulation) and a good bedside manner. Many of his former patients remarked on his "immaculate appearance" and his large, well-kept hands. These were equally capable of handling a coal shovel for hours at a time as they were of massaging bruised muscles or manipulating painful joints. His enormous strength was delivered with great care, and as patients recall he would "replace a disc," causing pain only for the briefest of moments.

The majority of his patients would have been local community members reflecting a wide range of occupations. Initially, his expertise was with sports injuries, but as the industries in this area were labor-intensive and many of the jobs manual, it was natural that he would see all types of work-related injuries. There are anecdotal accounts of local medical practitioners going to see him, which added to his fame, if not his growing lore.

Patients who needed attention for an injury may have been aware of the medical community's lack of success with the treatment of musculoskeletal problems. There may have also been a time delay between consultation and referral to the local hospital for the National Health Service (NHS) treatment.[2] Such delays could have kept patients off work for longer than they could wait. This factor of accessibility was cited by many of his patients as a reason for consulting Jack rather than the medical practitioner. A decision to go to Jack by low-paid workers and their families was not therefore a matter of "going private," but of getting quick results and getting back to work.

Eventually, the lease on his room at Station Road ran out and he moved back to his own home on Thomas Street. (It is not clear whether he voluntarily let the lease go so he could retire, or whether it would have been prohibitively expensive.) He no longer used the couch that he had previously, but now asked the patient to lie on the floor. With advancing age, he saw fewer and fewer people, until finally he would only admit those old patients whom he knew. Although he never refused to see patients earlier in his career, later he was known to peer through the net curtains of his front room, and if he could not recognize the caller, he would not open the door.

Although he described himself as a bonesetter, the methods he used were not restricted to manipulation. The regimen for the patient, nearly always the same, is indistinguishable from the methods used in the clinical sciences of today. A treatment session usually took about twenty minutes and was characterized by taking an oral history, physical examination (by manual palpation), premanipulation, manipulation (if any), and the posttreatment period.

Initially, he asked his patient the nature of the complaint, its history, and any complicating factors. Next, he examined the affected (exposed) area manually. He used his entire hand, including fingers, for this task. They would probe, knead, or lightly touch the skin in order to find out where the problem was located. If he found something, he would often exclaim, "That's it," or words to that effect, and either proceed to manipulate that area or use heat, massage, or a combination of both to first "loosen" up the area. Not all patients were manipulated, as this was often unnecessary, such as cases of strained or otherwise injured muscles. Problems affecting major joints and spinal joints would often be manipulated, but the circumstances always guided his approach. If he thought that the manipulation might be painful, he would tell the patients and ask them to bear with him, as it would only hurt for a short while. If the only treatment was to be massage of the area or some heat, he would proceed, talking with the patient all the time. His chatter, which covered all subjects, was continuous from the time he began the treatment phase until he finished. Undoubtedly, this was a way of relaxing patients by distracting their attention from the painful nature of their problem and its treatment.

The success of some techniques of manipulation depend on the speed and finesse with which they can be carried out, while others need the tacit cooperation
of the patient to receive the manipulation. When Jack was treating a spinal complaint in the lumbar region, he might press with his thumbs on the actual vertebrae itself until he heard a click or a crunch. There was the potential for pain, but
if done quickly enough, it would essentially be painless. In the neck, the preferred
method was to rotate the head in one direction and then suddenly rotate it a little more, but with increased speed. This frequently produces a crack from the
small joints in the neck vertebra. Provided this is done with enough care, there is
little pain and very little danger of injury. His ploy of always talking was often
distracting enough to stop the patient's resistance when the final part of the manipulation was carried through. Techniques of manipulation used for the major articulations were a different matter. In these cases, the limb or joint must be put
into a position that would permit the manipulation to be carried out without danger to the operator or further damage to the joint itself. These manipulations, especially if the joint was partially dislocated or badly bruised, could cause great
pain to the sufferer. Only Jack's great strength and finesse made the difference between success and failure.

The numbers of visits needed varied with the severity and chronicity of the
problem. If Jack could "catch it warm"—that is, right after the injury occurred—
only one treatment might be necessary. If the problem had been neglected by the
patient or had been treated unsuccessfully elsewhere, repeat visits might be in order. Apparently intractable problems that baffled other practitioners might be
miraculously alleviated by Jack in only one visit. Adhesions in some joints can
prove particularly difficult to treat, as there is more lameness than pain. His ability to identify the problem and manipulate it became his hallmark.

Clearly, there is a difference between manipulation and bonesetting, and there
were times when he set broken bones. One story tells of how he broke his own leg
while at work. He set it so well himself that when he arrived at the hospital, doctors there did not believe his story and wanted to know which doctor had set his
leg. This anecdote is another instance of his bonesetting activities augmenting the
myth surrounding him.

Jack was raised, worked, and died in the same community, though he had the
opportunity to leave. As a member of this community, he never turned his back
on it, even though his talent as a bonesetter could have allowed him a privileged
position elsewhere. Jack's activities as a bonesetter were extraordinary, not his character or temperament. His cultural values were firmly rooted in the community
that he lived and worked in, and these values would not have excused confrontation. Medical practitioners were known to visit him, so it may be supposed that
local exposure mollified any thoughts of professional resentment.

If a traditional bonesetter needed to be taught the manipulative method by one of his or her kin, or have had a history of such practices in the family, then Jack did not fulfill these criteria. This does not imply that he could not have been a bonesetter, only that his education was unorthodox even for a heterodox occupation because there was no obvious precedent in his family. A further deviation from the normal bonesetting family background occurred because he did not pass on his knowledge and experience to any of his own family members. In common with the Sweets of Rhode Island, Jack never appeared to exploit his patients. Perhaps his other work as a coal trimmer provided enough for him and his family to live on and the income as a bonesetter was a bonus. The amounts he charged varied from patient to patient. They always regarded the amount as reasonable, especially because many visited him only once or twice. However small the charge, the number of patients treated in the course of a week meant that his earnings could have added up over the years. If his income was substantially supplemented by being a bonesetter, it certainly did not show by any extravagance. He lived in the same house for decades and was not known to have a car or any other large expense. In all other respects, except for his activity as a bonesetter, his life was a model of normality. His upbringing, his marriage, his work in the docks as a coal trimmer, and in the broader sense his involvement with the community through church and sports were all intertwined. The fabric of life in the Port Talbot of the first half of the twentieth century is reflected in his own life.

The Bonesetting Experience

Patients' accounts are an important part of this study for two reasons. First, little is known of patients' interactions with this type of practitioner. Secondly, the chance to directly examine this bonesetter and his methods has, with his death, passed. But his beneficiaries, the patients, still recall their encounters with him. They are, in a sense, both participants and observers (albeit uninformed) of an empirical tradition that has been practiced for centuries. An oral history may, as Samuel (1982:141) points out, contain items that are unique to that one person. The patient accounts will provide direct access to the experience of their encounter with him. This cannot be obtained by observation, even if it were possible. The accounts should not be read as mere anecdote—even if the patients' recall may be less than perfect after many years—but as a narrative that adds a richness and perspective to the experience of pain and illness that might otherwise be lost.

Patterns of Complaint

What sort of disorders did Jack's patients present him with and how did he approach the assessment of these disorders? What were their recollections of the actual treatment session and were the patients already aware of their condition before they went to Jack?

The principal complaint that Jack saw was pain of the spine and appendicular skeleton with its associated muscles and joints. The assessment of the complaints was routine. Jack would ask the patient about the circumstances of the complaint and its associated factors while palpating the affected area at the same time. One patient recalled:

> RD: Well he felt it first. He was a clever man in the sense that he knew where your pain was and he would feel the leg and he would just gently come down. "How did you do this then, boy?" "Playing football." "Oh, it's a hard old game that." And he'd be there now saying, "Oh ye, what position do you play then?" And he's still there gently rubbing, and he's talking you off it. And the next thing . . .
>
> SL: What did he do?
>
> RD: Moved it. He said it was resting on a nerve.

This examination is in essence no different from the methods used by orthodox orthopedic practitioners. A history supported by an examination and other special tests is the prerequisite to formulating a diagnosis. Treatment follows the diagnosis, and the patient is reassessed to measure the outcome of treatment. Jack's clinical application is therefore entirely in keeping with current medical practice. While his estimation of the cause of his patients' problems may lack the morbid specificity of his medical counterparts who have access to a battery of special technologies, there is no doubt that his diagnostic methods were appropriate and relevant to the patient's problem.

Trauma played a significant role in producing some of the injuries, particularly in men. Football and rugby injuries were the most common. These types of acute injuries were usually seen quickly and followed a favorite phrase of Jack, where he liked to "catch them warm." A rugby player commented:

> BR: Yes. They'd go back to him a couple of times. Like my shoulder, I dislocated my shoulder and he put that back in. But with rugby injuries he never took long about it, if you went to him quickly when the injury was still warm or knew it was easy to put back in. If it was something which was out for about a week or a month or whatever it was I suppose it was harder to correct then because it had been there longer.

Community Knowledge

Many of the patients commented that Jack was so well known in the community that it was not necessary to ask anyone about him or what he did. As one patient put it:

SL: How did you know about him?

HN: Well he was just well known in Port Talbot. He was with the rugby players and I think it was just that everybody knew him. I don't think you ever talked about him consciously, but it was just that everybody knew him.

SL: So it was not really something to go and find out about?

HN: No, no.

SL: Did you ever tell your GP, or did your GP find out?

HN: No, I told my GP that I was going.

SL: And what did he say?

HN: He said that if he could help me in any way that it was unfortunate that he couldn't tell me directly himself to go there because officially he wasn't recognized but I know for a fact, he's dead now, but my own GP sent a lot of people there.

Most patients remember the actual treatment part of their encounter with Jack vividly. One patient recalls:

GJ: He sort of lifted my shoulder and he pulled my arm back and he sort of lifted my shoulder blade up. The pain was awful! And he sort of put his hand underneath. Aaah! It was awful. "I'm going to flatten this muscle down," he said. And then he did that and it was awful but indeed, it was very sore for the rest of the day, but it started improving, and I think it was only about three visits and I was right as rain.

SL: What did you expect though when you had gone there? Did you expect it to be painful or to be short or?

GJ: Oh I expected it to be awful!

SL: Did you?

GJ: Yeah, yeah. I went there in fear and trembling, you know.

SL: And it was indeed a bit painful?

GJ: Oh it was painful.

Another young patient, on dislocating his knuckle in a fistfight, put it more succinctly:

SL: When you were a fifteen-year-old schoolboy you must have been a bit frightened when you first went to Jack?

BR: No.

SL: You weren't?

BR: No. You knew straightaway what it was going to be like if you went down Jack's.

On one occasion, Jack advised a patient with inflamed joints to apply a poultice, made of flour mixed with water and vinegar, over the affected area. This was to be left on overnight. A patient recalls:

HJ: Oh, sometimes I never bothered with the doctor, I just went to Jack. As soon as he looks at it he says, "Oh, gout you got." But as soon as he got it worked out, "Oh," he said, "I can't do much for that. I tell you what to do," he said. "Go home now and mix plain flour in the basin and add warm water in it and add a spoonful of vinegar," he said, "and put it over that tonight." Do you know, it had gone by the morning!

SL: Had it?

HJ: It drew all the inflammation right out of it.

SL: This was applied almost like a . . .

HJ: Like a paste. And he said, "Put it right around it." By God, it was like it was gone in the morning. Dragged it out it did. Things like that, you know, Jack was up on everything to do with bones, there was not nobody could beat him on bones. Nobody.

His use of flour, water, and vinegar, advice on posture, correct breathing, and his own liniments all supported his bonesetting practice. These extra elements of treatment, however do not convert Jack into a folk practitioner with remedies for all ills.

Were the patients aware of the nature of their problem? What were their expectations for a cure? Some went to him with no prior expectations of cure but were confident that they would receive a sound opinion. Some patients who had been under investigation by their GP came with a "medical" diagnosis, but this was often tempered by their lack of success with biomedical treatments.

Those who visited Jack many times were used to describing their problems in commonsense, not pathological terms. Jack also described their ailments in commonsense terms. One patient came with a diagnosis of prolapsed intervertebral disc from his GP:

JA: I went to Jack Leyshon then and I told him I was going on holidays to Spain in the car. And then, well, he examined me.

SL: Then what happened?

JA: He said that the nerve had moved in my back and I've never had a pain since until . . .

SL: What did he actually do, do you remember?

JA: Yes. He laid me flat on my stomach, I laid on the bed and he pressed my back just here and he said, "Oh there it is." And he just pushed it in. I felt it going back.

SL: Did it hurt?

JA: Yes.

SL: So you went "Ouch!"

JA: Yes.

SL: But it was all over then?

JA: Yes.

This account contains all the elements discussed above: the history, examination, location, and identification of the pain's putative origin; a commonsense description; and, a manipulation with thrust. All this was accomplished within minutes of the first encounter between bonesetter and patient. The speed of events must have been strange to a patient who had been investigated for the problem at the local hospital and seen an orthopedic surgeon over a period of one year. That Jack so easily spotted the disc problem and corrected it within such a short space of time must have left him wondering what was wrong with the medical treatment he had received. This case illustrates the sense of medical failure and bonesetting success commonly encountered by persons with musculoskeletal complaints, epitomized by Paget's warning in 1867, illustrated earlier, that "if he can cure a case which you have failed to cure, his fortune may be made and yours marred."

Trust and Faith

It is clear that for the majority of his patients, Jack was a man who could be trusted. This is important for the patient in acute pain. They must at some stage have had enough faith in his abilities for him to carry out what was sometimes a painful manipulation. In addition there is a point when he had to get the patient to relax completely before making the final manipulative maneuver. At this point, patients must have made an active choice to be compliant or to resist him. A female patient's comment illustrates this faith:

CR: Yes. I had complete faith in him. It was as simple as that. What you've got to remember is that this man had enormous charisma, he really did. Once you had been to him a few times you were under his spell. I've never met a man with such charisma really.

Another describes this aspect as a "charismatic healing quality." Others were more down-to-earth in their descriptions particularly with regard to his qualifications:

SL: Again, this question of qualifications, it didn't matter to you that he wasn't qualified.

BR: No. He had qualifications. He had proven qualifications, not bits of paper that said that he had qualified in a college or in London, he had field qualifications, proven qualifications.

SL: By experience he was qualified.

BR: Of course.

The dominant attitude toward this particular bonesetter, by his patients, was one of trust. They had complete faith in his ability to locate the source of their pain and deal with it. The question of his qualifications was not a problem for his patients. His experience was the deciding factor. Conversely, patients expected their general practitioner to have the appropriate paper qualifications but did not trust or expect these medical practitioners to be able to deal with their problems.

For one patient, the experience of illness produced a profound reflection of the role of doctors and medicine:

JA: . . . I think I've learnt so much by people outside the medicine profession who treat a person with an illness, a doctor just treats an illness. And I don't think it's altogether the doctors' fault. I've got an idea that it's something in their training that might be lacking. Say you've got a spinal injury they treat the spinal injury, they don't treat the patient with the spinal injury. And I really believe that sincerely. In my case, it definitely happened in my case . . .

SL: But why do you think doctors don't have it or do you think that some doctors have it regardless of their training?

JA: Yes. Quite a few have it. All doctors aren't exactly the same but they've got to keep within a guideline, their training is such that they've got to keep within a rule book, I feel. But sometimes you've got to step over that to become patient/doctor related. Years ago it was called a "bedside manner." That's gone in medicine now and why I'm not quite aware.

SL: Do you think their training might train out that bedside manner?

JA: I think so to be honest. Please don't think I hold it against doctors as people. I hold it against the profession.

Remuneration

For most patients, the subject of payment was made at the end of a treatment visit. Many patients commented on Jack's reluctance to charge them a fee, preferring instead to say that they should make a contribution to his "electricity bill." The amount charged was seen by most patients as being very reasonable and affordable. Some regarded the amount as being nominal.

A patient, seen in 1962, recalls:

SL: Do you remember how much he charged you the first time?

RR Fifty pence.

SL: And did you think that was cheap?

RR: Yes. I mean if you were in pain it was cheap.

SL: And you only had to go the once anyway.

RR: Only once I was going.

One of his patients, a dock worker, was paid about £7.00 per week in 1954 which left him with £4/10s after deductions. His comments on the charge are illustrative of the need to return to work:

SL: What about . . . how much did Jack charge you for treating you then? Do you remember?

TH: It varied. Seven and six (7s 6d). It depends how long he was with you. But normally it was about seven shillings, ten shillings.

SL: Do you think that was reasonable then?

TH: Well it seemed a lot of money but I was also in a lot of pain. You know, you had to get well to earn money to keep the family going.

When he accepted money from satisfied patients, he may have done so with a sense of humility and because not accepting might have embarrassed the patient more. This aspect is best explained by one patient:

SL: If he had been very well qualified, do you think that would have helped or do you think that he would just have charged more and become more up-market?

GJ: Possibly he would have charged more but knowing Jack I don't think he would have charged more because he was a man of the people. He cared about people and he cared for people. I think he had a gift and it was a gift of God that he had, without a doubt, because this man was unique, absolutely unique in the way he dealt with you.

Charisma and Demeanor

Without exception, all patients reported good results from his treatment with no adverse reactions. Were these good results just a by-product of an extremely competent manipulator? Comments made by patients suggested that his manipulative expertise was just part of his success. It has been mentioned by a patient that he had a certain "charisma" but part of this concerned his hands. Many patients regarded these as very important. One patient recalls:

> GJ: I can remember that my first impression of him was that he was a fairly big man, and what I noticed was that when he held me his hands were soft and yet his fingers were extremely strong. He didn't have hard hands, you know like laborers' hands. They weren't hands like a laborer; they were more like a pianist's hands in their texture and yet they were incredibly strong!
>
> SL: What gave you the impression that they were strong?
>
> GJ: Well, the way he held me you know. The grip that he had. There was a tremendous grip there.
>
> SL: If you saw his hands, were they as soft and dull as mine . . . ?
>
> GJ: Yes.
>
> SL: . . . or were they calloused?
>
> GJ: No, they weren't calloused at all. Now he had worked in the steel works.
>
> SL: So he should have had calluses?
>
> GJ: He should have, but he didn't.

Again:

> LH: Well, he was a big man, must have been physically strong to work in the job he was doing. But what amazed me was that he was spotless clean always, well-turned out. His wife must have been a magnificent lady to look after him like that. And I never saw Jack like you see some of the coal trimmers—dirty and grimy. If you looked at Jack and looked at the others, you would never think that he was a coal trimmer.

In contrast to the last description of his size, the next patient recalls:

> JH: I was fascinated by the man—at one stage I even thought I would like to go in for that. His hands were so soothing and he was very relaxed. He was 5' 8" or 5' 9", say ten and a half stone, a good-looking man, hair brushed back, very clean appearance and quiet but the hands were very reassuring because the strength was there—that is what it was about.

This aspect of appearance expanded to include his demeanor as well:

SL: You said he was a very good-looking chap, always very clean.

JH: Yes.

SL: Did that add to his charisma, I mean was he charismatic anyway?

JH: I felt so. I felt that he had piercing eyes and he was a good-looking man. He had a presence about him . . . I'm quite sure that some people who went along to see him didn't have anything wrong with them! I can well imagine that because he had a charisma, a presence. There was, I don't know, perhaps an inner peace, he was a pretty self-assured man I think but without being in any way pushy. He was a quiet man but there was a self-assurance there I think.

One might question where this charisma came from. Was it a product of his up-bringing, his faith, his work, or his environment? For some, his skills were God-given but his natural ability was a "gift":

SL: Where do you expect his personality came from? Did it come from his Church or just from within himself, or from his father?

LH: I think it came from the Church and the environment he lived in. This is the peculiar thing, Jack was in more ways a very cultured man you know. In a sense he worked with the roughest of men, and I'm not speaking disrespectful of the dock-ers, but he worked in that environment.

But this interviewee while acknowledging that there was an environmental and re-ligious aspect to his gift, found that his particular talent was unique to him. He had asked Jack once where his talent came from. The reply may be the only clues we can gain directly from Jack himself:

LH: . . . And I used to say "Jack, you've got no academic background, you've got no scientific background in the broad sense, how do you do it?" And he said "It's a gift of God as far I'm concerned. It is a gift which I discovered quite accidentally . . ."

SL: . . . You say he discovered it accidentally, he never told you what the accident was that made him, did he?

LH: No. I asked him and he said that it had occurred accidentally in the early days.

An accidental discovery that he could manipulate joints and soft tissues is un-derstandable. To ascribe this discovery as a gift of God might indicate that he used his gift in a passive way, i.e., by allowing God to act through his hands. His religious devotion may have reinforced this belief. Perhaps this is a major factor in his unpretentiousness. A patient sums up this feeling:

SL: He was very gentle with his strength though with women and men alike?

LH: Very gentle. He had an uncanny knack of inspiring confidence. I can't describe it in a scientific sense. There are things in life that you can feel but you can't describe in an intellectual sense. And I had tremendous regard for Jack.

SL: If another one came along, would you be able to spot another Jack?

LH: Not in the modern world, no.

Could this description of the man account for a "charisma." Wilson (1975) cites Weber's definition of the term to mean "the gift of grace." Moreover this gift must be a quality that endows superhuman powers and must be recognized by others, making it a social phenomenon. Wilson (1975:x) differs from this orthodox perspective by saying:

> The paradox of charisma is precisely the attraction of faith in man, the element of personal trust that has in so many respects become either redundant or increasingly difficult in the modern world. It is the reassertion of faith in human virtues and dispositions that, if supernatural, yet are also apparently natural— natural that is, because not technological. They appear as uncompromised, either by the arduous effort that has to be undertaken to acquire them in everyday life, or by the conditions in which they were exercised. Faith is easier than empirical analysis, innate nobility a more congenial idea than cultivated learning, particularly when learning has turned away from the old, nineteenth century belief in the cultivation of inner resources to the modern demand for instrumental expertise and calculated skills for use in a rational system.

Emerging from the interviews was the discovery of a very different quality. The question of faith, trust, and charisma seem closely intertwined and difficult for some patients to articulate. Wilson's description puts the question of faith into sharp relief when matched with LH's feelings about this bonesetter.

From these interviews, I suggest that this bonesetter not only had special talents for this type of marginal practice gained over sixty years of practice but another, more indefinable quality approaching that of charisma. This quality complemented his private life and public work to such an extent that it is difficult to imagine him treating his patients without it. Patients describe a quiet, unassuming, self-assured man who could lead them through the healing encounter, reducing their fear and pain (figure 12.2).

Conclusion

A lasting legacy of this bonesetter, at least in the minds of his former patients, was the quality of care that he rendered. Defining this quality is difficult as it seems part of three related areas. First, there was never any doubt that the patients

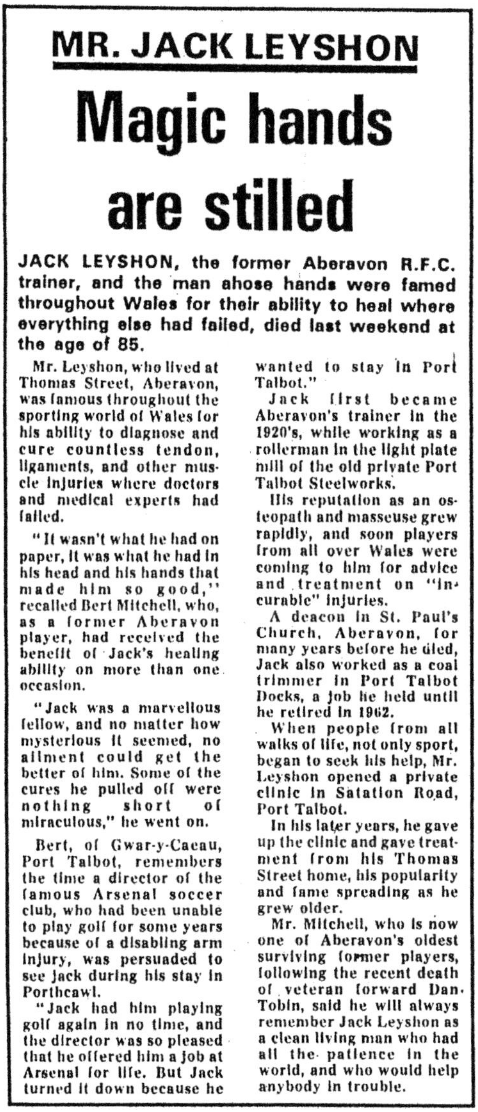

MR. JACK LEYSHON

Magic hands are stilled

JACK LEYSHON, the former Aberavon R.F.C. trainer, and the man ahose hands were famed throughout Wales for their ability to heal where everything else had failed, died last weekend at the age of 85.

Mr. Leyshon, who lived at Thomas Street, Aberavon, was famous throughout the sporting world of Wales for his ability to diagnose and cure countless tendon, ligaments, and other muscle injuries where doctors and medical experts had failed.

"It wasn't what he had on paper, it was what he had in his head and his hands that made him so good," recalled Bert Mitchell, who, as a former Aberavon player, had received the benefit of Jack's healing ability on more than one occasion.

"Jack was a marvellous fellow, and no matter how mysterious it seemed, no ailment could get the better of him. Some of the cures he pulled off were nothing short of miraculous," he went on.

Bert, of Gwar-y-Caeau, Port Talbot, remembers the time a director of the famous Arsenal soccer club, who had been unable to play golf for some years because of a disabling arm injury, was persuaded to see Jack during his stay in Porthcawl.

"Jack had him playing golf again in no time, and the director was so pleased that he offered him a job at Arsenal for life. But Jack turned it down because he wanted to stay in Port Talbot."

Jack first became Aberavon's trainer in the 1920's, while working as a rollerman in the light plate mill of the old private Port Talbot Steelworks.

His reputation as an osteopath and masseuse grew rapidly, and soon players from all over Wales were coming to him for advice and treatment on "incurable" injuries.

A deacon in St. Paul's Church, Aberavon, for many years before he died, Jack also worked as a coal trimmer in Port Talbot Docks, a job he held until he retired in 1962.

When people from all walks of life, not only sport, began to seek his help, Mr. Leyshon opened a private clinic in Satation Road, Port Talbot.

In his later years, he gave up the clinic and gave treatment from his Thomas Street home, his popularity and fame spreading as he grew older.

Mr. Mitchell, who is now one of Aberavon's oldest surviving former players, following the recent death of veteran forward Dan. Tobin, said he will always remember Jack Leyshon as a clean living man who had all the patience in the world, and who would help anybody in trouble.

Figure 12.2.   Jack Leyshon's obituary, April 24, 1980 (By kind permission of the Editor of the Neath and Port Talbot Guardian)

should consult him, even if some were apprehensive at first. At the risk of upsetting their medical practitioner, patients used him to treat their pain and disability.

Second the experience of the patient in relation to the bonesetter has highlighted the concept of "faith" and trust. Their encounter with him drew a profound respect for his abilities. As a man who shared the same community, work, and social interests, there was a common knowledge of who, where, and what he did in his other occupation as a bonesetter. Thus, he was accessible, local, identifiable, and successful in this other role. There was nothing to fear by going to him, no cultural divide nor punitive fees to find. These factors, added to his personality, made him trustworthy, reliable, and successful.

Third, the experience of the bonesetter with sixty years of bonesetting illustrates the nature of this type of practice. His remarkable hands gained that experience of how to examine, manipulate and reassure his patients. Romer's (1911:603-604) comments bear repetition, "A certain delicacy of touch is doubtlessly requisite to properly appreciate that lesion, whilst the correction of it largely depends on knack, but both can easily be acquired by experience and practice." If a personal apprenticeship with an established family bonesetter was helpful in learning the art, or even if this bonesetter had a natural talent, it was constant practice that honed it. Bennett's (1884:3) assertion "that the principles which they followed were sound, gained by experience and improved by constant practice; that they possessed, in the different parts of the country where they lived, the confidence of the people, though they were not educated in medical or surgical schools," sums up this experience.

Notes

I wish to acknowledge the family of Jack Leyshon and some of his past patients for their helpfulness in allowing me access to their memories of this remarkable man. I also wish to acknowledge the editorial assistance of Kathryn Oths, whose tenacity and skill has brought this contribution to fruition.

1. "North" refers to the North of England. Going North is a derogatory term insinuating that someone has sold out for money, i.e., they have gone from the (then) amateur Rugby Union code to paid Rugby League. The professional game of Rugby League was and still is well paid. Rugby Union is still played by amateurs but many clubs are now "professional," paying their players just like the league code.

2. It is remarkable that since I have worked in that same local hospital with direct referrals from local GPs, my waiting list was over 90 weeks! Such is the demand by GPs for effective treatment for low back pain. Jack is probably giggling to himself at the irony of it all.

References

Anderson, Robert T.
  1981   Medicine, Chiropractic, and Cast. *Anthropological Quarterly* 54(3):157–65.
  1987   The Treatment of Musculoskeletal Disorders by a Mexican Bonesetter (*Sobador*). *Social Sciences and Medicine* 24(1):43–46.
  1992   Spinal Manipulation before Chiropractic. Pp. 3–14 in Scott Haldeman, ed. *Principles and Practice of Chiropractic.* 2d ed. San Mateo, Calif.: Appleton & Lange.

Bennett, G. M.
   1981 [1884] *The Art of the Bonesetter: A Testimony and a Vindication.* First new edition. Tamor Pierston ed. London: Thos Murby.
Burgess, Robert G.
   1982   Personal Documents, Oral Sources, and Life Histories. Pp. 131–35 in Robert G. Burgess, ed. *Field Research: A Sourcebook and Field Manual.* London: Allen and Unwin.
Cooter, Roger
   1987   Bones of Contention? Orthodox Medicine and the Mystery of the Bonesetters Craft. Pp. 158–73 in R. Porter and W. Bynum, eds. *Medical Fringe and Medical Orthodoxy.* London: Croom Helm.
Cornwell, Jocelyn
   1984   *Hard Earned Lives: Accounts of Health and Illness from East London.* London: Tavistock Publications.
Crawford, R.
   1984   A Cultural Account of "Health": Control, Release, and the Social Body. Pp. 60–103 in J. B. McKinlay, ed. *Issues in the Political Economy of Health Care.* New York: Tavistock.
Darling, J.
   1911   Thomas v Barker. Mr Justice Darling's Summing-up. *The Lancet* 1:604–606.
Evans, J. L.
   1982   *The History of Taibach and District.* Port Talbot, England: Alun Books.
Hemmila, Heikki M.
   1997   Does Folk Medicine Work? A Randomised Clinical Trial on Patients with Prolonged Back Pain. *Archives of Physical Medicine and Rehabilitation* 78:571–77.
   2002   Quality of Life and Cost of Care of Back Pain Patients in Finnish General Practice. *Spine* 27(6):647–53.
Honigman, John J.
   1982   Sampling in Ethnographic Fieldwork. Pp. 79–90 in Robert G. Burgess, ed. *Field Research: A Sourcebook and Field Manual.* London: Allen & Unwin.
Hood, Wharton
   1871   On the So-Called "Bone-Setting," Its Nature and Results. *The Lancet* 1:336–38.
Hughes-Roberts, H.
   1935   *H. Meddygon Esgyrn Môn. Cyhoeddedig Gan Cyndeithas Eisteddfod, 1934.* Liverpool: Hugh Evans a'i Feibion.
Hywel, W.
   1984a The Anglesey Bonesetters. *Country Quest* (January):17–19.
   1984b The Bonesetters of Anglesey. An Unorthodox Genius and a Pioneering Nephew. *Country Quest* (February):15–18.
Janse, Joseph
   1976   *Principles and Practice of Chiropractic: An Anthology.* Lombard, Ill.: National College of Chiropractic.

Joy, R. T.
  1954   The Natural Bonesetters with Special Reference to the Sweet Family of Rhode Island. A Study of an Early Phase in Orthopedics. *Bulletin of Medical History* 28(3):416–41.

Keith, A.
  1918   Bone-Setting. Ancient and Modern. *The Medical Press*, November 13, 362–65.

Leng, P.
  1981   *The Welsh Dockers*. Ormskirk, Lancashire: G. W. & A. Hesketh.

Lomax, Elizabeth
  1975   Manipulative Therapy: An Historical Perspective from Ancient Times to the Modern Era. Pp. 11–18 in M. Goldstein, ed. *The Research Status of Spinal Manipulative Therapy*. NINCDS Monograph 15, Bethesda, Md.: National Institute of Neurological and Communicative Disorders and Stroke (NINCDS).

Mandelbaum, David G.
  1982   The Study of Life History. Pp. 146–51 in Robert G. Burgess, ed. *Field Research: A Sourcebook and Field Manual*. London: Allen & Unwin.

Marlin, Thomas
  1932   On Bone-Setting. *The Lancet* 1:60–62.

Marsh, Howard.
  1911   Bonesetting. *British Medical Journal* 1:1231–39.

Paget, James
  1867   Clinical Lecture on Cases That Bone-Setters Cure. *British Medical Journal* 1:1–4.

Romer, F.
  1911   Bone-Setting and Its General Principles. *The Lancet* 1:603–604.

Samuel, Raphael
  1982   Local History and Oral History. Pp. 136–45 in Robert G. Burgess, ed. *Field Research: A Sourcebook and Manual*. London: Allen & Unwin.

Smith, F. B.
  1979   *The People's Health*. London: Croom Helm.

Stephens, Meic
  1993   Dawn Y Meddyg Esgyrn I'w Gael Hyd Heddiw. *Western Mail*, January 2, 3.

Watson, F.
  1934   *The Life of Sir Robert Jones*. London: Hodder and Stoughton.

Williamson, W.
  1982   *Class Community and Culture. A Biographical Study of Social Change in Mining*. London: Routledge & Keegan Paul.

Wilson, Bryan R.
  1975   *The Noble Savages. The Primitive Origin of Charisma and Its Contemporary Survival*. Berkeley: University of California Press.

It Takes a Village
Reflections of a Modern-Day Bonesetter

MARC WEILL

RECENTLY, A COMPUTER ENGINEER of Czechoslovakian descent, whom I will call Stephen, came to see me. He had been in a car accident two months earlier and was bothered by what had become chronic pain in his right groin. He had already seen a number of orthopedic surgeons and spent two months in physical therapy, but he was experiencing no improvement. The conventional biomedical conclusion was that he had torn a groin muscle, with physical therapy the solution, and one physician recommended surgery. Stephen seemed not at all skeptical or resistant coming to see me when I spoke with him on the telephone. Later, he confirmed that in fact he held a deep suspicion of any type of alternative medicine. It turned out that his boss, Jacob, a biochemist with a doctoral degree from Oxford University, had suggested that Stephen call me immediately after the car accident, but it took two months for him to actually take that step. I had seen Jacob before for his lower back pain. Jacob is not only a brilliant scientist, but he is also extremely low-key. In addition to me, Jacob had been seen by a number of other Rolfers, so he was familiar with the practice. I say all of this because it would be hard for Stephen, despite his skepticism, to remain unpersuaded by Jacob to visit me at least once.

When Stephen came for his appointment, I sensed his skepticism immediately. In part, I suspected that Stephen was not looking forward to paying my fee, given that all of his other care was "free"—that is, covered by his company's health insurance. I knew then and there that I had a single session to validate myself and my approach to healing. If I were not able to do so, Stephen would have all of the evidence necessary to assume that he was right all along with his assumption that practitioners of alternative medicine are quacks who prey on people who are desperate and needy. I knew that disputing or challenging the conventional biomedical diagnosis of a torn muscle would be futile and it was not my place to do so. What I needed to do was quickly establish my own understanding of the problem, and then adequately explain what I intended to do about it. I had a hunch that Stephen, with his engineering background, did not have a lot of interest in hearing about the finer points of Rolfing theory and its philosophy of treatment, especially given that he was paying for this time. With a few basic tests, I determined for myself that there was no muscle tear. I had seen these symptoms before and confirmed what the problem was with some basic rotation tests. I felt I had a good understanding of the main problem and of how to go about relieving the pain. To correct the rotation, I would have to distract the femur from the acetabulum (hip)—which for a big guy like him is made easier with my electric table—and take advantage of the decompression to work some of the tissue and ligaments that were hard to get at directly. As the treatment progressed, I confirmed my original suspicion that he did not have a muscle tear.

The longest time I spent before treatment was letting Stephen tell me about the accident and the subsequent pain and how much he had done to get well (or pain-free, depending on how you look at it), although obviously to no avail. In fact, his pain had increased, limiting his social life and leading to his resignation that his recovery would be long and slow. Actually, I was his last resort, because Jacob, for whom he had great respect, suggested it. By the time I got my hands on Stephen—and I mean that quite literally, for I am, after all, a modern bonesetter—I knew that I had better produce some phenomenal results or Stephen's cooperation would not be forthcoming, and his belief that he had no alternative options would be confirmed. In directly working with his leg, I would be able to increase mobility and motility of the muscles of his leg and groin through releasing adhesions and increasing circulation to his affected areas. In Rolfing, the technique we use on a given area depends on the condition of the tissue and the client's ability to handle the intensity of the pressure as I move, shape, and sculpt the tissue into its proper alignment. Without Stephen's cooperation—in the form of his feedback through range of motion and resistance tests—I would be unable to effectively deliver results. If he felt hopeless or resistant, he would not divulge the level of detailed information that I required.

With most new clients, even when they are improving, they will keep coming back with the phrase "the pain is still there," despite the fact their range of motion and activity levels have substantially improved. If I do not get them to differentiate between their range of motion at an earlier point and their current range of motion (after treatment) they will end a session by saying, for example, that this side doesn't feel as good as that side, or something similar. My communication with my clients, and the ability for us to focus on the same treatment goals, is imperative. If I help them identify their initial range of motion, and then demonstrate that their range of motion is increasing substantially throughout a session, they will enthusiastically answer my questions because we have broken through their private conversation that all is hopeless.

This was essentially the strategy I used with Stephen, demonstrating how his ability to live his life could be enhanced by my Rolfing therapy. By showing some improvement in his range of motion, I was able to get Stephen to come back for a couple of subsequent sessions. It was after these subsequent sessions that I was able to elicit enough information from Stephen that convinced me that the car accident was not the actual source of the problem, but rather just a proximate cause that made the problem obvious.

On his initial visit, following my usual diagnostic routine, I took a lengthy medical and life events history, then observed Stephen's structure by having him stand, in his underwear, at all angles, and walk around the room. His posture was defined in certain ways that gave me important clues. Stephen had a big, rugged, muscular body with an outward rotation in his right leg. The turn out on his leg was extreme for a short-term injury. Little by little, over the sessions, it came out that Stephen practiced martial arts and competitive dancing and had previous problems with his right hip. With his European background and penchant for athletic activity, I inquired if he had played soccer, and indeed he had done so heavily, which accounted for the rotated kicking leg.

It was only after the fifth session, and after Stephen was back to doing martial arts, that he brought his wife along and she made it clear to me how much he had doubted the value of the therapy at the beginning. As a client, Stephen's doubt and resistance to trying something outside of the predetermined choices for therapy is not that different from the norm in U.S. society. Stephen even may have been a little less resistant, given that Europeans have traditionally had a wider range of treatment options available to them. Clients from other societies often have exposure to a wider variety of treatments, although this does not always help build their relationship with me. No matter who the clients may be, I first have to establish precisely what their previous treatments have been and then find out all of their assessments, judgments, and criticisms of previous practitioners and their work. I find it important to also inquire if any family, friends, or others they know have been treated by alternative practitioners and what thoughts they have about those treatments. If by chance anyone of significance in their lives was ever injured, hurt, or taken advantage of by an alternative practitioner, my job of getting their compliance or assistance in making my treatment work is much, much harder. I also understand that most people's frame of reference for healing modalities includes medications (anti-inflammation, pain pills), surgical procedures, and/or physical therapy. I have, therefore, the responsibility to demonstrate to the clients' satisfaction the effectiveness of Rolfing or manual manipulation for their particular problem, when indicated, and sometimes as a complement to what they are doing elsewhere.

As the contributions to this volume show, manipulative therapies have a long and effective history as a part of healing practices. These therapies are part of medical systems throughout the world. At times, they are more a part of the formal institutional system of care, and at times they are less a part of that system of care. In our own society, the United States of the third millennium, various forms of manipulative therapies are alive and well, although by and large (with the exception of biomedical physical therapy) they are outside the formal system of care. In a small way, I hope that this chapter can add to the cross-cultural literature on manipulative therapies and healers.

What Is Rolfing and How Did I Come to Practice It?

Let me start with what Rolfing is not because, unfortunately, the term often carries pejorative implications due to false or misleading presentations of it by the media. Rolfing is *not* the separating of muscle from the bone and it is *not* always painful. Rolfing *is* a gradual realignment of the body in gravity so that a body works with the tensional forces of gravity rather than against them. In a Rolfing session, the Rolfer use his hands, knuckles, and elbows to shape the muscles, ligaments, tendons, and fascia into a more balanced posture to support the correct kinesiological position. Throughout a series of sessions, the Rolfer works with the client to discover where restriction and holding patterns in the tissue are located and how they are affecting the ease of motion of the patient.

I came about this line of work by facing my own health crisis when I passed a kidney stone while attending law school. I made radical changes to my diet and my career path at that time. My first training was in body-oriented psychotherapy and later as a certified nutritionist. Following that I became a certified massage therapist, but was dissatisfied with my ability to produce the results that I knew I would be capable of with the correct training. A personal experience with being Rolfed convinced me that Rolfing could produce the kind of dramatic results I sought, so I furthered my learning at the Rolf Institute in Boulder, Colorado.

Every patient who can benefit from Rolfing usually has pain or difficulty, and this implies inflammation. To the biomedical practitioner's mind, any work done on tissue that is already inflamed will inflame it more. I have found that I can balance a patient's Ph sufficiently using nutrition and biochemistry to reduce this inflammation. Some clients do not follow my nutritional advice and end up feeling exhausted and achy for up to two or three days after a treatment, especially if they consume alcohol, salt, coffee, or anything that increases their dehydration. So my recognition of the limits of structural therapy alone—that is, that a patient requires a certain biochemical integrity for the Rolfing to hold—along with my previous training in nutrition and physiology have led me over the years to expand my practice to include homeopathy, herbs, supplements, and numerous electrical devices (e.g., the Vega machine[1]) to assist me in speeding up the results that I could not accomplish with Rolfing alone (see Fitzgerald 2003 for one of my client's case history, which illustrates this point).

Some Basic Issues in My Practice

In the remainder of this chapter, I want to reflect a bit on my own practice. This is not intended to be an academic treatise on the practice of a modern alternative healer. I am quite sure that if an ethnographer were to spend a month or so with me, she would observe much that goes on in my practice and in my interaction with my clients that is outside of my conscious awareness. Instead, this is my view of some of the basic issues that I deal with every day in practicing my art.

I Often Get Really Hard Cases

In our society, scientific biomedicine is the dominant medical paradigm. This is true not only theoretically but, perhaps more importantly, institutionally. It is easy to see a physician for a problem. Sometimes it is easy to see a lot of physicians for a problem, but finding an alternative healer can be difficult. Referral often comes through the client's social network (see below).

The point I want to make here, however, is that I often see cases only after they have progressed to a point where the client is feeling helpless and hopeless, despairing of finding relief. We have seen this already with the case of Stephen, who only came to see me after he had been informed that the only alternative to his continuing pain was surgery. An example of this is Bell's palsy, a condition in which there is loss of muscle control on one side of the face, which causes that side of the face to droop. The condition can be emotionally crippling, especially in a society placing so much emphasis on facial beauty. I have seen four Bell's palsy patients, two of whom were actually referred to me by physicians. They had tried any number of other treatments. Part of their motivation for continuing was due to the fact that their problem had no apparent cause and, more importantly, no predictable relief. Three out of the four cases were resolved within three to five sessions with no relapse or further complications. The fourth case discontinued treatment and over a year later still has the condition.

In my assessment, I focused on emotional triggers to the condition that seemed to be present in all of the cases. My treatment, regardless of these emotional triggers, focused on manipulation of their facial muscles and their jaw and neck. The youngest of the clients, a twenty-three-year-old woman, had been repeatedly struck in the face by a violent boyfriend. Another, a thirty-year-old man, was a particularly hardworking scientist whose daily stress level probably contributed to the facial disfiguration. The third had been in a car accident and had a previous history of alcohol abuse.

All three were surprised by the sudden onset of symptoms. All three of these patients had been through several rounds of testing for the viral agent that biomedicine defines as the cause of Bell's palsy. The most obvious case (to me) of ignoring other factors going on in the client's life was that of the twenty-three-year-old woman. When she came to see me, I noticed that her lower jaw was slightly displaced to the left. I asked her straight out if she had been hit in the face; she looked shocked, thinking that I knew something that she thought was private and had no relationship to her condition. Her physician had not asked about any trauma, even though the abuse had been going on for months.

These three cases illustrate the point that those who end up seeking my help are often those who have exhausted their other options.

People Need Relief

I raised this point in my discussion of the case of Stephen, and it is a central theme that runs through my practice. My clients may have heard from their physicians that the only thing that will help their situation is a drastic intervention, something to which they are unready to commit. Or they may have heard from their physicians (as in the case of Bell's palsy) that there is nothing that can be done. But above all, my clients are coming to get relief. Because I am a Rolfer, the most common problems for which people seek my services are carpal tunnel syndrome and lower back pain. One of the questions that I have to deal with in these cases is the accuracy of the original diagnosis. Some people will have self-diagnosed with the enormous amount of health information available in our society, but they may or may not be correct. Many people will have exhausted their patience with biomedicine and seek relief from me, which in some ways I find advantageous. If a client has seen a good orthopedic surgeon, then the obvious causes and surgical treatments have been ruled out and I can go on to looking for other causes and trying other interventions. At the same time, as in the case of Stephen, I have to prove quickly that I know what I'm talking about and offer some relief, or my client probably will not return more than a second time. Carpal tunnel is the easier problem to deal with because there is usually an upper-rib compromise that responds quickly if the rib and its misalignment are correctly identified. It actually is rare that the wrist itself is to blame, although everyone else has already looked at and worked on the wrist.

Usually, working on the ribs at their attachments near the spine is the best place to give immediate relief. At this point, my client gains my trust quickly because he directly can feel the result.

Rib manipulation for carpal tunnel can be difficult, however, because a lot of clients cannot figure out why it is that I am working on their ribs when they have a pain in their wrist. If I were to launch immediately into a treatise on how Rolfers understand the musculoskeletal system, however, they would be out the door in a flash. What I have to do, therefore, is balance my offering of symptomatic relief with my education of the client.

In lower back pain, there can be any number of reasons for the problem, and I usually have the advantage that some physician has gone through a workup and ruled out the dangerous problems. Because previous diagnoses and treatments have not been effective, I have the opportunity to inquire about other things that may seem, to the client, unrelated to back pain. Some examples of this are leg length discrepancies, gastrointestinal problems, inappropriate dominant postures throughout the day, bad shoes, and a seemingly insignificant trauma to the system, such as missing a step going downstairs and coming down too hard on one leg. It is not uncommon for the client to have no memory of such incidents, or to be un-aware of how everyday activities can affect the system. But these problems are usu-ally pretty easy to spot on examination, especially when the really bad possibilities have already been ruled out. A realignment of their bones can be accomplished pretty quickly, with attendant relief for the pain they are experiencing. The prob-lem is, however, that this may not resolve the problem, especially if they have been misaligned for years. The longer they have been misaligned, the harder it is to fig-ure out all the compensations and unwind them in as simple a way as possible. This can become discouraging for the client, when their pain goes away only to come back again.

The image of the permanent fix that uses surgery and/or medication sur-rounds us every day, implying that there are quick and permanent cures for just about everything. All of this leads to educating clients that their bodies in most cases went out of balance with small event after small event, and that the straw that broke the camel's back (so to speak) was not any more significant than the one-hundred-plus other events that weakened the structure in the first place. If the pain goes away only to come back again in a differing intensity or locale, clients may often believe that I am not doing my job. My job is to continue to gather data during each session, with questions designed to narrow down the potential causes. They have to understand that I am not questioning their memories or attention to detail, but rather that I am trying to zero in on the true cause so that I can treat it. Without obtaining relief in the short term, however, I will never get to the place of treating the real problem.

Clients' Beliefs and Resistance

With either carpal tunnel or lower back pain, the client usually does not understand why I do not want to start working on the exact place where the pain is located. With carpal tunnel it is often quite easy to get quick relief (if the client has not had the wrist pain for much more than one or two months) by working with the neck and shoulder girdle on the arm with pain. Clients will usually feel improvement in the form of pain relief or tension going out of the affected hand at the moment I am working. In most cases, I never have to work on the affected wrist. This begins to teach clients the difference between symptom and system. The same usually holds true for pain in a foot or leg, for which I rarely have to touch their foot or lower leg, and most relief comes from manipulating their sacroiliac joint and realigning the pelvis. As a result of these experiences, it becomes easier to have clients understand the concept of referred pain and go to the root cause of their pain and discomfort.

This step is necessary before I can go on to talk about factors outside of the musculoskeletal system as being part of their imbalance, such as nutritional deficiencies. It is an easier step for clients to understand how their physical use of their body at work or play has an effect on their symptoms. But this is not always the case when their use of their body involves what seems to them as nothing related to their current pain. It can also be difficult to ask them to go back in their memory to old childhood injuries that they assume have nothing to do with their current problem. The more I probe about anything that they assume has nothing to do with the complaint/symptom, the more I must be in a good relationship with them to establish that my skills can deliver in the new areas on which I am suggesting we must focus.

I must constantly use a two-pronged approach to treatment and education. If I am not constantly demonstrating that I can produce some immediate relief, then I may not get another opportunity to establish the additional trust and get clients to explore additional, and perhaps more profound, causes of their problem. At the same time, there is the danger for both the client and me to believe that the relief of the symptom amounts to a cure. I have to remind clients that getting rid of a symptom is a little like putting duct tape over a warning light on the dashboard of their car. Yes, that pesky light does not bother you, but you may be masking damage to the system that will be even worse. Clients are easily seduced by the "one problem/quick cure" emphasis in our health culture. They are resistant to changing their beliefs in this regard. As a practitioner, I also am not immune to this influence. It is not uncommon to prefer treating at a basic level of signs and symptoms to the immediate satisfaction of the client and oneself. But many problems are long term and require a more profound alteration in patterns of living, something that can be daunting to the client.

Communication

In a sense, much of what I am talking about in my practice as a modern bonesetter revolves around the flow of information, of communication between my clients and me. At the same time, there is a much larger system of communication and information flow in which I am embedded. As a healer/alternative practitioner, I am living and practicing in a larger community that becomes a functional village due to the unusual nature of the highly interactive environment in which I live. I recently started working with a new client from New Zealand whose job as a professional photographer brings him to new places as a normal part of his life. When I asked him who referred him, he said that he had read about me on the Internet, and several posted comments on my services caused him to call. This is no different than what has occurred in the past, in that direct referrals account for about 90 percent of the new clients I encounter. But I have discovered through the Internet that, just as in a small village, your reputation will precede you. Communication in forms that I only dimly understand establishes clients' expectations, which I must discover and clarify if I am to assist them in any way.

If I were a traditional bonesetter in a small village and I had established myself by productive work, people from another village might eventually seek me out if their local bonesetter was unable to heal them. It is not that different in the global village of which San Francisco is a part. When clients call my office requesting help or information, my first goal is to connect with them, establishing a relationship with a clear exchange of information about their needs and my services and abilities. All of this is necessary if their first visit—our first physical meeting—is to maximize the possibility of achieving the outcomes they desire. And I cannot even presume that a client and I are speaking the same language.

In small villages, we assume that we all speak the same language and have a commonality of thought because of our common experience. In any village, these assumptions are based on years of interaction and memories involving family and friends, and the stories of how they were helped by the healer. This is what establishes a healer's credibility. In the modern village of San Francisco, there are both similar and drastically different processes at work. The city itself is relatively small in terms of alternative practitioners, and we are under constant scrutiny by the biomedical as well as alternative community. There are the normal competitive pressures involving both one's personal reputation and one's financial stability. Because the community I practice in is so small and visible, I feel the pressure to perform above the level of the average practitioner. I am also under financial pressure to produce results that are immediate and perceptible because clients can vote with their pocketbook. Insurance is not bearing the expense, so if clients do not get the result they want, not necessarily what I think is best, they will not return, much less refer their family and friends.

As I have already noted, it is often the really hard cases that end up in my office. One of these was Tom, a sixteen-year-old boy suffering from severe exhaustion (possibly chronic fatigue syndrome) and asthma. He was in such a state of exhaustion that he had been forced to drop out of high school. Despite prolonged treatment within the biomedical system, he failed to respond. When Tom came to me, I immediately saw a strong desire to get better and get back to school. As with all clients, the hardest part of working with him and his parents was creating the belief that, along with manual therapies, changes in behavior and eating habits—in fact, adopting dietary practices that are neither appealing nor socially valued—could help him in his treatment goals. After six months of difficult work, taking two steps forward and one step backward, we succeeded in completely reversing all of his symptoms. Tom has reentered school and is returning to a normal adolescent life. But even with the school, family, and client acknowledging the change, the larger medical community refuses to recognize the improvement. The mother wanted to set up a meeting with the boy's doctors and me, but they had no interest in hearing how he was better or in following up on his case. When something seemingly impossible occurs, physicians, in my experience, nearly always provide an explanation that makes it sound as though there were a misdiagnosis in the initial evaluation, and that the alternative treatments, therefore, had no validity.

I use this anecdote to illustrate the difficult nature of treating patients with methods neither normally accepted nor convenient within our social milieu. People sometimes think that alternative practitioners have it easier because of a lack of peer review, but it must be kept in mind that people can vote with their pocketbooks when you give them a treatment protocol that is oftentimes expensive, inconvenient, socially unacceptable, and directly against the advice of dominant biomedical practitioners. The only way to achieve success is to stack result upon result in ways that directly improve the lives of those we seek to help, even if it contradicts their entire mind-set. There are only very small margins for error when everyone has you under scrutiny and can easily label you a quack or charlatan. All this leads to the conclusion that, regardless of the success of treatment, one's reputation can easily be made or lost by any one patient articulating his or her negative feelings, whether or not these are accurate reflections of their symptomatic relief.

Conclusion

I hope that I have been able to provide the reader with a sense of my work as a modern bonesetter. I understand that I have only been able to touch on some issues, and that many (such as the actual nature of my manipulative therapies, and the fact that I use nutritional and other strategies routinely to supplement those manipulative therapies) have only been mentioned in passing. Instead, in this chapter I have emphasized how I see my main work as a healer interacting with my clients and the larger institutional systems of healing of which I am a part.

If anything has come through regarding my philosophy of healing, I hope it is my belief that symptoms can point the way to the door to awareness for a client. I must correctly identify and treat the problem for this to occur, not merely chase after symptoms, no matter how satisfying that might be for both the client and me. This approach to healing is difficult because it requires that I continually learn and update my skill level in a society in which there is relatively little support for what I do. I must develop and maintain a network of practitioners who support me and whom I support in this process of continuing education. It is infinitely more satisfying to me intellectually to explore the links between symptoms and basic, underlying imbalances in life than to just dole out symptomatic relief. The most satisfying part of this work is that an increasing percentage of patients are understanding that their healing goes well beyond the level of symptomatic relief, and they are excited to discover the links between their current symptoms and not only the recent injury, but previous injuries or patterns that contributed to their symptoms.

Note

1. The Vega machine, developed in Germany, is a bioenergetic testing device that includes a galvanometer. The device records the change in skin conductivity after the application of a small amount of voltage. Its operation is based on the theory that disordered electrical charges are the first sign of pathology in the body.

Reference

Fitzgerald, Randall
  2003 Personal Journey: The Case of the Dizzy Dame. *Alternative Medicine* Jan/Feb.

Index

Page numbers in italics indicate figures, tables, illustrations, or photos.

About the Authors

Robert Anderson (M.D., D.C., Ph.D. anthropology, UC–Berkeley), an anthropologist-physician who is also trained as a chiropractor, is professor of anthropology at Mills College and chair of the department of sociology and anthropology. He served as director of manual medicine at the San Francisco Spine Institute at Seton Medical Center from 1988 until 1992. A prolific author in the fields of medical anthropology and manual medicine, his most recent book, *Alternative and Conventional Medicine in Iceland—The Diagnosis and Treatment of Low Back Pain* (2000), was published by the Directorate of Health in Reykjavik, Iceland.

Hans A. Baer (Ph.D. anthropology, University of Utah) is professor of anthropology and sociology at the University of Arkansas at Little Rock. He has been a visiting professor at Humboldt University in Berlin, University of California–Berkeley, Arizona State University, and George Washington University. Baer has conducted ethnographic research on Hutterites in South Dakota; the Levites (a Mormon sect in Utah); African American spiritual churches; osteopaths, chiropractors, and naturopaths in the United States and the UK; sociopolitical and religious life in East Germany; and conventional and alternative HIV clinics. A prominent medical anthropologist, his books include *Encounters with Biomedicine: Case Studies in Medical Anthropology*; *Critical Medical* (with Merrill Singer); *Medical Anthropology and the World System: A Critical Perspective* (with Merrill Singer and Ida Susser); and *Biomedicine and Alternative Healing Systems in America: Issues of Class, Race, Ethnicity, and Gender*. Baer has served on the editorial board of the *Medical Anthropological Quarterly* since 1996. He presently is completing a book titled *The Taming of a Popular Health Movement in the United States: From Holistic Health to Complementary Medicine* to be published by AltaMira Press.

H. Vincent Black (L.Ac., California Acupuncture College) is owner and head practitioner at the Four Winds Health Center in Tucson, Arizona, for ten years, founder of the North American Tang Shou Tao Association (NATSTA), and director of the NATSTA Research and Development Committee. As the founder of the NATSTA and director of research and development, Black traveled to Taiwan and mainland China to research traditional internal kung fu and Traditional Chinese Medicine (TCM) between the late 1970s and the 1990s. He studied traditional internal kung fu and traditional bonesetting with his teacher, Master Hsu Hong Chi, from the late 1970s until his untimely passing in 1994. During his travels to China, he also studied with a number of other TCM and kung fu masters, including Liao Wu-Ch'ang, Yu Wen Tong, Zhong Jao Bao, Share K. Lew, and Xie Pei Xi.

Ian Coulter (Ph.D. sociology, London School of Economics and Political Science) is a medical sociologist and public health professor in the School of Dentistry at UCLA. He also holds an appointment as a senior behavioral scientist at RAND and as a research professor at the Southern California University of Health Sciences. He is also a graduate of the Harvard program in educational management (IEM) and from the RAND/UCLA Center for Health Study Policy. He is a past president of the Canadian Memorial Chiropractic College. His main field of scholarship has been in the area of complementary and alternative medicine. For the past three years, he has held an NIH grant for an evidenced-based practice center for complementary and alternative medicine and is currently funded to conduct a qualitative study of integrative medicine. A leading figure in the social science of chiropractic and of health policy, Coulter has published over forty articles and two books on chiropractic care.

Servando Z. Hinojosa (M.A. anthropology, UCLA; Ph.D. anthropology, Tulane) is currently an assistant professor of anthropology at the University of Texas–Pan American. He earned a doctorate in 1999 and has conducted cultural anthropological research among highland Mayas of Guatemala since 1991, focusing on various dimensions of reproduction, spiritual knowledge, dance, and bonesetting. Recent works of his include *"The Hands Know": Bodily Engagement and Medical Impasse in Highland Maya Bonesetting* (*Medical Anthropology Quarterly*, 2002) and *"K'u'x como vínculo corporal en el cosmos"* (Estudios de Cultura Maya, 2002).

Eric Jacobson (Ph.D. anthropology, Harvard) trained in Rolfing with Ida Rolf in 1972. He is also trained in psychotherapy and has maintained a private practice in Rolfing and psychotherapy in the Boston area for over thirty years. His dissertation in medical anthropology examined the psychiatric aspects of classical Tibetan medicine as practiced in refugee communities in northern India, with special attention to depressive and anxiety disorders. He is currently lecturer at the Department of Social Medicine and a member of the Placebo and Healing Research Group at the Osher Institute, both at Harvard Medical School. Current research activities include the study of clinical reasoning in Tibetan medicine, a clinical trial of the placebo response in acupuncture, and a brain-imaging study of meditators.

Norman Klein (D.C. Cleveland Chiropractic College, Los Angeles; Ph.D. anthropology, University of Oregon), chair and professor of anthropology at California State University–Los Angeles, is a cultural anthropologist whose research into alternative medicine included becoming a doctor of chiropractic. He specializes in medical and applied anthropology with a focus on integrative medicine. Most recently, his interests have turned to anthropological film. Selected works of his include *Culture, Curers, and Contagion* (Chandler and Sharp, 1979) and the film *East Meets West: Traditional and Orthodox Medicine*.

Jennifer Minor (M.A. anthropology, Northern Arizona University) is a cancer research training award fellow and medical anthropologist with the Office of Cancer Complementary and Alternative Medicine at the National Cancer Institute. In addition to receiving her chiropractic degree, she has studied Traditional Chinese Medicine with H. Vincent Black since 1995, completed fieldwork in China on musculoskeletal therapy in traditional Chinese medicine in 2001, and is a bodywork therapist specializing in Tuina, craniosacral therapy, and Thai massage.

Isaac K. Nyamongo (Ph.D. anthropology, University of Florida) is a senior research fellow and director of the Institute of African Studies at the University of Nairobi, Kenya. His research interests include health care systems, malaria, reproductive health, and research methods. He has published in various journals including *Tropical Medicine* and *International Health, Social Science and Medicine, Bulletin of the World Health Organization, Field Methods*, and *African Study Monographs*. His most recent publications include "Assessing Intracultural Variability Statistically Using Data on Malaria Perceptions in Gusii, Kenya" (*Field Methods*, 2002) and "Health Care Switching Behavior of Patients in a Kenyan Rural Community" (*Social Science and Medicine*, 2002). He serves on the editorial board of the journal *Field Methods*.

Simon Leyson (D.C. Anglo-European College of Chiropractic; M.Phil. health care services, University College, University of Wales, Swansea) is a practicing chiropractor and has worked in his native Wales for the last twenty-five years. He was editor of the *Journal of European Chiropractic* from 1986 to 1999. He researched and wrote an ethnography of a local bonesetter for his graduate degree. His current academic interests are broadly centered on the medical humanities and, in particular, the phenomenology of pain. Leyson has done anthropological fieldwork in his native Wales.

John O'Malley (Ph.D. chiropractic and osteology, Royal Melbourne Institute of Technology University) is a chiropractor in private practice in Christchurch, New Zealand. He earned a B.Sc. in neurophysiology at the University of Canterbury and a chiropractic degree (B.App.Sc.) at the Phillip Institute of Technology, now a part of the Royal Melbourne Institute of Technology University (RMITU). He was awarded his Ph.D. in chiropractic in 1998 at RMITU. He is an active member of the New Zealand Chiropractors Association. He spent a total of two years in the Philippines from 1986 to 1994. During this time, he conducted fieldwork among urban poor communities, learning the techniques of a group of indigenous healers, the *hilot*.

Kathryn S. Oths (Ph.D. anthropology, Case Western Reserve University), professor of anthropology at the University of Alabama, is a medical anthropologist who has done fieldwork on chiropractic in the United States and bonesetting in Peru, following twelve years of full and part-time work as a massage therapist. She has conducted research on topics including medical treatment choice and health outcomes; reproductive health; gender, ethnicity, and health; domestic violence; and complementary and alternative healers. Her most recent publications include "Setting It Straight in the Andes: Musculoskeletal Distress and the Role of the *Componedor*" (in Koss, Leatherman, and Greenway 2002) and *Social Status and Food Preferences in Southeast Brazil* (Ecology of Food and Nutrition 2003).

Susan Walkley (M.A., Columbia University) is completing her Ph.D. in applied anthropology at Columbia University and is currently conducting research on the treatment of back pain. Her master's thesis was entitled "A Modern Affliction: The Experience of Stress in New York City." She has taught anatomy and physiology, palpation, living anatomy, perspectives on medicine, anthropology of the body, and medical anthropology at New School University, Marymount Manhattan College, and The Swedish Institute. She has been a licensed massage therapist in New York City since 1994 and plans to complete her certification in structural integration in the summer of 2004.

Miranda Warburton (Ph.D. anthropology, Washington State University), an anthropologist with the Navajo Nation for fifteen years, is currently a bodywork therapist specializing in Chinese medicine, specifically Tuina and craniosacral therapy. She also teaches Thai massage and craniosacral therapy at Northern Arizona Muscle Therapy Institute, Sedona, Arizona.

Marc Weill (ReUnion Center, San Francisco), is a certified advanced Rolfer and nutritionist with over twenty years of clinical experience in the Bay Area. He taught massage therapy at the Boulder School of Massage from 1980 to 1986 and later received his training at the Rolf Institute in Boulder, Colorado, under Ida Rolf. He currently integrates several modalities into his bodywork practice, including photon stimulation therapy, Vega testing, thermography, and darkfield microscopy. His work was recently featured in an article in *Alternative Medicine* (Fitzgerald 2003).